Troubled in the Land of Enchantment

Troubled in the Land of Enchantment

Adolescent Experience of Psychiatric Treatment

Janis H. Jenkins and
Thomas J. Csordas

UNIVERSITY OF CALIFORNIA PRESS

University of California Press
Oakland, California

© 2020 by Thomas J. Csordas and Janis H. Jenkins

Library of Congress Cataloging-in-Publication Data

Names: Csordas, Thomas J., author. | Jenkins, Janis
    H., author.
Title: Troubled in the land of enchantment : adolescent
    experience of psychiatric treatment / Thomas J.
    Csordas and Janis H. Jenkins.
Description: Oakland, California : University of
    California Press, [2020] | Includes bibliographical
    references and index.
Identifiers: LCCN 2020001564 (print) | LCCN 2020001565
    (ebook) | ISBN 9780520343511 (cloth) |
    ISBN 9780520343528 (paperback) |
    ISBN 9780520975019 (epub)
Subjects: LCSH: Adolescent psychotherapy—Residential
    treatment—New Mexico. | Adolescent psychiatry—
    New Mexico. | Psychiatric hospital care—New
    Mexico.
Classification: LCC RJ504.5 .C78 2020 (print) | LCC
    RJ504.5 (ebook) | DDC 616.89/140835—dc23
LC record available at https://lccn.loc.gov/2020001564
LC ebook record available at https://lccn.loc
    .gov/2020001565

29 28 27 26 25 24 23 22 21 20
10 9 8 7 6 5 4 3 2 1

Contents

Illustrations and Tables

TABLES

Acknowledgments

The collaborative project of which this book is the outcome was funded by National Institute of Mental Health Grant no. RO1 MH071781–01, "Southwest Youth and the Experience of Psychiatric Treatment," Thomas J. Csordas and Janis H. Jenkins, Co-Principal Investigators. Our logistically complex, geographically dispersed, and emotionally strenuous ethnography in New Mexico benefited greatly from the contributions of skilled and intrepid doctoral student fieldworkers Bridget Haas and Whitney Duncan. Child psychiatrist Michael Stork, MD, and clinical psychologist Mary Bancroft, PhD, artfully and empathically accomplished the work of conducting research diagnostic interviews. Elisa Dimas's assistance with recruitment of research participants was invaluable. Back in California at our UC San Diego research offices, graduate students Heather Hallman and Allen Tran worked intensively on the first phase of data organization and preparation, and later conducted fieldwork (not reported in this volume) with a comparison group of nonpatient adolescents. In addition, many UCSD graduate and undergraduate students assisted with the extensive task of interview transcription and data entry, including Jessica Hsueh, Nofit Itzhak, Jessica Novak, Celeste Padilla, Marisa Peeters, Leah Retherford, Amy Rothschild, Ellen Kozelka, Farah Bishay, Nicholas Locke, Mania Mgdysian, Cassidy Shapiro, and Shayna Orensztein. Alexis Burnstan, Alexandra Pryor, and Giselle Sanchez assisted with final preparation and submission of data tables and figures.

We are grateful to the colleagues at the following institutions who have invited us to speak about this research as we have developed it over the course of several years. Each of these occasions afforded us the opportunity to advance our analysis and benefit from many astute questions and insightful observations: the Resident Members' Seminar at the Institute for Advanced Study in Princeton; Seminar in Medical Anthropology of the Departments of Global Health and Social Medicine and of Anthropology at Harvard University; Conference on Critical Research on Culture, Psychiatry, and Mental Health at Harvard University; Mind, Medicine, and Culture Seminar in the Department of Anthropology at UCLA; Department of Comparative Human Development at the University of Chicago; Humanities Institute and Institute for the History of Production of Knowledge at New York University; Yankelovich Center for Social Science Research at the University of California San Diego; Institute of Anthropology at the University of Copenhagen; Department of Anthropology at the London School of Economics; École des Hautes Études en Sciences Sociales in Paris; Conference on Emotional Experience in Narratives of Depression at Freie Universität Berlin; Workshop on Phenomenology of Depression at Durham University UK; Conference on Psychiatry, Religion, and Healing at Westfälische Wilhelms-Universität Münster; Department of Anthropology at Universität Osnabrück; Interdisciplinary Center for Intercultural and Indigenous Studies at the Pontifical Catholic University of Chile in Santiago; Proyecto Oferta Terapéutica Religiosa para Fármaco-dependientes at El Colegio de la Frontera Norte in Tijuana; Instituto de Ciencias Antropológicas at the Universidad de Buenos Aires; Department of Sociology and Anthropology at Tel Aviv University; and School of Political and Social Inquiry at Monash University. In addition, we are pleased to have been able to present findings from this research on more than one occasion to the meetings of each of the following associations: the Society for the Study of Psychiatry and Culture, the American Anthropological Association, and the Society for Psychological Anthropology.

We are immensely grateful to Medical Director David Mullen, MD, and the other highly skilled and dedicated health care providers at the Children's Psychiatric Center who supported this research and provided useful feedback during presentation of our findings and interpretations. Our heartfelt thanks go to the wonderful circle of family and friends who have been the lifeblood of support during the many years of doing this massive project and writing this book. Particular thanks to our two children, now adults, for the many occasions and long periods of being relocated to New Mexico, away from their home and friends. Living as a family in the research project house during the first year of the fieldwork, their presence helped to ground us during particularly arduous periods of ethnography. Hearty thanks to our daughter for her comments and keen editorial eye for the final wrap. Thanks also to Bridget Haas (ethnographic research team member), who provided feedback and clarifications of terms we deploy in particular parts of the book. We thank UC Press for the editorial expertise of Kate Marshall and the production work of Enrique Ochoa-Kaup and Emilia Thiuri. Thanks as well to our expert indexer, Amron Gravett. We also thank the three peer reviewers for feedback of value in revisions. Finally, we are indebted to all who participated in this research by allowing us extended time together in homes, neighborhoods, and clinical settings. Learning about your life experiences has been an anthropological privilege and challenge. We are deeply grateful.

Prelude

New Mexico is a place we have known for nearly three decades now, returning for various lengths of time for collaborative research in which each of us has individually been involved, on topics including Native American healing, refugees from political violence, and adult and child mental health. Our first extended sojourn there together—two anthropologists, one pregnant—was in 1991, when we lived in a silver spray-painted cabin with marginal plumbing, a couple electrical outlets, and heat from a woodstove. The silver cabin was situated high among ponderosa pines in the foothills of the serenely imposing Chuska Mountains, referred to in the local community of Crystal as the Navajo Alps. Crystal was where our anthropological forebear Edward Sapir had once worked and where we first observed the Navajo practice of setting a table with a big cylindrical carton of Morton salt instead of a puny shaker.

Our second sojourn—two anthropologists and two six-month-old twins—was in 1992 at the beginning of the "mystery illness" outbreak that was killing people in the Navajo Nation. We learned a lesson in perspective when friends and our children's pediatrician in the East warned us not to go, and friends on the reservation said that the problem was no big deal since, in any case, it was centered in an area more than a hundred miles away. "After all, it's always something, like last year when there was a grasshopper infestation." We set out with the understanding that we would turn around if the CDC had not identified the disease vector by the time we reached Albuquerque, and when we awoke in Albuquerque to the news that the illness was due to hanta virus spread by deer mice, we knew what to avoid and what to clean out before moving into our double-wide trailer. We proceeded to initiate our summer's work. Initial setup, however, was not without incident. It had nothing to do with infected deer mice but instead with an ominous arrangement of bones appearing on the front stoop that, while the subject of contestation between us, was identified unequivocally by a close Navajo friend as calling for a protective ceremony.

Our third sojourn was in 2006, when the four of us—our children now almost fourteen years old—lived in a small house in downtown Gallup with a four-foot-long stucco Gila monster sculpted into its exterior walls, across the street from a reputed crack house and close to the town's newly refurbished public plaza. Occasionally one or the other of our children accompanied one or the other of us to one of our ethnographic sites, where their common sense was evident in certain situations, like the time we were photographing in a locale where questionable security became apparent to our daughter, who insisted, "Mom! Get *over* here!" We listened to the whistles of trains a few blocks away, passing all through the day and night on the trunk line connecting east and west coasts, and traveled each day to the hospital where we were working with troubled youth who, at the time, were the same age as our own children.

This was difficult fieldwork not because of the typical anthropological requirement of becoming fully immersed in the milieu, but because the work required engagement with difficult and often painful life situations at the edge of experience. The extremity of life conditions faced by the children, clinicians, families, and healers could be overwhelming for all involved. For us, the process of engaging these persons and conditions entailed a daily roil of empathy, contradiction, exhaustion, and immediacy. As reflected in what follows, we are grateful for the opportunity to present our results in this ethnographic monograph.

CHAPTER I

Land of Enchantment, Land of Pain

SCENES FROM THE FIELD

In late winter, as the New Mexican sunlight gleamed in the subfreezing wind chill, I (coauthor JHJ) first met Taciana at the Children's Psychiatric Center (CPC), in a small room that is part of the larger pueblo-style residential facility. Taciana had been admitted the previous week, and this was her first hospitalization. Slight and remarkably soft-spoken, she seemed younger than her stated age of fourteen years. She had agreed to meet to learn more about the research we were doing on how young people come to the hospital. After I explained our work and ensured she understood that we were not part of the treatment team, she gave her permission to be included in the study. Without hesitation, she plunged into a long and commanding narrative:

> I am Zuni. I come from the other side of the mountains. I come from Zuni. I came here because bad things happened to me and some people told me I could come here to rest. People could take care of me. This is my first time coming here, or in trying to commit suicide. I hate myself. Because I hear voices, like voices telling me what to do or "hang yourself, do it, become like one of us."

She explained that it seemed like hanging herself was "worth it" and tried it. She had no idea how long she had been hanging before her father found her. He told her that she needed help, so she went to her school counselor and told him that she was "having trouble dealing with anger" and wanted help. The counselor told her that "there were some real nice people at a hospital who can help." Taciana continued her story about why she had come to the hospital:

T: For depression and I was dealing with a lot of things like my grandpa, when he passed away, I was sad because he meant a lot to me, and when he was gone, you know, I stopped going to school and I started smoking [marijuana] and I started ditching school, and I thought that was a really good thing to do, but when I talked to my brother, my oldest brother, who lives in [small town], he said I'm hanging around the wrong people and I don't have to do that. And he was getting, you know, angry because he hates seeing me following the wrong footsteps, and he told me, "You have to follow the light. You have to look for the light so you have to get out of your trouble." And I told him, "Well, I am going to a place where it is really going to help and I am volunteering to go." And I've been here at the hospital and it's really helping me . . . and I'm really glad I came.

J: Ah. So, you came to get help and to try to get away from the wrong crowd.

T: Yes. And my childhood was really bad back then because there was a lot going on, a lot of drinking in the family, and I didn't have enough time to sit down with somebody and talk with them about my problem. So, I've been dealing with it ever since I was five. When my grandpa died, I started seeing him and I thought I was going crazy, so I told my grandma about it, and she sat down with me and she said, "OK, let's talk." So I told her, "I'm seeing uncle, he's coming to me, asking me questions about whether I want to live or die. And I told uncle I wanted to live, I want to move on with my life." And back then I was moved from my mom and my father, and two social workers came to my house and told me that I needed to be removed from their house, because I wasn't getting the help that I needed at home, and there wasn't enough support, like, um, enough food at the house, or money that we needed. So they told me that there was a family where you could be loved and that I was going to go there. So, I said, "OK, that sounds nice. I'll go."

At the time she moved into this foster home, she was five years old. She told me how she was removed from her family home:

Because my mom wasn't taking care of me like a parent should. She was leaving me outside when they were drinking, and there was a lot of fights going on, and when they were fighting, you know, the fighting would just get worse and worse. And I would get involved like Mom telling me to go outside, and I would be outside for a long time, so there was a neighbor that called the social workers, and they came to the house, picked me up, and we went to a home [foster family], and I was there for about two years . . . from [that] home I went back to the other foster home. That home I didn't like because I was abused.

Sexual violence and ravaging of her bodily and psychic integrity had occurred three times in Taciana's young life. Narrating these events, she paused to wonder: "I was saying, 'Why *me?* Why does it have to be me?' Because I'm the youngest? Is it because I'm the youngest [that] I have to be raped all the time?" The first rape occurred when she was ten years old, during a family party in her neighborhood. She decided to go back home to her trailer to get her sweater, but when she turned around to leave she encountered a young male by the door. She began to scream, but he grabbed her mouth and threw her down on the bed. Taciana continued to try to scream but, she told me, she had no idea what was going on. The young man raped her as she continued to try to scream. After he left, she wanted to go to urinate but could not because her "private was hurting, [so] I just took a nap and I was sleeping." Her foster mother entered the trailer and, seeing Taciana, asked why she didn't want to return to the party. She replied that she just wanted to take a nap. She narrated that she was scared to tell what had happened because she was afraid that the perpetrator, Taciana's foster mother's grandson, would lie and say nothing had happened to her.

T: So, I told her I just wanted to stay in the trailer. [My sister was there and said,] "You *have* to go down there." I told her, "I don't want to." And then she slapped me, and every little thing I did wrong she would hit me with her hand, or with a washcloth, and I would always cry. I was depressed at that home. And that day we had a meeting with the social worker. I was scared to tell her, but I just said, "I *have* to tell her." So, I was brave enough to tell her what had happened.

J: I'm glad you are here [at the hospital], that you could stay. You must be a very strong person to have gone through all these terrible, terrible things, and to have the strength, and the goodness to be able to sit here with me, and to share your story, because I feel very much just how difficult this is. So, it is a great honor to be able to talk to you.

T: Yes. You are welcome.

At this point in our encounter, the end of the first ethnographic interview, my mind raced with thoughts of what had happened to Taciana and what would happen next. I began to imagine how I would rearrange one of the bedrooms of my home so she could stay with my family. As an ethnographer with training in psychiatry and working in the field of mental health for over two decades, I felt flustered. Nothing like this had ever crossed my mind, even though, in my fieldwork in the homes of poor families, I had had innumerable encounters marked by pain, anguish, and uncertainty about the future. I thought of all the practical and ethical reasons why taking in this young girl could not possibly work. Why was I even thinking like this? Then, as I was leaving the hospital, I stopped dead in my tracks in the snow, frozen with the full-blown realization that ethnographic counter-transference had been activated: at the time, my own daughter was also fourteen years old.

Five months later, I (coauthor TJC) met Taciana at a residential treatment facility where she had been living for three months following her discharge from CPC. This was not a first-rate university hospital but a for-profit residential facility with poor management, supervision, and quality of care. A number of our interlocutors had been placed in this facility at one point or another in their trajectory as patients. They typically compared it with CPC and said they experienced this residential center as harsh, as a place of blame, punishment, and stigmatization. Taciana's experience (further described in chapter 5) was that the facility was neither supportive nor therapeutic. In fact, several years following Taciana's stay, the number of assault and battery calls at this treatment center had risen dramatically, with reports of teens smoking marijuana, getting into fights, or having sex. The New Mexico Children, Youth, and Families Department determined that the facility could no longer keep children safe or provide an adequate level of treatment, and it was permanently closed in April 2019.

Familiar with Taciana's first interview and the way in which JHJ had been compelled by her situation and her engaging personal presentation, I was eager to get to know her. Rather than leading with her Zuni identity and background, however, by this time Taciana's narrative was in an entirely different cultural idiom of misogynistic victim-blaming, neoliberal individual responsibility, a medicalized discourse of diagnosis, and a constricted pragmatics of therapeutic working, processing, and coping:

> I'm here [at the residential facility] because I fucked up my life. I did it to myself. I can't really do anything right. I need to use my coping skills. . . . Right now, I'm working on my depression, my anger, my hallucinations, and my self-harming. I have [processed] with a lot of stuff and I do coping skills and I also call my mom if I need help.

Her mom in this narrative is her caregiver in treatment foster care. Taciana was eager to be discharged to the caregiver's family and was looking forward to their visit on the following day. Meanwhile she was having difficulty with the peer environment after an internal move to a different unit: "I was there for about two months and I started messing up. A lot of girls started hating me and they started lying about things and I started getting mad. And I started cutting and I started banging my head, and I started trying to hang myself again." She defined banging her head against a concrete wall of the facility as a "coping skill" she had learned by watching others do it at the facility.

Taciana's initial cultural and personal narrative was framed by "being Zuni" and being a person who had had a series of "bad things" happen *to* her. Now, it had been radically transformed into a narrative of the silencing and erasure of violation, shaped by the neoliberal discourse of individual responsibility whereby she was a girl who "fucked up my life." Nevertheless, she retained attachment to Zuni culture and her Zuni family, keeping a wooden prayer stick, a dried corncob, and cornmeal to protect her in moments of crisis and prevent her from lashing out at others. She proudly described the Zuni dancing deities as well as her own fluency in the Zuni language and knowledge of Zuni songs. My encounter with Taciana, like my coauthor's, produced a compelling moment, but this one had to do with a self-discovered practice that symbolically bridged the world of Zuni traditional healing and secular therapeutics. She had a stress ball that she sometimes squeezed, and on one particularly fraught day she found herself holding it in one hand while she held her ritual corncob in the other: "I had this feeling. Like I'd gotten lifted up or something. I got this feeling, went down my body, like something good touched me. I just squeezed them, [and felt] something touching me. So that's why I do it every morning before I wake up. It just gives me a better day every day."

Taciana's agency, identity, and reflectiveness in dealing with extraordinary conditions are critical to understanding her lived experience and her hope for a better day, as well as the possibility of her having a life beyond the hospital and the world of treatment. Overall, and as we develop further below, we will not represent her experiences—nor those of our other interlocutors—either as reducible to "bad parenting" (as one psychiatric colleague said) or as summarily "tragic," "sad," or "depressing" (as some anthropology graduate students have said). Such characterizations only invite us to turn away and are not responsible characterizations of these young people, as troubled as they may be, nor are they apt for the intricate life experiences we explore in this book.

CONCEPTUAL ORIENTATIONS: LIVED EXPERIENCE, INEQUALITY, AND ENGAGED STRUGGLE

Our challenge in this book is to engage the lived experience of adolescents who have been inpatients in a psychiatric hospital, their trajectories through the mental health treatment system, and their hopes for having a life in the face of extraordinary conditions of precarity and affliction. Our theoretical framework is grounded in the interrelations among lived experience, power and inequality, and engaged struggle that concurrently structure subjectivity, sites of care, and sites of harm. "Lived experience" is central to our concern with immediacy and inter-subjectivity as wellsprings of meaning and plays an important role in contemporary phenomenological anthropology (Jackson 1996; Csordas 2008, 2013; Katz and Csordas 2003; Duranti 2010; Kirmayer 2008; Desjarlais and Throop 2011; Jenkins 2015a; Ram and Houston 2015). It is a powerful yet redundant phrase, for isn't all experience lived? In fact, the apparent redundancy is itself a reminder that all experience is first and foremost "lived," whether it is mundane or remarkable, in dreams or in everyday life. And in any case, are we as anthropologists even interested in any kind of experience that is not lived? There are three reasons that we choose to foreground lived experience.

First is our long-standing theoretical commitment to the primacy of experience as the starting point of ethnographic investigation (Martin 2009, 2010; Biehl 2013; Jenkins 2015a; Csordas 2002, 2015; Haas 2017; Csordas and Jenkins 2018), rooted in the fields of psychological and medical anthropology. This could not be clearer than in the argument by Arthur and Joan Kleinman that made explicit the theoretical prerequisite for medicine and anthropology to foreground experience qua experience: "What is lost in biomedical renditions—the complexity, uncertainty and ordinariness of some man or woman's unified world of experience—is also missing when illness is reinterpreted [by anthropologists] as social role, social strategy, or social symbol . . . anything *but* human experience" (Kleinman and Kleinman 1991: 276, emphasis added). To be of value, this approach demands attention to the *interpretation* of experience in contextual specificity without losing sight of the *immediacy* of experience in its bodily specificity.

Second, empirical attention trained on lived experience inevitably involves the workings of power and thus provides a window onto critical points of intersection. This line of thinking stems from a theoretical framework developed for the reciprocal production of subjectivity on the one hand and structural-institutional inequalities on the other. To be more precise, concentrated into this formulation are "extraordinary conditions" (Jenkins 2015a) that are constituted by personal experiences of bodily alteration that, in the present case, are culturally diagnosed as forms of mental illness on the one hand, and as sociopolitical and institutional conditions and forms of violence and adversity—including poverty, misogyny, racism, and abuse or neglect—on the other. These dual sets of conditions are reciprocally produced as interlocking sets of extraordinary conditions. The former set of conditions can be defined as illnesses, syndromes, or disorders; the latter set of conditions can be defined as forces of structural violence as formulated by Paul Farmer (2004a). Both kinds of conditions might come to feel "ordinary" in the sense of becoming routinized, recurrent, or expectable. However, as experiential modes of suffering and conditions of social pathology, they are not properly regarded as either unusual or normative conditions but rather as matters of well-being and social justice that can best be addressed by development of critical sites for engaged listening, care, and social change.

Third is the human capacity for struggle as a fundamental human process of vigorously engaging possibility, a capacity shared by children and adolescents, as well as by those who are living with conditions diagnosed as mental illness. "Recognition of struggle goes beyond the useful and increasingly prominent notion of individual resilience in the face of affliction. When we analytically elevate the study of struggle, we see beyond the usual conceptual categories of analysis and see instead a fundamental human process that comes to light as a product of an anthropological approach trained on lived experience" (Jenkins 2015a: 2). How do people with serious mental illness struggle, and how do children and adolescents struggle, particularly those living with disorienting and disturbing features of illness experience? Such people do in fact struggle, and however disabling their affliction, it is seldom the case "that the human capacity for striving is eclipsed" (Jenkins 2015a: 94–95).

Guided by these conceptual orientations, we have three primary aims in this book. First is to contribute to a corpus of ethnography grounded in experiential specificity and to a body of anthropological thinking on subjectivity[1] understood as a relatively enduring but circumstantially transformable structure of experience (Jenkins 2015a; Csordas and Jenkins 2018; see also Biehl, Good, and Kleinman 2007). A second goal is to produce knowledge of value to clinicians who treat troubled youth or who are responsible for developing treatment programs, whether in outpatient or residential care settings. A third goal is to present ethnographic and empirical documentation of potential value for those who design, implement, and assess health policy. Though policy is not our area of expertise, we feel there is potential value in examining what is happening on the ground as policies and institutional arrangements play out in the daily lives of our interlocutors. Restrictive cutbacks in funding for mental health services, which we witnessed over the course of this study, have only been exacerbated by an ever-increasing constriction of health care for the poor and disadvantaged.

In the next sections of this chapter, we first consider the concept of "adolescence" in relation to mental health. We then provide an overview of the ethnographic setting and state of New Mexico, including the clinical setting from which we launched our work. Finally, we describe our study and introduce descriptive characteristics of the youth, their kin, and their households.

ADOLESCENCE AS CULTURAL AND HISTORICAL NOTION

The category of adolescence has not been universally recognized across cultural contexts and historical periods. It is a cultural rather than a natural category, though based partially on biosocial characteristics of development. That is, though puberty is a biological event marked in part by the onset of the capability to reproduce, it is ritually marked in many societies by a ceremony that meets a criterion of a sacrament as defined by anthropologist Robert R. Marett (1933), namely the cultural consecration of a culturally perceived "natural" process. What comes before and after puberty is widely variable across and within cultural settings and historical periods, but social adolescence is often conceptualized in relation to reproductive capacity and includes preparation for a wide range of marital arrangements across cultures (Schlegel and Barry 1991). As is the case with adolescence, mental health and illness are categories as much cultural as natural and are not easily defined, especially since so much is at stake in terms of social stigma placed upon those diagnosed. Clinicians are often rightly hesitant to impose diagnoses on children or teens, due to developmental fluctuations as well as the instability of psychiatric diagnostic categories within and across cultural contexts. Recognizing that our work on adolescent mental health takes place at the intersection of these not entirely stable categories introduces an inherent element of caution and critique, and requires us to consider what we mean by adolescence in relation to mental health and illness.

Philippe Ariès (1996) provides a European history of the family over the past six hundred years, claiming that in medieval times the "ages of life" included a period of adolescence lasting from the age when a person can beget children until one is no longer able to reproduce. In France, the only words available were those referring to childhood, youth, and old age, leaving no room for adolescence, which was conflated with childhood at least in linguistic usage (1996: 23); and in the seventeenth century both English and French were lacking words to distinguish little children from bigger ones (1996: 25). Ariès writes that "even when a vocabulary relating to infancy appeared and expanded, an ambiguity remained between childhood and adolescence on the one hand and the category known as youth on the other. People had no idea of what we call adolescence, and the idea was a long time in taking shape" (1996: 27). The "first typical adolescent of modern times" was a type which appeared in France in the years around 1900. By this time the notion of youth was collapsing into adolescence, and by the end of the First World War there was a clear sense of generational opposition between the younger troops at the front and the older generations in the rear: "From that point, adolescence expanded: it encroached upon childhood in one direction, maturity in the other. . . . Thus, our society has passed from a period which was ignorant of adolescence to a period in which adolescence is the favourite age. We now want it to come early and linger in it as long as possible" (1996: 28). In wealthy countries adolescence became the "privileged age" of the twentieth century, an era which "recognized itself in its adolescents" (1996: 29).

In the United States, the concept of adolescence received an influential formulation in the two-volume work published in 1904 by the psychologist G. Stanley Hall. Hall wrote about biological and social development, promulgating racist evolutionary views in his description of the variations among puberty initiation ceremonies in savage tribes, classical civilizations, medieval knighthood, and Christian confirmation. He devoted considerable attention to negative features of adolescence in chapters on "Diseases of Body and Mind" and "Juvenile Faults, Immoralities, and Crimes," which included statements like "Again with children as with savages, truth depends largely upon personal likes and dislikes" (Hall 1904, vol. 1: 351). The attitudes of this influential psychologist most certainly penetrated popular consciousness, though by midcentury a major compendium on *The Adolescent* (Seidman 1953) made no explicit reference to Hall's specious and by then outmoded work.

One lasting element of Hall's legacy is his characterization of adolescence as a period of *Sturm und Drang,* a phrase borrowed from the early German Romantic movement's emphasis on emotional intensity and turbulence. When Sigmund Freud visited the United States on Hall's invitation, he was teaching about the power of an inherent conflict between opposing instinctual forces of sexuality and aggression on the one hand and social needs to live together on the other. Based on this, Anna Freud elaborated the idea of adolescence as a period of internal disharmony between these forces and needs (Adams 2005: 4). Anthropologists suggested caution in generalizing this conclusion about adolescence too far. Margaret Mead (1928) pointed out that emotional turmoil was not inevitable in adolescence, offering the counterexample of a relatively relaxed and carefree adolescence in Samoa. For her this argument supported the possibility of critically examining aspects of our own culture supported by taken-for-granted categories presumed to be universal and/or biologically invariant. Ruth Benedict (1938) explained that in our society adolescent turmoil could be accounted for as part of a specific cultural configuration in which there is a discontinuity of expectations when behavior interdicted among children becomes expected of young people as they mature. Unlike in some other societies, our cultural institutions do not adequately support young people undergoing such role transition, and in fact they are negatively sanctioned if they cannot manifest the new behavior spontaneously or, on the contrary, manifest it too belligerently. Nevertheless, this notion is so ingrained in North American society that such behavior appears naturalized, expected of adolescents who often conform to expectation. The teenager in turmoil, trapped between childhood and adulthood, reappears in popular culture over the decades in figures of the rebel without a cause, stranger in a strange land, girl interrupted, failure to launch.

We are uncertain even whether to refer to this period as adolescence, the teenage years, the second decade of life, youth, or emerging adulthood.

In contemporary anthropology the concept of adolescence has received a notable amount of attention as a stage in the life course at which identity is consolidated and people approach full cultural membership (LeVine 2007; Lowe 2003; Suárez-Orozco and Suárez-Orozco 1995; Csordas 2009), but which is also fraught with challenges to well-being that anthropology can contribute to understanding in a way relevant to mental health policy and practice (Burton 1997; Dole and Csordas 2003; Lester 2011; Meyers 2013; Jenkins and Haas 2015; Duncan 2015, 2018). This literature is too voluminous to fully cite here,[2] but we can capture its flavor by considering two special issues of the journal *Ethos* devoted to adolescence. The first, edited by Alice Schlegel (1995), included work from two major anthropological predecessors of our project, the Adolescent Socialization Project and the Harvard Adolescence Project. This collection was organized around the questions, considered across cultures, of the overall movement from childhood dependency to adult autonomy and responsibility; the "naturalness" of adolescent revolt against authority and the question of continuity or discontinuity between generations; the management of adolescent sexuality and, in particular, the recent claims of adolescent girls to control their reproductive lives; delinquency or conformity and the relative influence of peers, lovers, and parents; and the social roles of adolescents, including training for adult occupations and a sense of competence in life. The second collection, edited by Eileen Anderson-Fye and Jill Korbin, explored adolescence as a developmental period of becoming more aware of and engaged in the surrounding social world in the context of the contemporary historical period of unprecedented social change and globalization that constitute a significant challenge for young people (Anderson-Fye and Korbin 2011; Korbin and Anderson-Fye 2011). Contributors observe that the concept of adolescence as a time of storm and stress has been supplanted by talk of the dangers and risks in youthful social behavior. Notably, the majority of contributions are based on ethnographic work in the United States.

We are convinced that these two sets of works do not represent simply two different sets of interests but demonstrate a shift in emphasis, within anthropology over this fifteen-year period, from concern with socialization and development to concern with health and well-being. In general, we can say that if anthropology lagged behind psychology and sociology in addressing adolescence, within the anthropological literature on adolescence there has been a lag in addressing mental health in particular. An important contribution by Fabrega and Miller (1995a) is an exception that proves the rule. Writing at the same time as the volume by Schlegel that we have just considered, they likewise emphasize the biocultural basis of adolescence, and also endorse the idea that the contemporary form of adolescence is a product of capitalist industrialization and market development, the stresses and strains of which generate "adolescent psychopathology." They apply a historical and comparative perspective to anorexia nervosa, dissociation disorders, and social aggression among adolescents and argue for the importance of the interactions among historical and structural forces, experiential meaning, and psychobiological/biomedical changes. Late or not, the turn by anthropologists to adolescent mental health in terms of how social conditions create a precarious situation for contemporary youth constitutes a recognition of the urgency of the situation.

ADOLESCENT MENTAL HEALTH

The fields of child psychiatry and psychology have not been immune to changes over this period. In this arena as well, two prominent reference works on adolescent mental health in the United States can serve as a touchstone for our ethnographic departure. The volume edited by Van Hasselt and Hersen (1995) is framed as the first thorough treatment of the subject against a background of more general books on adolescent development and adjustment. It opens with a chapter recognizing the cross-cultural and historical variation in the concepts of adolescence and mental health, and that the fields of adolescent psychiatry and psychology are "recent creations of Western biomedicine" (Fabrega and Miller 1995b: 4). Fully half of the book is devoted to themes of biological and intellectual development, social interaction and family environment, diagnosis and assessment. The chapters on specific disorders are organized according to a format that includes description of the disorder, historical background, clinical picture, course and prognosis, complications, epidemiology, familial pattern, differential diagnosis, and clinical management. Appearing ten years later, a volume by Gullotta and Adams (2005) is framed in terms of a development since the middle of the twentieth century, when the influence of psychoanalysis was waning. Over the course of several decades the orienting "buzzwords" became family and social justice, giving way in the 1990s to genes and the decade of the brain, and in the opening of the twenty-first century to biopsychosocial theory and evidence-based practice (2005: xvii). The editors accept this development without critique or consideration of its consequences, and the chapters on individual disorders are organized around the idea that clinical treatment should be directly based on evidence derived from research studies. Authors discuss each disorder in terms of risk and resiliency factors, and examine treatment and prevention strategies in terms of research evidence about what works, what might work, and what does not work.

Changing clinical concerns over this relatively brief span of time can be seen in the disorders that receive chapter-length treatment in the two books. The 1995 volume includes gender identity and impulse control disorders, which are excluded from the later work; the 2005 volume includes pediatric bipolar disorder and obesity, neither of which had achieved diagnostic currency at the time of the earlier work. However, perhaps the most consequential change across the two volumes, acknowledged by Gullotta and Adams to be due to the influence of bureaucratically managed health care, is the overall reconceptualization of concern with mental health as concern with *behavioral health* (2005: xvii). This is evident in the 2005 volume's relative emphasis on cognitive behavioral therapy and psychopharmacology. It is also evident in a dual perspective that results in separate sections, one with chapters on diagnostic entities such as depression, post-traumatic stress disorder, and conduct disorder, and another with chapters on behavioral categories such as violence and delinquency, substance abuse, sexual offenses, and gang behavior. Indeed, whereas in the 1995 volume suicide and sexuality are the only "special topics" to receive separate chapters, the 2005 volume includes chapters on ten separate problematic behaviors. Finally, it is worth noting that in the earlier book substance abuse is treated as a disorder while in the later book it is a behavior; and in the earlier book suicide is included as a special topic while in the later book it is a disorder.

From our standpoint, one advantage of the shift within the health sciences toward the "behavioral" is a relative decentering of exclusive focus on psychiatric disorders and the highlighting of features of the social environment and what can be described as problems of living. The disadvantage is that behavior is construed in such a way as to exclude attention to experience. Thus, for example, emphasis is placed on the external or surface features of violent behavior without analysis of the immediate circumstances and meaning of violence, on the management of anger without nuanced examination of the experience of anger, on the recommended forms of treatment without description of how patients experience that treatment, and on promulgation of coping skills without appreciation of what it is like for troubled adolescents to "cope" on a daily basis. Moreover, because available evidence focuses on discrete disorders and behaviors, Gullotta and Adams recognize that "little attention has been given either to bridging the experience of young people from the residential to the community setting" or to discussing co-occurring disorders (2005: 631).

The work we present in this book is focused precisely on the experience rather than the behavior of children with co-occurring problems as they move along a trajectory into and out of residential treatment and inpatient care. Our dual concern with lived experience and with equitable access to treatment is exemplified in two complementary intellectual undertakings in which anthropology has a critical stake. First, the contemporary anthropological approach to childhood, influenced by *child standpoint theory*, aims at an account of society from where children are socially positioned and in which they are not passive social "others" but agentive participants in social life, hence co-constructors of knowledge and, by extension, of knowledge generated by research (Alanen 2005; Fattore, Mason, and Watson 2016; Hunner-Kreisel and Kuhn 2010; James 2007; Mayall 2002; Wells 2015). In particular, anthropologists have taken up the idea that "children have agency and manifest social competency" (Panter-Brick 2002: 156; see also Bluebond-Langner and Korbin 2007: 243). This is put to the test in the case of severely troubled youth under conditions defined as structural violence (Farmer 2004a; Jenkins 2015b), but by no means is it canceled out by their troubles.

The second relevant intellectual undertaking is addressing the inequality of exposure to adversity that threatens the mental health of children and youth. As a matter of social justice, this inequality is a central concern of this book. To take but one factor that affected many of our interlocutors—food insecurity—there is empirical evidence for relationship among hunger, poverty, and the mental health of adolescents. A large national survey of youth thirteen to seventeen years old found that "the association between food insecurity and mood disorders was strongest in adolescents living in families with a low household income and high relative deprivation" (McLaughlin et al. 2012: 2). The World Health Organization (2013) reports that with respect to the global prevalence of mental disorders among adults, at least 50 percent of disorders are developing by age fourteen. As we will see, that is precisely the mean age of those in the present study. Taken together, understanding how youth make sense of and engage in their illness, and understanding the intergenerational effects of socioeconomic disadvantage and structural violence on mental well-being, are essential to describing the lived experience of struggle (Jenkins 2015a, b).

Accordingly, we are concerned with equitable access to services and treatment as advocated by the movement for global mental health (Patel 2005; Becker and Kleinman 2013; Opakpu 2014; Kohrt and Mendenhall 2015; Kirmayer et al. 2015; White et al. 2017). This interdisciplinary field is only in the initial stages of being extended to children and adolescents, both with respect to scholarship and with respect to actual funds committed for relevant programs (Patel et al. 2007a, b; Lu, Li, and Patel 2018; Kieling et al. 2011; Kohrt et al. 2008, 2010; Floersch et al. 2009; Jenkins 2015b; Jenkins and Stone 2017; Jenkins, Sanchez, and Olivas-Hernández 2019). Yet recent reports suggest that serious mental health difficulties are common among children and adolescents, with approximately 20 percent being affected worldwide (World Health Organization 2005, 2012: 6; Bird 1996; Verhulst 1995; Ford, Goodman, and Meltzer 2003; Kessler et al. 2005). Working toward global health equity in adolescent mental health and well-being requires continued input from anthropologists focused on the lived experience of youth in treatment such as we present in this book. This is true not only from a methodological standpoint, but also in the pragmatic sense that the United States contains under-resourced regions like New Mexico, regions currently posing challenges of inequity and offering inadequate services that are no less of a concern for global mental health than in what are often classified as "low- and middle-income countries" (cf. Jenkins and Kozelka 2017).

THE ETHNOGRAPHIC SETTING

New Mexicans call their state the Land of Enchantment (map 1 and figure 1). It is a land of historical depth where the ancient ruins at Chaco Canyon lie close to the lands of the Jicarilla Apache people, and the sheer cliff dwellings of Bandelier National Monument lie close to the government's Los Alamos National Laboratory. It is a land that inspires an awe of nature (figure 2), home to the massive grandeur of Mount Taylor, the sacred southern mountain of the Diné people; the startlingly jagged peaks that serve as a badge of identity for Las Cruces; and the Sandia Mountains that preside over Albuquerque so loomingly close that an airliner once crashed into them near the site of the present-day tramway to the park near their summit. The tree-lined Rio Grande is a ribbon-like oasis flowing hundreds of miles as it bisects the state

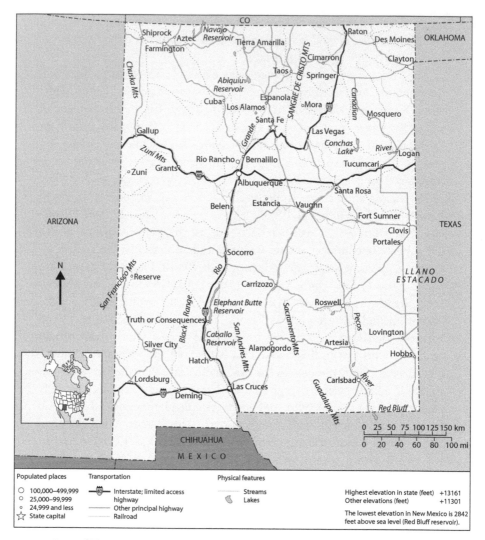

MAP 1. State of New Mexico. Source: Nations Online Project, fair use (www.nationsonline.org /oneworld/map/USA/new_mexico_map.htm)

from north to south, serving as the state's aorta and making it possible as a phenomenon of human geography. The banks of the life-giving river are also home to the heritors of the Anasazi, their Pueblo communities marked by gaudy roadside casinos and mesmerizingly elegant galleries of indigenous pottery, with quiet back streets where clusters of crosses have been placed at the base of chain-link fences to commemorate untimely deaths. It is a land where Mexican food can be ordered "Christmas

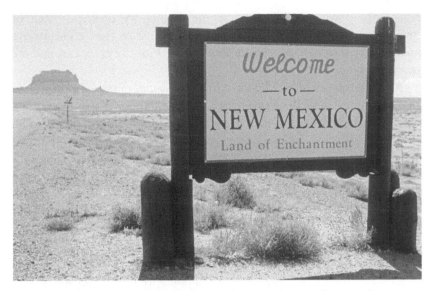

FIGURE 1. Welcome to New Mexico. Source: Shutterstock (www.shutterstock.com /image-photo/welcome-new-mexico-sign-10228129)

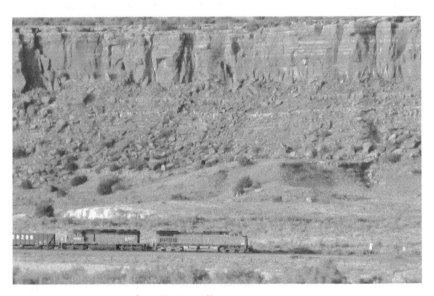

FIGURE 2. Train en route from Zuni to Albuquerque.

style," the I-want-it-all answer to the mandatory question "Red or green?" that refers to the diner's preference for red or green chile (always spelled with the "e") sauce made from peppers ideally grown around the town of Hatch.

Albuquerque is New Mexico's sole major city, situated centrally in the state along the Rio Grande. Its 2010 population of 545,852 for the city and 887,077 for the metropolitan area had by 2019 grown to an estimated 558,000 and 903,000, respectively. The metropolitan area accounts for nearly 45 percent of the state's total population. The city is a magnet, attracting people from everywhere else in the state who come for entertainment, shopping, health care, or to visit relatives. Albuquerque is divided into quadrants by the north-south rail line that runs just west of Interstate Highway 25 and east of downtown, and by the east-west Central Avenue. The Northeast Quadrant, nestled up against the Sandia Mountains, is relatively affluent and characterized by the elegant ranch houses of the "heights" along with the University of New Mexico (UNM) campus, the Sandia Peak Tramway, and the grounds for the annual hot air balloon fiesta.

The Southeast Quadrant includes Kirtland Air Force Base and Sandia National Laboratories, but is also known for residential neighborhoods referred to by many of our interlocutors as the "War Zone" of violent crime, gang activity, and drugs. The poverty in parts of the War Zone and other neighborhoods of southeast Albuquerque is marked by over-crowded households, food insecurity, crime, dangerous neighborhoods, and often violence. Many businesses in the area have been abandoned or boarded up, including a motel on Central Avenue reminiscent of the Route 66 glory days (figure 3). Photographed by JHJ in 2016, it was destroyed later that year by arson and was subsequently demolished. Meanwhile, the city government had begun to strategically counter the locally common War Zone rubric by posting signs designating the area as the "International District." This has been criticized by local residents who claim that the zone is the place that "saved" them from being home-less since it was the only place in the city where they could rent an apart-ment, having been ejected from their home and either being below the age of eighteen to rent legally or not having any record of employment. Sometimes ambivalently and sometimes with vehement loyalty they use alternate referents, calling the area "my home" or, in a play on the state's motto, the "land of entrapment."[3]

The Southwest Quadrant is a locus of the diverse Latinx/Hispanic population and home to the National Hispanic Cultural Center; it

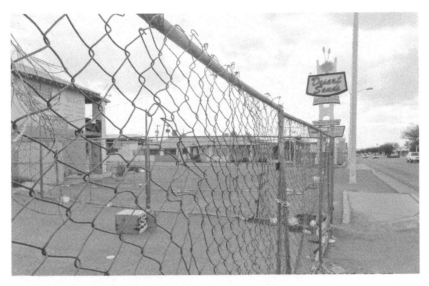

FIGURE 3. Abandoned motel, Albuquerque.

includes the areas of Barelas and the South Valley, the latter a relatively poor area with a reputation for crime and gang activity. The Northwest Quadrant (figure 4), an area of rugged volcanic landscape, includes the old colonial central plaza, the Indian Pueblo Cultural Center, and the relatively affluent North Valley. The latter includes, outside the city limits, the sprawling suburb of Rio Rancho with its inclination toward fundamentalist megachurch Christianity and conservative politics, as well as the smaller communities of Corrales and Bernalillo, which are relatively more inclined toward a holistic lifestyle and liberal politics.

Civic life is organized on its north-south axis by the Rio Grande and on its east-west axis by the nationally prominent UNM campus and the downtown business district, within which is nested the touristic "Old Town." Two Tiwa-speaking pueblos lie along the Rio Grande near the city, the Sandia Pueblo just to the north and the Isleta Pueblo just to the south. These two communities differ in demographic profile: Isleta has a population of approximately 3,000, out of a total of about 4,500 enrolled members, while Sandia's population is around 4,500, though enrolled members number only about 500. Each pueblo has its own tribal casino.

Las Cruces, the state's second-largest city, is part college town, with its state university campus; part military town, with the White Sands Missile Range, Fort Bliss, and Holloman Air Force Base nearby; and far

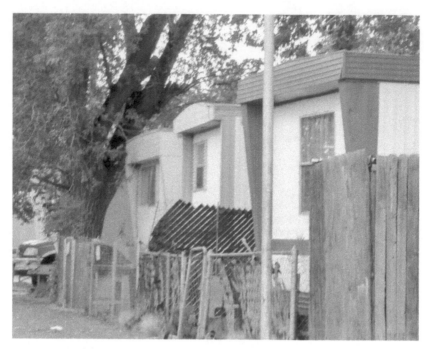

FIGURE 4. Neighborhood in northwest Albuquerque.

enough south that it is oriented as much toward El Paso, Texas, as toward Albuquerque. It is also where Billy the Kid once escaped from jail. The state capital, Santa Fe, is noted for the hotels, restaurants, craft shops, and outdoor Native American jewelry vendors of its central plaza, the museums and art galleries of Canyon Drive, and an upscale zen spa on the outskirts of the city. Away from these attractions are the grittier and less well-off homes and neighborhoods where one can see stucco walls covered with graffiti or painted with colorful murals depicting, for example, a dying young man cradled *Pieta*-style by his mother (figure 5), or memorial crosses next to a garbage can and over-turned shopping cart (figure 6). Española is a small town with no iden-tifiable center but a proud tradition of Spanish colonial heritage—not Latino, not Hispanic, Chicano, or Mexican, but *Hispano,* or sometimes *Spanish*—where local vineyards support the art of traditional Iberian wine making and where the population endures record-setting rates of heroin addiction. Gallup, sometimes called the "Indian Capital of the World," is a city of barely twenty thousand with an ethnic mix of indig-enous Navajo and Zuni, long-term communities of Hispanics and

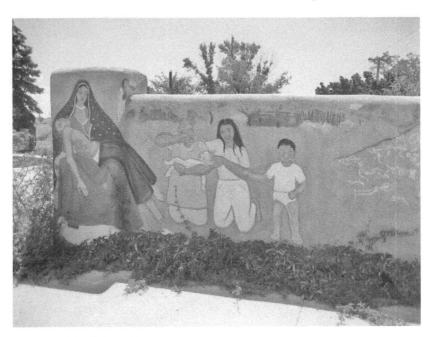

FIGURE 5. Mural, Santa Fe.

Anglo-Americans, and a more recent Arab immigrant community. It is the home of the annual Gallup Inter-Tribal Indian Ceremonial with its rodeo, arts and crafts exhibits, and Indian Queen competition, but also the site, in a barren area just outside of town, of a gathering place called Hairspray Alley where inhalant addicts share their mind-melting highs. Alamogordo and Roswell are slightly larger. Smaller towns include Grants, Las Vegas, and Belen, each having just over or just under ten thousand people, with broad horizons in the literal sense and narrow ones in the metaphorical, where the Chamber of Commerce and the Catholic Church are blocks away from the crack house and meth lab.

According to the 2010 United States Census, the total population of New Mexico was 2,059,179. While the ethnic/racialized categories of census data are widely contested and fraught as cultural and political categories, the 2010 census reports Hispanics or Latinos as accounting for the largest single bloc (46.3%), followed by non-Latino generically "white" (40.5%) and American Indian (8.5%). The latter demographic includes twenty-three federally recognized Indian tribes in the state, comprising various groups of Pueblos, Navajos, and Apaches. Economically, New Mexico is one of the poorest states in the nation. According

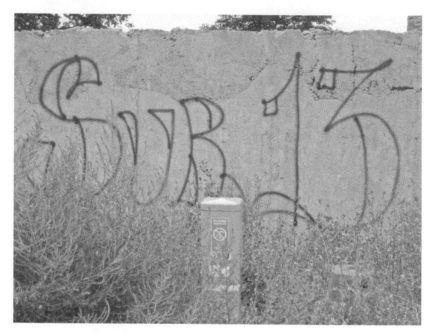

FIGURE 6. Gang graffiti by Sur 13 (across the street from the mural in figure 5).

to the U.S. Statistical Abstract, as of 2008 the median household income was $43,508 (forty-fourth among the fifty states), and the proportion of persons living below the poverty level was 17.1 percent (fifth highest among the states). In 2011, New Mexico ranked as one of two states hardest hit by child poverty, with a rate of 30 percent; only Mississippi ranked worse, with 32.5 percent (Macartney 2011: 6). Relatedly, home foreclosures have also been inordinately high. Along with poverty and dispossession comes the presence of violent gangs, with one antigang website listing 178 in the Albuquerque area. There are serious drug problems across the state, particularly with heroin and methamphetamine use. Statewide, while heroin received most notice in New Mexico, by 2017 overdose death rates ranked the same for methamphetamine as for heroin. Data from 2018 (New Mexico Department of Health) show that death by methamphetamine has become more common than fatal heroin overdose. Prescription drug overdose has also taken a significant toll, particularly in rural areas of the state.

This Land of Enchantment is the ethnographic terrain of our research project on adolescent mental health, called Southwest Youth and the Experience of Psychiatric Treatment (SWYEPT). Our work was inspired

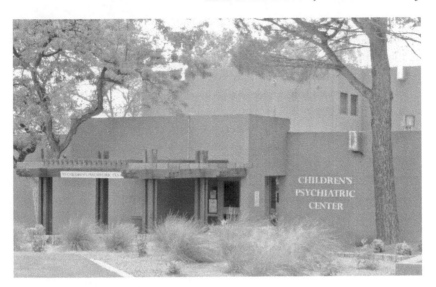

FIGURE 7. Children's Psychiatric Center.

by the opportunity to observe the development of an inpatient psychiatric unit for adolescents within a hospital that was being built by the Indian Health Service to replace a deteriorating facility in the Navajo Nation. Realizing the importance of a richly contextualized understanding of the life experience of the troubled youth we encountered, we also recognized that such problems extend across all ethnic groups, social strata, and geographic locales, and oriented our work to take that observation into full account. Accordingly, we chose to base our study at the Children's Psychiatric Center of the UNM Medical Center in Albuquerque (figure 7), the premier public facility in the state and the recourse for troubled youth and their families from a wide range of communities.

Our work included ethnographic observation and interviews with staff in this clinical environment but cannot be described simply as a "clinical ethnography." Our intent was to develop an understanding of adolescent and family experience not only while the youth were hospitalized, but over time and across settings, as an element of developmental trajectory, course of illness, and transformation of how they interpreted their situations. In order to achieve this intent, we conducted ethnographic observation and interviews in their homes and other institutional settings in which they might be placed. Thus, while our work goes beyond the clinical ethnography and into the community, when we identify New Mexico as our ethnographic terrain we do not intend a general ethnography of the state and its communities. To be precise, ours is what is referred to in anthropology as a problem-oriented rather than a community-centered ethnography. The latter has as its prototype and ideal type the study of small indigenous villages, largely in what currently is often termed the Global South, ones that can perhaps even be surveyed end-to-end from a strategic vantage point and where much social interaction is face-to-face and public. Such a setting requires a different mode of ethnographic engagement, a different degree of mobility, and even a different kind of temporality from the study of a problem or social phenomenon that transcends the boundaries of locality. Put another way, our ethnographic focus is not a particular geographic locality, community, or clinical setting but the challenges and experiences of a diverse group of young people—in this case, severely troubled young people—and their kin who live under conditions of structural violence (Farmer 2004a) and social and psychological precarity[4] (Jenkins 2015a).

THE HOSPITAL AND THE HEALTH CARE SYSTEM

Located at the quiet northern edge of the UNM campus, adjacent to the medical school, CPC is a Southwestern-style compound surrounded by an adobe wall high enough to create a sense of enclosure but not high enough to prevent someone from climbing out. The front door of the main two-story building is the only official entrance, and its modestly sized lobby accommodates incoming patients as well as visitors and staff passing through to their offices. Beyond the lobby are two parallel hallways with administrative, records, and clinician offices, with more of the latter on the second floor. A staff lounge is at the end of the main corridor, near the locked door to the compound's courtyard, which includes a cafeteria/school/activity building and six free-standing patient cottages. Each cottage includes a small lobby/reception/living area with an adjacent glassed-in staff conference room, an administrative office, and two hallways of patient rooms. An outdoor recreation area with a basketball court is set near the back wall of the compound.

As a university medical school's teaching hospital, at which the attending psychiatrists are faculty in the Department of Psychiatry and which accepts patients from throughout New Mexico, CPC defines the center of gravity in the child mental health care system. As the current medical director summarized, it is "the de facto state hospital for kids." It was formerly named (and is sometimes still referred to as) the Children's Psychiatric Hospital (CPH), founded in 1978 with an orthopsychiatry orientation. A book edited by two of its leading psychiatrists, pooling the collected experience of CPH clinicians, described the hospital's philosophy and program through the 1980s (Hendren and Berlin 1991). The authors understood the development of CPH as part of a trend toward expansion of hospital-based care in which child and adolescent psychiatric inpatient treatment had evolved from an initial focus, in the 1920s and 1930s, on custodial care of autistic, postencephalitic, and schizophrenic patients to multimodal treatment units with long-term, psychodynamically oriented programs whose therapeutic goals were complex and far-reaching; the first medical director of CPH was himself a psychoanalyst (Hendren and Berlin 1991: 4).

On admission children were assigned to one of the six cottages, each with the capacity for nine patients, based on their chronological and developmental ages and their treatment needs. Milieu therapy including modalities of individual, group, and family therapies along with psychopharmacological treatment was provided by a team consisting of cottage clinician, attending psychiatrist, cottage program manager, child-care workers, nurse, social worker, teacher, educational diagnostician, and recreation therapist, augmented as needed by allied therapists including occupational therapist, speech/language therapist, adaptive physical education teacher, art therapist, music teacher, and children's librarian (Kerlinsky 1991: 95; Stearns 1991: 116). The on-campus, state-accredited Mimbres School merged behavioral and psychodynamic concepts as an integral aspect of the treatment program, using comprehensive assessment methods to develop an individual education plan for each student and utilizing teams of a teacher and two child-care workers in each classroom. Behavioral management was based on a "level system" in which consistently acceptable behavior was rewarded by advancement to successively higher levels, each of which granted a greater degree of independence and autonomy within the cottage and school (Cavalluzzo 1991: 163–67).

During this period, CPH prided itself not only on its treatment program but also on a carefully cultivated approach to culturally sensitive inpatient care for adolescents. Indeed, the book by Hendren and Berlin is in large part focused on Hispanic and Native American patients. Their discussion draws on numerous case vignettes of cultural barriers to clinical understanding, conflicting assumptions, cultural differences in family organization and dynamics, recognition of witchcraft or evil spirits as causal explanations of affliction, and accommodation of indigenous healing by Hispanic *curanderas/curanderos* or Native American traditional healers, with virtually no attention to the third major group, the Anglos. The university's department of psychiatry at this time also included an anthropologist as a regular faculty member. The director of CPC during our research recalls that UNM psychiatry residency training during the 1980s included participation in a sweat lodge ceremony and a presentation by a Navajo healer on cultural and spiritual themes relevant to mental health.

Hendren and Berlin defined the typical "length of stay" for acute-care inpatients as thirty to sixty days, that for intermediate-term care as one to six months, and that for long-term inpatient treatment as longer than three to six months (1991: 7–8). They typically anticipated providing intermediate-term care for patients diagnosed with depression, conduct disorder, or cyclothymic disorder; intermediate- to long-term care for patients who had been physically or sexually abused; and long-term treatment for patients with borderline, narcissistic, and antisocial personality disorders, as well as for those with eating and panic disorders (1991: 76–77). At the outset the key challenge is to develop trust, which Hendren and Berlin say usually takes place "shortly after the 'honeymoon'— the testing period of 1 to 2 weeks" (1991: 79), though this is also a function of cultural barriers and the nature of the family's engagement. Already at this period, however, the book's editors recognized the impending future impact of criticism that inpatient care was being overused, of a strong movement toward community-based mental health services, and that managed health care as a means of controlling cost was the fastest-growing trend in modern health care, with great potential for affecting the length of time they would have to work with each patient. They write: "Unfortunately, most managed health care organizations resist providing mental health care, impose severe coverage limitations, and rely on risk-sharing physician-'gatekeepers' to reduce specialist referrals and inpatient treatment. Thus, managed care not only leads to limited psychiatric benefits for the population served, but also raises ethical dilemmas for physicians and administrators who participate in these rapidly growing organizations" (Hendren and Berlin 1991: 268).

In the intervening decades, changes within the field of psychiatry and within the economics of health care have combined to affect the treatment program and the typical length of stay at CPC. The treatment program has evolved in a direction typical of many psychiatric institutions, away from psychoanalytic and insight-oriented therapies and toward cognitive behavioral approaches and, more recently, dialectical behavioral therapy. The impact of managed care has been profound. At the beginning of our study in 2005, New Mexico had become the first state to contract a health care management company, called Value Options, to administer all its Medicaid insurance payments. From a statewide New Mexico perspective, a series of articles based on ethnographic study of mental health professionals (Willging, Waitzkin, and Lamphere 2009; Kano, Willging, and Rylko-Bauer 2009; Willging and Semansky 2010; Watson et al. 2011) examines the pragmatic, institutional, community, and policy effects of the behavioral health care reforms of which the operations of Value Options were emblematic, including attitudes toward evidence-based therapy and culturally competent treatment among health care providers in the state's "safety-net institutions," the concept of "wrap-around services" provided by multi-institution "clinical homes," and the institutional emphasis on promoting "recovery" from mental illness.

Their findings are fully in accord with our observations and interactions with staff at CPC in indicating that this was a period of severe contraction of services, indeed a period that lasted the duration of our project. The prevailing philosophy of Value Options was that extended inpatient treatment is therapeutically ineffective and economically extravagant. As payment for both residential treatment and day treatment was approved with decreasing frequency, the average long-term stay in a residential treatment center (RTC) declined from one year to thirty to sixty days. The approved length of short-term stay for acutely distressed patients declined to between five and ten days, not even the length of Hendren and Berlin's "honeymoon period" during which basic therapeutic trust was expected to become established. From the standpoint of CPC clinicians, this meant that patients were often being discharged to disorganized family environments, which did not provide sufficient opportunity for their condition to stabilize, or to less intensive levels of care for which they were not prepared. Accordingly, clinicians perceived an increasing frequency of adolescents being discharged too soon, and ending up hospitalized again too soon, creating as a commonplace the category of a "revolving door" of discharge and readmission for patients whose clinical need was extended residential treatment (this is further discussed in chapters 2 and 5 and in the book's closing remarks).

The restrictions on length of stay also meant that the apportionment of beds within the cottage system had to undergo radical reconfiguration. More beds had to be allocated to acute care for the institution to remain financially viable, and during the course of the research one of the cottages was switched entirely from residential to acute care, leaving only one cottage operating on the significantly reduced residential length of stay. One cottage that had been dedicated to girls who were in legal trouble was closed when lack of support for that program rendered it unsustainable and when the state applied pressure to admit more violently aggressive girls for whom the hospital's capacity to care was limited. No residential care was available in the two cottages dedicated to treatment of younger children. Thus, in this short span of time, under the regime of managed health care, CPC had gone from three residential and three acute cottages to one residential and four acute cottages. Finally, a day hospital program at CPC, one of the critical intermediate steps in the continuum of care between outpatient and inpatient treatment, had recently been eliminated. Reports by clinical leadership were that the medical director at Value Options did not "believe in" this level of care and simply did not approve any requests for it, necessitating the program's closure. Given the degree of retrenchment forced on CPC, the central pillar of adolescent inpatient care in New Mexico, it can come as no surprise that a number of other facilities simply ceased operation during this period. This most certainly rearranged the kinds of trajectories through the system possible for patients, but that in itself is a story beyond the scope of the present work.

In 2009 the state contract for health care management was assumed by a new company, Optum Health, regarded by clinicians as even more restrictive. According to CPC clinical staff, Optum was even more restrictive in the context of a greater severity of the state's budgetary problems, during the Great Recession. There is concern that Optum, in tandem with state actors, collaborated to reduce spending for behavioral health care through budget cuts. The situation was one of ostensible deniability and finger pointing, with no one taking direct responsibility. Ethnographic interviews show that these changes were experienced as having ambiguous but observable effects, undermining staff morale and contributing to demoralization and a crisis of faith among clinical staff. Moreover, there was concern that this situation could affect therapeutic relationships by opening up the possibility of undermining patients' faith in the process, while at the same time inspiring some clinicians to resist the powers that be in the form of a restrictive health care system. These changes were doubtless exacerbated by everyday stresses and ethical challenges among those committed to the best-quality treatment across the mental health care system, from the frontline community health clinicians described by Brodwin (2013) to those we encountered in a specialized children's psychiatric facility.

Nevertheless, and increasingly as intensive data collection for the research project was winding down, CPC was attempting to adapt to explicit expectations mandated by the state to implement evidence-based treatments such as cognitive behavioral therapy and dialectical behavioral therapy, to adopt cost-effective and cost-efficient practices, and to allow funds to be shifted more into outpatient services as they shortened inpatient stays at both the residential and acute levels. The new emphasis was to be on "wrap-around community-based services" that in theory would provide a protective cocoon with coordinated and seamless transitions from one level of care to another. These levels refer to intensity and cost more than to types of treatment, and are understood to constitute a "continuum of care" through which patients may pass as their conditions and circumstances evolve. Thus, a crisis can result in a youth going into a highly secure acute inpatient hospital unit, which is the most intensive level of care. A patient determined to be somewhat less disturbed can be placed in an RTC with a structured treatment program, or in the more socially oriented therapeutic living arrangement of a group home. In therapeutic foster care the child is placed with a family in which the parents have received special training as well as additional professional and financial support to provide care, often for more than one troubled child in addition to their own children. Day or partial hospitalization provides at least four hours per day of out-of-home educational, counseling, and psychotherapeutic interventions for patients and their families. In-home therapeutic services are intensive, crisis-oriented, family-oriented, and relatively brief (two- to five-month) interventions. Finally, at the least intensive end of the continuum is outpatient treatment, in which patients and/or their families meet one or more times per week for psychotherapy and medication management (Hendren and Berlin 1991; Stroul and Friedman 1986).

While this continuum is quite logical from a clinical standpoint, from the standpoint of young people the transition to and from different levels (in either direction) adds to what is often already a significant degree of residential instability. On more than one occasion they may have changed domicile, going from one caregiver to another, one school to another, or one community to another. Among these youth, it is not uncommon for a patient to go from home to acute inpatient care, to an RTC, to outpatient treatment living with a relative, to treatment, back to acute care, and so on. A study of 225 randomly selected adolescent psychiatric inpatients determined that approximately 30 percent of hospitalized youth had experienced a high rate of residential instability, meaning five to twenty domicile moves (Mundy et al. 1989). Although treatment may be necessary, the resulting series of disruptions in the subjective experience of the "rhythm of life" (Jenkins 1997) may itself become a countervailing force against recovery. Our interlocutors were often quite able to compare the treatment facilities in which they had been placed, sometimes with respect to general criteria such as whether the food was better or worse and whether the staff members were mean or nice, but also with respect to whether they felt relatively more or less safe, whether their peers were supportive ("I made friends there") or hostile ("They were all gangsters"), and whether they felt the treatment they received was helpful or not. It is worthy of note that among the facilities experienced by the youth and their families, CPC was most often mentioned in a positive light (see also chapter 5).

Among the adaptations being made during the period of our study was recognition that the clinical role was changing. Compared with previous clinical work based on an operating toolkit of therapeutic practices deployed on the basis of the underlying dynamics and situations that led to hospitalization, the new regime required clinical tasks to be largely constricted as matters of practicality and therapeutic ethics. Primary tasks were clinical assessment and stabilization in preparation for an anticipated discharge to familial homes or other residential facilities. The imposed changes required the streamlining, if not industrialization, of the flow of patients and overall hospital environment. Staff were being initiated into expeditious and standardized diagnostic and assessment practice so that decisions could be made about each patient within one to three days: standardized rounds quickly specified diagnoses, focal treatment issues, and discharge plans, while standardized treatment programming and behavioral management systems had staff efficiently circulating from one unit to another. Psychotherapy was not abandoned, but there was a trend toward shorter, three- or four-session interventions. Medication was not used more than in the past but was perceived to be initiated a bit sooner and titrated somewhat more actively in relation to length of stay. A track system was created, with track A for children with developmental disabilities, track B for children exhibiting more commonly encountered types of psychiatric distress, and track C for acutely psychotic children in need of intensive supervision and monitoring. In recognizing that the new norm of five- to seven-day stays not only required efficiency but is associated with "revolving-door" recidivism, the pragmatic approach was to "teach them [patients] more skills" of emotion regulation to help keep them out of the hospital longer. The slack was supposed to be picked up by community support agencies, which would provide a full range of wraparound services so that the hardest-to-treat and most complex cases could be maintained in the community. As it happened, the program is widely understood not to have been adequately funded, there were gaps in the continuum of care and the continuity of care, and otherwise qualified agencies were not being certified because they lacked one or another of the required forms of care.

In addition to providing patient care, CPC was thus attempting to maintain a capacity to advocate for its patients to receive needed treatment and also to advocate for itself, if not for resources at least for not having to provide care without resources. A scenario of such advocacy was when a patient with a *DSM* (*Diagnostic and Statistical Manual of Mental Disorders*) Axis II diagnosis was denied treatment because such disorders are typically defined as chronic and therefore ineligible for coverage, even though the young person was undergoing a behavioral episode that by clinical criteria requires hospitalization within twenty-four hours. We wondered whether the problem could be resolved by the newly passed federal Affordable Care Act that prevents insurance companies from denying coverage based on "preexisting conditions," but the status of what the law would really mean and how it would affect practice at CPC was uncertain.

The hospital was also attempting to maintain a capacity for outreach to (1) the community at large, which was insufficiently informed "of what we do and what we target in doing so" and found both access to the hospital and consistent communication with it complicated and frustrating; and (2) the medical and mental health community, who wanted diagnostic consultation and psychological testing/screening from CPC in cases with complex clinical presentation. Staff carried out this agenda in the face of specific systemic constraints. Because families who provide treatment foster care resist increased pressure from insurance companies to accept patients with more severe problems, some children stay at CPC beyond what insurance recognizes as "medical necessity" and is willing to pay for; at the same time, because of the mandate to shorten stays, some leave CPC before they should and hence, without adequate community services, end up readmitted. Because the state wants children with specialized needs who in the past have been sent to facilities in other states to now be treated in New Mexico, CPC experiences pressure to take them in; yet because of having to scale back residential treatment, they have had to become "more of a generalist program," even less capable than before of providing specialty residential treatment such as that required by autism spectrum disorders. Residential treatment had, in part, given way to acute care—where the work, in the words of one therapist, was to "put out fires and arrange for placements"—while retrenchment in the system had made placement increasingly difficult because, as another said, "we have less places we can refer to, and I feel like the kids are kind of boxed in and their families are too."

In this context, the following remarks from one of the clinicians participating in the research indicate a sense of how some staff perceived the role of CPC and its perception within the community:

> I think a lot of the time people in the community are so disempowered they don't even know what is out there and if you can get a pamphlet and say, "Oh yeah, I've heard of this hospital"—but if one is not connected with an actual person I think it is much less likely that there is going to be any flow there because there really has to be a name and a face. Like I said, so many of the guardians and parents [who] come through our doors don't seem to know how to get access to services, how to advocate for themselves and their children, and it is intimidating—I can't even imagine. . . . I know people come in here like "Oh my god" they have to deal with doctors and therapists and nurses and you know case managers, you know everybody else that works at this very, it's a very thick onion [*laughs*], there are lots of layers to peel, and I would be overwhelmed frankly if I had to deal with all these people coming in here. So I always try to put myself in the parent or guardian's place and as a parent myself I can identify with how they might feel, walking in[to] the system, dealing with all of these layers, reminding myself what would that feel like coming into this system, so that's kind of how I tie into thinking it'd be nice if we could reach out in a more formal systematic way that I don't really think occurs, you know, it's not really criticism, just something that is lacking . . . and then it wouldn't be so frightening and overwhelming, especially for people from poorer communities that are already so disempowered, the people that come in that are economically challenged, and then there are cultural barriers and it just goes on and on, you know, so I think there is quite a bit of work to be done and we need to bridge all the gaps that are out there.

Such statements reflect awareness of the intimidating institutional edifice that a hospital like CPC can represent and the value of putting a human face on the process of accessing the treatment it offers, an awareness that exists simultaneously with the increasing impersonalization imposed on the treatment program by the managed care regime.

Likewise, the legacy of sensitivity and awareness of cultural factors in psychiatric treatment remains, though attenuated in comparison to the period described by Hendren and Berlin. Assessment of patients includes identifying cultural and spiritual beliefs that may affect treatment, but this is without the former level of explicit attention or incorporation of sufficient time to fully address cultural specificity or to integrate families into the therapeutic process. Clinical staff know that Native American families, Navajo and Pueblo, ask for ceremonies to complement treatment. They provide passes for children to attend such ceremonies and make accommodations for healers to perform ceremonies at CPC, are cognizant that Hispanic and Mexican immigrant families sometimes have recourse to *curanderas/curanderos,* and that a range of families have an interest in herbal or energy therapies and other forms of alternative treatment—the CPC pediatrician, in fact, shares an alternative-medicine perspective and recommends that patients take regular doses of omega fatty acids. There is also awareness that some cultural groups, particularly Navajos, are traditionally not expressive to outsiders and face logistical and transportation problems in coming to participate in their child's treatment. Here again the managed care regime is an obstacle, since it requires more than the typical week of approved acute care to develop sufficient trust for a young person to begin to express extreme distress or suicidal intent. As one clinician said, "if you're not saying it in a managed care regimen, it's simply not there, it's treated as if it's not there," and so additional treatment time will not be approved. With a sense of frustrated urgency, the CPC clinical leadership articulated a more widespread critique of the inability to deal with chaotic circumstances and multiple levels of concern created by short lengths of stay in terms of an "industrial production line of psychiatry . . . health care providers providing interchangeable widget-like psychopharmacological services to 'consumers,' a business model which is not the language of medicine."

With an eye toward our study's relevance for adolescent mental health care policy, we must observe that the institutional climate has not improved in the ensuing decade since we heard this statement. The mental health care system, with its human-made scarcity of mental health services generated by the conjoined complicity of state government and corporatized managed health care systems, is more a part of the problem of structural violence than of the solution to the problems of mental illness and emotional affliction. A 2018 report by the U.S. Department of Health and Human Services Office of Inspector General focused on New Mexico found that beyond the flagship Children's Psychiatric Center at UNM the state has a significant shortage of behavioral health care providers. Most of the state's licensed behavioral health providers serving Medicaid managed care enrollees work in behavioral health organizations, which cannot always ensure timely access for enrollees seeking behavioral health services (Chiedi 2019). The report came in the wake of a "behavioral health crisis" in the state in which a dozen nonprofit agencies providing mental health and substance abuse treatment had been cleared of fraud charges, but only after being shuttered for two years. The disruption in desperately needed services for the state's most vulnerable citizens has been described by Willging and Trott as reflecting "a deepening pattern of systemic failure, top-down reform, and corporate profit in New Mexico's behavioral health care system" (2018: 231). They show how repeated rounds of reform in three successive gubernatorial administrations and a distortion of provisions in the Affordable Care Act undermined a system "enmeshed in a complex web of privatization, bureaucratization, and the intrigues of pubic stewards and corporate actors" who are influenced by neoliberal ideologies of transparency, accountability, and quantifiability (2018: 232).

Given their need to rely on such a therapeutic and institutional milieu, it is all the more important to provide insight into the lived experience of those struggling with mental illness. Meanwhile, we must not neglect to portray clinicians' sense of their encounters with patients in terms of what they perceived as gratifications and disappointments. Some of these issues were bureaucratic, and the disappointments had most often to do with denial of insurance coverage for what they regarded as adequate care. Among the gratifications was that felt when, in 2011, the last of CPC's long-term patients, a girl who had been in residence for two years, was finally found an alternative placement. This was the result of having a system in place in which CPC staff could advocate for patients and challenge denials of coverage under the regime of managed care, and required multiple meetings with representatives from the hospital, the state, child services, the insurance company, and treatment foster care. The complex, year-long negotiations over who should take responsibility included a recognition that care of troubled children is a social problem requiring that staff, despite influences beyond their control, "try to provide a practice which we feel is ethically, legally, clinically still consistent with our mission and values here." Another staff member expressed pride in having persisted in advocating up the chain of command within the social work system, all the way to the director's office in the state capitol, to successfully place a young man in the custody of his older sister, while at the same time expressing frustration over what appeared to her as an ethos of disaffection, a loss of moral compass, and a culture of risk taking that seemed increasingly evident among youth.

On the therapeutic side, for one staff member the most satisfying scenario was one in which the patient's family was fully engaged and truly "got it" in terms of their child's experience, while most frustrating was facing the time restrictions imposed by insurance companies. Another recalled being gratified by working with a boy diagnosed with schizophrenia who was able to return to school and in having been recognized as a reliable person to call by another who had been suicidal, while expressing disappointment at having worked with one girl whose mother was totally uninvolved except to sabotage therapy and with another who falsely accused him of putting his hand on her leg. The hospital director recounted an instance of relief upon encountering an unexpected success:

> I saw one young man—I went out to eat with my family, and he was a waiter, and he had been working at this restaurant for several months. I had worried (that) he would be either dead or in jail by now, but he wasn't. He was doing better than I would have predicted. Sometimes you get surprised. It's not as bad as you think.

Another therapist recounted that

> I had one seventeen-year-old, this was an older child, she said, "The placement worked out, I finished high school, and I got into college." And I thought, "Wow! How exciting is that?" I don't hear a lot of, or see a lot of, letters or notes or calls like that. It's a success story, you know—she had been placed in a TFC [therapeutic foster care] family, it worked very well for her, she got to finish high school and she was a bright girl, but bipolar. She had a good relationship with mom but it was maybe meshed, there was just a lot of stressors in the family at the time, but it was nice to hear follow-up later on—she went from our acute hospital to our RTC unit, stepped down to treatment foster care, and is now going to be going to college, you know— that was months ago that I heard from her.

Such vignettes of success are vivid for clinical staff not only because they are less common than might be hoped, but also because it is typically beyond their resources and available time to determine what becomes of the young people who are discharged from their care. The prospect of learning some of their stories was part of why CPC staff were favorably disposed to the research project, for this is precisely our concern.

SOUTHWEST YOUTH AND THE EXPERIENCE OF PSYCHIATRIC TREATMENT

Our study was an examination of cultural meaning, social interaction, and individual experience, with the long-term goal of producing knowledge of broad use to those concerned with the treatment of adolescents who are living with one or more conditions of mental illness. Our work began in 2005, with ethnographic and clinical data collection continuing through 2011 (for SWYEPT methods, see the appendix). We arranged to work intensively with three CPC therapists who referred patients to us aged twelve to eighteen whom they judged as not so severely cognitively disabled or developmentally impaired as to be unable to participate in interviews, and not so emotionally fragile or clinically vulnerable that their participation would be unduly stressful. All participants entered the project as inpatients at CPC, and their initial interviews often took place in the hospital. It was rare for a participant still to be there at the time of the second and third ethnographic interviews, though it was not always the case that they were at home, since it was not uncommon for them to be placed instead at another residential facility.

Over the six-year course of the study, we recruited sixty-one young people as participants. As is typical in research with people whose lives and living situations are often unstable, fourteen of them were lost to follow-up from the study because they either had moved elsewhere and could not be located or were unresponsive despite numerous and repeated contacts by our research team. By the end of the study, forty-seven adolescents had completed the research procedures sufficiently to be considered in our final analysis. As shown in table 1, they include twenty-five boys (53.2%) and twenty-two girls (46.8%) whose ages ranged from twelve to seventeen (with a mean age of 14.7 years).

Specification of ethnicity is complicated. The most simplified (and anthropologically unsatisfactory) description is that the youth were distributed primarily among "Anglo/Euro-American" (twenty, or 42.6%), "Hispano/Mexican/Latinx" (sixteen, or 34.0%), and a smaller number of "Native American" (seven, or 14.9%). Table 1 reports only the primary ethnic label endorsed by each youth. Using an overly generalized version of ethnicity/race that is commonly reported in health and sciences literature, the "mixed" ethnic backgrounds included four Native American and Euro-American, two Hispanic and African American, two Hispanic and Euro-American, one Hispanic and Native American, one Hispanic and Asian, and one Euro-American and African American. While this approximates the census demographic data for New Mexico, we were interested in cultural and ethnic distinctions among research participants that are nuanced and subtle. Dual and hybrid ethnicity is not uncommon, but the classification in table 1 does not do justice to the difficult process of attributing a dominant ethnicity to a number of Anglo-Latinx participants. Without question, any listing by ethnic identity preference is inevitably oversimplified. This is because it is not possible to summarize ethnic self-descriptions with precision. A full account cannot not be "collapsed"

TABLE 1 GENDER, AGE, ETHNICITY, AND HOSPITALIZATION STATUS OF
ADOLESCENT PARTICIPANTS (N = 47)

	n	%
Gender		
Male	25	53.2
Female	22	46.8
Age (years)[a]		
12	4	8.5
13	7	14.9
14	8	17.0
15	10	21.3
16	14	29.8
17	4	8.5
Ethnic identity preference[b]		
"Anglo"/Euro-American	20	42.6
Hispano/Mexican/Latinx	16	34.0
Native American	7	14.9
African American	1	2.1
Chinese American	1	2.1
Other	2	4.3
First hospitalization		
Yes	14	29.8
No	33	70.2
Admitting incident		
Recurrence of psychiatric symptoms	20	42.6
Suicide attempt/threat	16	34.0
Legal/police involvement	10	21.3
Other	1	2.1

[a]Mean age: 14.7 years.
[b]See specification of ethnicity and hybridity in text.

in a data table but instead would include an extensive number of combina-
tions and permutations that would require multiple pages of description.
Categories of ethnic identity preference are often fluid and occasionally
idiosyncratic, blending understandings and imaginings of how to self-iden-
tify. That said, some of our interlocutors were decisive or prosaic in their
descriptions (e.g., I am "Zuni," "Mexican," Native American," "Anglo,"
or "Guatemalan"), while others were ambiguous in their descriptions.

Indeed, we can describe the idiosyncrasy, variation, complexity, and
diversity of perspectives and societal positions in the social environment of
New Mexico as characterized by a "hyperdiversity" of cultural identities

(Hannah 2011). In such an environment, what emerges is a "shattering of culture" (Good et al. 2011) in any conventional sense, and certainly as utilized by the U.S. Census Bureau or as commonly deployed in publications within many of the health and social sciences. These authorities typically conflate and obscure matters of social race, political geography, and cultural ethnicity. Among our youthful interlocutors, for example, there is one boy who identifies himself as "Anglo" yet has a Mexican father and a mother with Irish ancestry. To complicate things further, his household includes three siblings from different biological fathers of different ethnic backgrounds who have all come and gone. For another example, one girl identifies as "Guatemalan" even though her mother is of Chinese origin and her last contact with her father (born in Guatemala) was over a decade ago. She simply likes the "idea of being Guatemalan" because "it's different than the Mexicans and other Hispanics around here." Nevertheless, although ethnic hyperdiversity is deeply embedded in the social fabric of New Mexico, our ethnographic observation is that ethnicity appears to be less consequential than issues of household instability, poverty, and social marginality.

Cultural processes, however, are profoundly significant with respect to all of these issues, particularly in relation to gender, social interaction, narrative, expectation, complaint, and interpretation. Some anthropologists have abandoned the concept of culture, apparently unaware of the acknowledgment over a century ago that the concept incorporates aspects of human life that are inherently complex, variable, fluid, contradictory, paradoxical, and messy. Gender, for example, is hardly reducible to "biological sex" and, like many cultural processes, exists on a continuum rather than as a binary or category. Certainly, culture/cultural processes are not reducible to variables or factors that can be quantified, and so it is unsurprising that the concept is either misunderstood or sidestepped in much of psychology and psychiatry. In contrast, for contemporary anthropologists who make use of the concept, culture is conceived as an intricate and multimodal process of meaning-making in the substantive and tangled weave of social, political, economic, psychological, and biological processes. Building upon formulations pioneered in cultural anthropology over a century ago (Sapir 1932; Hallowell 1955), the concept of culture remains critical in an ethnographic approach to experience, because

> culture is not a place or a people, not a fixed and coherent set of values, beliefs or behaviors, but an orientation to being-in-the-world that is dynamically created and re-created in the process of social interaction and histori-

cal context. Culture has more to do with human processes of attention, perception, and meaning that shape personal and public spheres in a taken for granted manner. What do we pay attention to and how? What *matters,* and what does not? (Jenkins 2015a: 9)

Also critical for a cultural analysis is the question of *who* matters and who does not. Do persons living in poverty and subject to racial, ethnic, and class inequities *matter?* Problematic gender binaries notwithstanding, does the near-universal cultural and political devaluation of girls and women—misogyny—mean that girls and women don't matter, or that they matter "less"? Certainly, from the standpoint of mental health, inequities of cultural and social "mattering" contribute significantly to the disproportionate numbers of girls and women who live with depression and anxiety-related disorders (Jenkins and Good 2014).

In addition to the political and legal debates at national and global levels about equitable access to health care, there is a moral issue aptly formulated by Sarah Willen (2012) as a matter of "deservingness." This idea has broad relevance across categories of those subjected to inequitable treatment, such as in the analysis by Bridget Haas (2019a) of how asylum seekers are subjected to "categories of deservingness and moral personhood" that are intersubjectively negotiated in relation to moral economies of care. Moreover, as Steven Parish (2014) has argued, the ways in which persons are conceptualized are integral to making moral experience possible. We cite these ideas about "mattering" as key to the core of this book insofar as the struggles of our interlocutors described herein are largely invisible to or discounted by the broader public.

In terms of religious identities of the cohort, we note that overall, religious identity was not particularly strong. The ways in which the teens identified themselves in relation to religion (per the Achenbach self-report—see appendix) are interesting: fifteen (32%) said they had "none" (with many specifying they consider themselves as "atheist"), and another sixteen (34%) left that question blank or "unspecified." For the minority that did report a religious identity, nine (22%) listed Catholic, three (7%) Native American, and two (5%) Protestant. In terms of the degree to which they considered themselves "religious," responses were twenty-one (45%) for "somewhat," fifteen (31%) for "not at all," and eleven (24%) responded that "yes" they thought of themselves as religious. The two sets of questions do not map onto one another in an entirely even fashion, but they do provide an overall indication that the majority of these youth did not endorse a religious identity or think of themselves as religious.

In terms of sexual identities of the cohort, we do not have quantified data because this was not a specific question for any of our research protocols. However, in narrative statements volunteered by the youth, we found that in most cases it was possible to record how adolescents identified themselves, with the majority saying they were "hetero" or "straight," followed by a substantial number of teens who identified as bisexual, and a smaller number who said they were "gay," did not know yet, or were "working on it." Given that some were relatively young (twelve to fourteen), it is unsurprising that sexual identities were indefinite or unknown. One of our interlocutors, however, took her participation in the research project as an opportunity to request that we (JHJ and the girl) meet in a coffee shop, rather than her home, for a second ethnographic interview. As we arrived, she was keen to find a quiet corner with no other customers around. Having achieved this, she began by explaining to the ethnographer that she had designs on "getting out" of New Mexico and going to college. She next bent low over the table and whispered that she wished to tell something she claimed she had not yet told anyone, saying, "I am gay. No, actually, I'm a lesbian. But I think it sounds better if I say 'gay.'" She asked for and received extra assurance that this information would not be transmitted to her mother. It was reassurance, because we stressed at the outset—and throughout the research as seemed indicated—that all information that the youth provided was never shared with parents, clinical staff, or anyone else not part of the immediate research team.[5]

Table 1 also shows that while this was the first hospitalization for fourteen (29.8%) of them, the vast majority (thirty-three, or 70.2%) had been hospitalized previously. Among these thirty-three who had been hospitalized more than once, thirteen had been admitted twice and eight had been admitted three times; the maximum reported was eleven times, though for some these were consecutive admissions from one facility to another rather than discrete episodes. Six youth had been first hospitalized as early as eight years of age and two at ten years. The mean number of hospitalizations, including the one during which we met them, was 2.87. Moreover, during their participation a number of young patients were readmitted, not always to the same facility, after having been discharged from CPC. The reasons for which they had been admitted to the hospital at the time we met them and asked them to participate in the study were recurrence of psychiatric symptoms for twenty (42.6%), suicide attempt/threat for sixteen (34.0%), and legal or police intervention for ten (21.3%); in one case the admitting incident was ambiguous. When police were involved they often gave the parents a choice between jail and hospital for their adolescent. Parents typically preferred the hospital, which in the prevailing cultural milieu was less stigmatized than incarceration.

Table 2 is based on data from the Adolescent Health Survey (see appendix) and describes the basic demographic characteristics of participants' families and households. Slightly less than half of the study participants (twenty-two, or 46.8%) lived with two caregivers (in households with two caregivers, both those individuals were not necessarily biological parents of the adolescent participant), while approximately a third (seventeen, or 36.2%) lived with a single caregiver (all but one of them female), and eight (17.0%) lived with multiple caregivers. Parents/guardians were typically employed either full or part time (thirty-six, or 76.6%), while a minority (eleven, or 23.4%) were unemployed. The leading parent/guardian occupation types reported were skilled labor (twenty-seven, or 38.0%), professional (seventeen, or 24.0%), and service industry (fifteen, or 21.1%). Even among those making minimum wage or higher, many (but not all) of the overall household incomes were affected by reduced employment (e.g., half-time), and significant caregiver responsibilities meant that they were living below or barely above the official poverty line. Household size ranged from small, at two to four people (ten, or 23.2%); to medium, at five people (eighteen, or 41.9%); to large, at six to eleven people (fifteen, or 34.9%). Dwelling size varied considerably, from between one and three rooms (twelve, or 28.6%), to four or five rooms (sixteen, or 38.1%), to six or seven rooms (ten, or 23.8%), to eight or more rooms (four, or 9.5%). A substantial proportion of the youth had biological parents who were were divorced or separated (twenty-two, or 54%), while the parents of significantly fewer were married or living together (eight, or 19.5%), and for several of the adolescents one or both parents were deceased (four, or 9.7%); seven youth (17%) did not know the marital status of their parents. Occupation, employment, and household size indicate a relatively broad range of socioeconomic status; the substantial minority of parents and guardians in professional employment indicate that while poverty and economic hardship are definitely in play, the class position of the families is not uniform, as is to be expected in the population served by the premier public adolescent psychiatric facility in the state.

Table 3 provides information on school, drugs, and gangs, derived from the Adolescent Health Survey. These data indicate that the majority of these hospitalized youth (80.9%) were attending school when they entered the study, but only two-thirds (63.2%) were at their expected grade level. There was a broad range of academic achievement as expressed in grades

TABLE 2   KIN/HOUSEHOLD CHARACTERISTICS OF ADOLESCENT
PARTICIPANTS (N = 47)[a]

	n	%
Number of parent/guardian caregivers		
Two (mother/father/stepparent)	22	46.8
One (female)	16	34.1
One (male)	1	2.1
Multiple	8	17.0
Parent/guardian employment status		
Full- or part-time	36	76.6
Unemployed	11	23.4
Parent/guardian occupation[b]		
Skilled labor	27	38.0
Professional	17	24.0
Service industry	15	21.1
Works at home	4	5.6
None/unemployed	8	11.3
Number of people in household		
2–4	10	23.2
5	18	41.9
6–11	15	34.9
Number of rooms in house/apartment		
1–3	12	28.6
4–5	16	38.1
6–7	10	23.8
8+	4	9.5
Status of biological parents		
Divorced/separated	22	53.7
Living together/married	8	19.5
One/both parents deceased	4	9.7
Don't know	7	17.1

[a]Not all participants completed all items on the Adolescent Health Survey (Resnick, Blum, and Harris 1989). N may be less than 47 for some items; percentages are based on number reporting for each item.
[b]"Works at home" refers to housekeeping in parent/guardian's own home; "service industry" includes such labor in the homes of others.

reported, ranging from A (23.1%), to B (30.8%), to C and below (25.6%), with a minority reporting that they did not know their grades (20.5%). In general, attitudes toward school were mixed, ranging from liking school quite a bit or very much (40.5%), to liking school very little or somewhat (33.3%), to hating or disliking school (26.2%). A substantial proportion

TABLE 3 SCHOOL, DRUGS, AND GANGS IN THE LIVES OF ADOLESCENT
PARTICIPANTS $(N = 47)^a$

	n	%
In school at start of study		
Yes	38	80.9
No	9	19.1
At expected grade level (if in school)		
Yes	24	63.2
No	14	36.8
Current grade ranges		
A, A–	9	23.1
B+, B, B–	12	30.8
C+, C, below C	10	25.6
Don't know	8	20.5
Feelings about going to school		
I hate/don't like school	11	26.2
Like school some	14	33.3
Like school quite a bit/very much	17	40.5
I worry about how I'm doing in school		
Not at all	12	27.9
Very little/somewhat	11	25.6
Quite a bit/very much	20	46.5
I worry about getting beat up in school		
Not at all	25	58.1
Very little/somewhat	12	27.9
Quite a bit/very much	6	14.0
Gang involvement		
Not involved/no friends in gangs	17	39.5
Friends in gangs, not me	19	44.2
I spent time in gangs	7	16.3
There are drugs at school		
Not at all/little	8	20.0
Some	9	22.5
Quite a bit/very much	23	57.5
There is drinking at school		
Not at all/little	22	55.0
Some	4	10.0
Quite a bit/very much	14	35.0

[a]Not all participants completed all items on the Adolescent Health Survey (Resnick, Blum, and Harris 1989). N may be less than 47 for some items; percentages are based on number reporting for each item.

of adolescents expressed being worried about being at school quite a bit or very much (46.5%), while others expressed worrying very little or some-what (25.6%) or not at all (27.9%). Worries about getting beat up at school were not pressing for most, with a minority worrying quite a bit or very much (14.0%), a slightly higher proportion worrying very little or somewhat (27.9%), and the majority not worrying at all (58.1%). With regard to gangs in school, those who reported that they had spent time involved with gangs were a notable minority (16.3%), while those who had friends in gangs but claimed not to be involved themselves were a substantially higher proportion (44.2%), with slightly fewer (39.5%) reporting neither personal involvement nor any friends in gangs. Higher levels of drug use (57.5%) than alcohol use (35.0%) at schools was reported by some adolescents. Others reported observing no use or smaller percentages of use (20.0% for drugs and 55.0% for alcohol).

Against the background we have provided in this opening chapter, the data we have gathered afford a number of complementary perspectives in the following chapters that allow for the presentation of textured case studies of young people's experience over time (see particularly chapter 4), while also analyzing a range of thematic domains common to their experi-ence. We have been able to juxtapose the experientially rich but unevenly elaborated accounts of cultural meaning and social interaction in our nar-rative data with data from standardized instruments that present a system-atic and comparable but relatively shallow profile of participants' distress, symptoms, and patterns of behavior. We are able to examine the words of adolescent psychiatric patients in relation to those of their parents. The narratives are often poignant, revealing, and disturbing tangles of lives on the edge of endurance and capacity. There are narrative shifts in self-positioning of the teens (e.g., one day "my parents don't understand," and the next "I can't wait to get out of here so I can be with my 'real' family" [gang]). In the course of our work with youth and parents, we have also gone through shifts in our own experience of ethnography that range from sympathy to incredulity. Throughout what follows, we have endeavored to remain as faithful as possible to the lived experience of those who chose to speak with us as well as to the interpretive task of anthropology.

CHAPTER 2

Coming to the Hospital

How do these youth and their parents understand the way they came to be hospitalized at this particular moment in their lives? This question is a critical point of entry into the challenge of describing their lived experience. However distressed they may have been prior to their admission at CPC, and however disrupted their lives may already have been, entering the psychiatric hospital is a significant rupture in their everyday experience. It is the beginning of a separation from family members, only to become surrounded by professional caregivers who work within a distinct treatment protocol and quotidian institutional regime. From a research standpoint, the admitting incident is the one experience held in common by all the project's participants. It is a methodological bottleneck passed through by all forty-seven youth in the study—from disparate parts of the state, with different diagnostic and demographic profiles, different family experiences and ethnic backgrounds, different histories of prior treatment and hospitalization, and different trajectories that we have attempted to trace. Thus, it is incumbent upon us to elucidate the ways in which youth and parents talked about how they came to be there at the moment when they encountered members of our research team.

How they got to the hospital may be consequential for how young people engage treatment, and their accounts of how they got there could be valuable background information for treatment providers who want to anticipate the kinds of predicaments the adolescents are facing as they enter inpatient treatment. Hospital admission is certainly a prime event in which we can observe their lives in the context of extreme disruption that may involve an entire family and creates a critical interaction with the mental health care system and sometimes law enforcement. Finally, the accounts of coming to the hospital afford insight into a young person's awareness and articulation of their own experience in the form of telling a story, to formulate a *narrative* about what happened and why. Invoking the idea of narrative brings us into a field of narrative theory and narratology that includes work on self and illness in medical anthropology and the medical humanities (Kleinman 1988b; Ochs and Capps 1996, 2001; Hydén 1997; Mattingly and Garro 2000; Shimazono 2005; Kokanović and Flore 2017; Woods 2011, 2012). We can specify what attending to narrative can tell us about the lived experience of this particular group of troubled young people. To be precise, there are "two competing views on the relationship between narrative form and lived experience. The first view holds that the narrative is a linguistic or cognitive form used to reconstruct human reality. . . . By contrast, other authors promote the view that the relationship between narrative time and lived time is continuous or even homologous" (Shimazono 2005: 21, 22). In the first view, narrative and lived experience are distinct, and narrative is imposed on experience after the fact; in the latter view, narrative and lived experience have the same form, and life unfolds as a story.

These alternative understandings of narrative are relevant to our analysis in two ways. First, the narratives offered by these young people about how they came to be hospitalized were often given in response to an ethnographic interview and were not stories that emerged in the course of everyday lives or that young people necessarily tell one another or their family members. Thus, they are reconstructions situated outside the flow of the everyday. Second, and at the same time, they reflect the very ability and willingness—or, in some cases, an urgent insistence—to relay stories of events that have a distinct place in the fabric of their troubled lives. This observation is reinforced by the fact that not all the youth respond with anything like a developed story. The accounts they provide are sometimes hardly elaborated and do not necessarily have all the elements that typically constitute a narrative, including a plot with beginning, middle, and end or characters with motivations.

To be precise, the accounts we elicited of being hospitalized range in degree of elaboration from giving a *minimal reason* to offering a *fleshed-out narrative*. Some of the young people are laconically concise in their responses, in a way that is, if not dispassionate, markedly matter-of-fact.

The least elaborated responses are those such as "I'm here for fighting" or "for running away" or "for a suicide attempt" or "for threatening somebody with a knife" or "for anger problems and to be put on medication" or "for anger problems and because I smoke weed" or "My grandparents died. . . . I just went in saying that I was depressed." In instances that are notably spare, there may well be a story behind such truncated presentations, which in themselves afford a very limited narrative purchase on lived experience. With even a minimal degree of elaboration, elements of lived experience become observable through word choice, expressive style, contextual features of the social situation, and nuances of interpersonal relationships. Ethnographically, we anticipate surprises (for interlocutor and ethnographer alike) when presuppositions and taken-for-granted ideas are subject to spontaneous questioning, puzzlement, or moments of silence. Our analyses likewise attend to emotion, expressed both through narrative content and by vocal qualities of voice including tone and prosodic elements of speech. Finally, we attend to narrative processes of struggle evidenced by actively engaged communication of personal suffering and the places, persons, and situations that are perceived as foreclosing or fostering the possibilities for having a life.

Before considering more fleshed-out narrative accounts of coming to the hospital, we offer several illustrations of minimally elaborated reasons for the current hospitalization:

> Just because I have been a troubled kid . . . like not listening in school and never doing what I am told and for drug abuse, doing drugs.

This boy deploys the overarching category of "troubled kid"—not an illness or diagnosis—to account for his hospitalization, with a concise enumeration of criteria that qualify him for that category. Or consider another brief example, from a girl we recorded, that provides minimal reasons for the hospital admission and in which there appears a less marked matter-of-factness in the abbreviated narrative form:

> Well, just a lot of stuff. I had tried to run away. Um, uh, arguments, just in fights, just I had lost control, I guess. And I was depressed and angry all the time. It was a unanimous decision between me, my therapist, and my mom.

As in the preceding example, this girl invokes an overarching category unrelated to an illness or diagnosis, with the idea of having "lost control" subsuming a number of specific criteria. She includes narrative elements of running away and getting in fights as well as the affective components of depression and anger. She emphasizes that the hospitalization was based on a unanimous decision that indicates an element of agency on her part, along with the inclusion of the language of psychiatric disorder. Another girl unequivocally invoked a particular psychiatric disorder with narrative concision:

> Um, I'm bipolar. And being bipolar is really hard because sometimes I get really out of control and all, I go all manic or I go into depression. I'm here for basically being bipolar and the things that I do when I'm bipolar, being manic and stuff.

Spare as it is, and focused as it is on the reasons for hospitalization, this girl's account has narrative elements in referring to "sometimes" getting out of control and "the things that I do" on such occasions. She not only cites a particular illness, but taps into a distinction between being and doing, with recognition that bipolar is a condition but that it is characterized by certain types of action/behavior. The affective reference to the illness being "really hard" opens onto the theme of *struggle,* rather than symptoms, as central to the lived experience of mental illness (Jenkins 2015a), and even in such a brief account we can infer that this is a struggle not only with the illness but also with its consequences, including the fact of hospitalization. In another example, a boy gave the following reason for his hospitalization:

> You know why I think I went up there [to the hospital]? It's 'cause I quit my medication. I just stopped it. Cold turkey. And then I lighted up again. I ran away. Actually, I went nowhere. I just stood outside the door. I was talking to Mama Tia. I was screaming at that cat. The police came. My mom called them.

This boy gives no motive for quitting his medication, but he makes a clear causal link between quitting and the admitting incident. The narrative suggests a "vexed agency" in which quitting medication is no more a considered act than is becoming "lighted up" and out of control outside the door. In other words, one can infer a paradoxical relation between his *recognition* that one act led to another and his apparent lack of *motivation* for going off his medication. Likewise, there are paradoxical relations between running away and going nowhere, and in both talking to and screaming at Mama Tia the cat without an explicit reference to any affect associated with his screaming. Finally, there is both narrative elegance and poignant matter-of-factness in the narrative's conclusion: "The police came. My mom called them." For a final brief illustration, a girl explained her hospitalization like this:

> Well, I have depression and I hallucinate also. I don't remember what really happened, but I've heard that I overdosed on my prescription drugs. And I was cutting my arm. 'Cause I was hallucinating. . . . Before I went to the hospital I just remembered talking to my mom on the couch, just watching TV. And then I just remember waking up in the hospital. . . . When I went to CPC they said that when I get angry, I black out sometimes [epilepsy]. So I'm thinking that's what happened.

Aside from the matter-of-fact acknowledgment of depression, hallucination, cutting, getting angry, and blacking out, the critical narrative element is that this girl "heard" about her overdose and hospitalization as if in a secondhand report, making her own inference after the fact about what happened. Rather than a vexed agency, her narrative is characterized by a sense of spontaneous occurrence, with even less expression of motivation and agency for overdosing than the boy in the preceding example gave for going off his medication.

These brief accounts still say little about the complexity of individual cases, and we do not intend them to do so, which is why we gave no more background than whether the speaker was a boy or girl. The purpose in presenting them is to make the point that even minimally elaborated narratives afford a degree of insight into the immediacy of lived experience in the context of a particularly salient event, admission to the psychiatric hospital. Even from these brief narratives we can conclude that our young interlocutors have something of consequence to say about their experience. Beyond that, we must be prepared to address language, intersubjectivity, and empathy as conceptual portals for engaging the struggles embedded in the process of coming to the hospital.

How we read and understand these accounts depends in part on how we understand *language,* including narrative language. We have noted that narrative can be viewed either as reconstructing reality or as continuous with lived experience, and in some circumstances it can be both. Likewise, it is inadequate to conceive of language only as a public medium that shapes, constructs, or distorts a domain of experience that remains private and even inchoate, such that we only ever have access to language and never to experience or the subjectivity that underlies it, and such that language becomes not only a framework for experience but also a kind of cage for it. We prefer a warmer theory of language, one closer to the assertion by Heidegger in his "Letter on Humanism" that "language is the house of being" (1978 [1947]). Language can, again in Heidegger's terms, not only conceal but also "disclose" experience if it is understood not in abstract, mentalistic terms but as a kind of bodily secretion imbued with intersubjectivity. It is in this sense that language is the form of, borrowing a phrase from Merleau-Ponty (1968 [1964]), our "sonorous being," the meaningful sounds that we can feel emanating from our chest, throat, and head when we speak or tell a story.

Intersubjectivity, in general but specifically with respect to trying to capture the experiential immediacy of such an event, does not allow us to answer the question "What is it like to be someone else?" but instead allows us to ask the question "What is it like for someone else to be?" (cf. Linger 2010). The first question implies that what we want to know is what it would be like *for me* to be another person; the second is about what it is like for that person to be her, himself, or them. Ethnography is predicated on intersubjectivity not as overlapping or penetrating the being of the Other but as the aspect of consciousness that inherently includes "the possibility of being in the place where the Other is" (Duranti 2010). This necessarily is an inferential process because it is based on engagement and intuitive listening rather than our identity with that person; intersubjectivity is not shared subjectivity, but as Merleau-Ponty (1962 [1945]) observed, the recognition that an interlocutor is "another myself." It is also inferential because a person is unlikely to be able to respond to a direct question about what it is like to be him/her/them, and because such an answer in any case would already be in the register of reflexivity and not immediacy.

The question of intersubjectivity in interpreting narrative—an aspect of what we will call narrative intersubjectivity—is closely bound up with the idea of *empathy,* a topic recently revisited in anthropology and philosophy. Authors from both disciplines (Hollan and Throop 2008; Ratcliffe 2012) observe that much current debate on empathy revolves around whether interpersonal understanding is primarily theoretical, a cognitively based processing of others' observed behavior based on a tacit but organized body of knowledge; or simulated in an implicitly mirrored or explicitly reenacted form based on an embodied experiential ability. This parallels the debate we mentioned above about whether narrative is a reconstruction of reality or whether there is an embodied continuity between narrative time and lived time. It may not be a coincidence that similar questions can be asked about the structure of narrative and the structure of empathy. If it is not the case that narrative is the ideal vehicle of empathy, at least we can posit the possibility of a narrative empathy to go along with the idea of narrative intersubjectivity.

Anthropologists are concerned with how (and in what forms) empathy exists across cultural, social, and economic contexts as well as with its role in ethnographic methodology, where empathy is "approximating the subjective experience of another from a quasi-first-person perspective" and "a first-person-like perspective on another that involves an emotional, embodied, or experiential aspect" (Hollan and Throop 2008: 387, 391). Hollan observes that not only the capabilities of the empathizer but "the imaginative and emotional capabilities of the person [are] to be understood as well" (2008: 475). From the side of philosophy, Ratcliffe (2012) distinguishes between mundane empathy that presupposes a shared or mostly shared world and radical empathy that recognizes a variable sense of belonging to a shared world. For Ratcliffe, radical empathy is predicated on a phenomenological stance that recognizes reality as constituted by a horizon of possibilities that can become constrained and foreclosed, but also altered in structure or transformed. In the present case, ethnographic description of adolescent experience encountered in sites of care and subject to forms of harm entails fluctuating between trying to imagine oneself in the place of another and interacting with another from one's own positionality. Also embedded in the challenge of ethnographic empathy is the reach to grasp our interlocutors' often strikingly engaged *struggle* as central to their being (or wishing *not* to be) in a world constituted at once by anguish, abandonment, oppression, cruelty, love, care, and compassion (Jenkins 2015a). This, in turn, requires awareness that ethnography affords situated standpoints for an apprehension of experiential epistemologies (Harding 1991, 2015) and invites engagement with a feminist ethics of care (Lindemann 2006).

HEARING NARRATIVES OF CRISIS AND HOSPITALIZATION

Having established our mode of engaged listening in terms of language, intersubjectivity, and empathy, the bulk of this chapter is about those of our young interlocutors who not only had relatively more elaborated admission narratives but whose parents/guardians also offered narratives of the same event. How do these narratives do their cultural work? They do so by highlighting a scenario of disruption. In fact, there is a theory of narrative process that precisely fits this scenario. This is Todorov's (1969) idea that any narrative goes through five stages: a situation in equilibrium, disruption of that equilibrium, recognition of the disruption, an attempt to remedy the disruption or repair its damage, and arrival at a new equilibrium. Todorov was describing an elementary structure of narrative in general, but this structure is particularly amplified and poignantly vivid in the case of severely troubled adolescents. We adopt this understanding of narrative structure/process with the express recognition (1) that equilibrium is a relative and, in the present ethnographic case, an arguably oxymoronic term since the quotidian "equilibrium" preceding hospitalization is marked by fragility and instability; (2) that the disruption of equilibrium comes in the form of exacerbation of instability wherein our interlocutors perceive and respond to an event of urgency or a crisis that ruptures expectable daily routine (e.g., suicide attempt, arrest by police); and (3) that the "new" equilibrium is achieved only by hospitalization, and this equilibrium is no less fragile than the initial one, a temporary respite from further disruption or urgency. We will go so far as to say that this model (or elements of it) is self-evident across these admission narratives.

Examining these narratives allows us to take a critical further step toward the lived experience of psychiatric hospital admission by adding the element of family intersubjectivity, juxtaposing parent and child accounts from cases in which both sides are relatively well elaborated. To be precise, while we have referred to narrative intersubjectivity between the ethnographer and interlocutor, in these admission narratives there is also a narrative intersubjectivity within the family. Again, to be precise, if we allow that a story is "what happened," and a narrative is the "account of what happened," the fundamental feature of narrative intersubjectivity would be whether or not the youth and parent/guardian are "telling the same story." At a minimal level, in the terms we have introduced from Todorov, there would be concordance between the youth and parent/guardian in recognizing a disruption of equilibrium and an attempt to restore equilibrium.

Noteworthy in addition to this narrative intersubjectivity is the interplay within the individual narratives between *description*, which can be quite concrete and matter-of-fact, and *reflection*, which can be quite insightful and narratively rich in these accounts. Also of import for lived experience are modulations of temporality. This is so in two senses. First, as an event the hospitalization may be experienced as something that happens over the course of hours or as the culmination of a process that takes place over days, weeks, or months. Second, even though hospitalization is a profound rupture in the fabric of everyday life, it may not be the first such rupture insofar as a significant proportion of the youth had been hospitalized and separated from their families previously. In addition, not only does each event have a distinct character based on the circumstances, individual actors, and illness processes involved, but the narratives of different youth/guardian pairs often share motifs that are elaborated in very different ways. In an overarching sense, these narratives can be understood in terms of a distinct set of temporal schemas. In order to make this observation as phenomenologically lucid as possible, we have identified six such temporal schemas: *The Precipitating Event; Last Trigger, Last Straw; Three Days in a Row; In the Revolving Door; Kill or Be Killed;* and *Clinical Volunteers.* Note that at this stage of our analysis we are not yet concerned with psychiatric diagnosis or family definition of the young person's problem (chapter 3), nor with their experience of treatment or medication (chapter 5).

THE PRECIPITATING EVENT

These narratives describe relatively discrete episodes that led directly to a hospitalization, and the disruption of equilibrium typically has to do with an act of aggression or transgression. This does not mean that the episode occurred "out of the blue," without context or a history of emotional disturbance and psychiatric treatment. What the following instances of Mariana and Scott show is a narrative style shared by both youth and parent that brackets the event as if it were a discrete or isolated episode.

Mariana was a fourteen-year-old Mexican-American girl who lived with her mother, her mother's husband, her maternal grandfather, an older sister (eighteen), an older brother (seventeen), and a younger sister. Her family had recently moved into a small adobe house in a Spanish-speaking neighborhood southwest of Albuquerque, having relocated from the War Zone neighborhood. Her mother had a long history of gang involvement (since age eleven), including "running" the gang. When Mariana was nine years old, her mother was sent to prison for aggravated assault. Around the same time, Mariana began having negative experiences of not only seeing but now also hearing a longtime imaginary friend she called "The Man." The voice she heard was mean to her, telling her to hurt herself and others, berating her, and even instructing her to kill herself. For a couple of years she lived, in succession, with her aunt, her grandmother, and her stepfather, who raped and beat her. During that time she tried to hang herself and also stabbed a schoolmate/bully with a pair of scissors because she was sick of him making fun of her and her mother. Voices in her head caused her to became more agitated and scared, until she was placed in inpatient care at age twelve. Following discharge, Mariana tried to commit suicide again because she thought her mother and sister didn't love her. She describes her most recent hospital admission at CPC below, and her mother's narrative follows:

> *Mariana:* Well, what happened [then] was I was at school and I had a shoelace in my pocket and a boy wanted to see the shoelace. So, I let him see it. I didn't know he was gonna start choking people with it. And he blamed it on *me.* He said I made him do it. And I told him that sometimes I think of choking people and he went and told them [the cops], so that's why I was [taken] in the psychiatric hospital. I told him, 'cause he asked me, "Before you went to the hospital did you think about choking people?" and I'm like, "Yeah," and he's all, "Well, I feel like choking people right now." And I was like, "OK." And then he just started choking people and I was like, "Oh, my God." And then he had the nerve to tell them that I made him do it. And then he told them that I was thinking about choking him . . . I went to them [the cops] 'cause I didn't want to get in trouble. And I still got in trouble! They read my notebook and I have all kinds of personal stuff in there and they wouldn't let me see my mom 'cause I didn't want to see her 'cause I was scared. I didn't want to get in trouble, have her yell at me. I was just like, "God, I don't want to see her right now." And they were like, "You don't have to see your mom." And I was like, "OK." So, we were just, like, they had me in the back room and then, like, my mom was in the front room cussin' them out 'cause she wanted to see me. So, when I was walking out, I hugged my mom and they were like, "Well, you can't hug your mom because you requested not to see her." And I was all, "I can, I can hug my mom if I want to" . . . sometimes I feel really, really angry and I write down in my book. Um, it had some awful stuff in there so they—that's the whole reason probably why I went to CPC 'cause I've had that book for, like, two years. Four years. I've never seen my notebook since. They [police] won't give it back to me.

> *Mariana's mother:* I guess one day she took a shoestring to school and told this little boy, "Have you ever thought about choking anybody?" And I don't know exactly what the conversation was like, but I know that it consisted of choking somebody and a shoestring. And the little boy went and choked some of the kids and they—'cause Mariana told him and they know that she has a mental disability and they, they put a 504 plan into place and they didn't really explain it to me. He read it to me and when I came home—I should have read it before I signed it. But I trusted him, the vice principal or whatever he was. And when I came home the paper was saying that they were having problems with her but I was never informed of any problems whatsoever. And then when this incident happened, because the 504 plan

was in place, they pulled her out of school. . . . They had her in the office. The cop was questioning her and questioning her. And then when I got there, the cop—I don't know what the cop told her, she was so scared she didn't want to see me! And I was like—I told the cop, I said, "I know my rights. I have every right to be in there. She don't want it, it doesn't matter what she wants, she's a minor child." Well, anyways, to make a long story short, the little boy said that she made him do it and she was held accountable for his actions. And she was kicked out of that school for the rest of the year. So, um, she told them that she felt homicidal and I'm sure she did . . . but, you know, like I told 'em, "You can't hit people and get away with it. You gotta let stuff go." And she just, I guess she told 'em, "I feel this and that," and sometimes I noticed that to get out of trouble she says things, she'll make up something . . . but I told her, "You know, you need to get it right. Don't make up stuff. This is very serious stuff. You know, [when you get older] they can put you in jail for this." And, she just looked at me and I told her, "You know, you gotta think of every aspect of every situation. You're old enough to make your own choices. You know regardless of the conversation—if it was just like a consensual conversation between both of you and you were just telling how you feel, because of what's wrong with you, they blew it all into craziness" . . . so, it was just a really big thing. They put her in the hospital.

This is a case in which the narrative focuses on a discrete event that results in a hospital admission, Mariana's second. Between her admission narrative and her mother's there is substantial concordance, but also ambiguity over who instigated the choking event at school, and over what the relationship was between Mariana and the boy, since, as Mariana said, they "weren't really that much of friends." Mariana attributes her hospitalization as much to the discovery of "awful stuff" she had written in her journal, which she says was never returned to her, as to the shoelace incident itself. Twice, with reference to the police and her mother, Mariana indicates a concern that she not "get in trouble." While Mariana indicates that she did not want to see her mother because she was scared of being in trouble, her mother indicates that the police told Mariana something that made her scared of seeing her mother. The warmth between them is poignant in the image of Mariana trying to hug her mother but being led away in handcuffs to the hospital. Her mother's own issues with the police, having been imprisoned herself, were evident in her complaints about not having been adequately informed about Mariana's 504 behavioral management plan at school, about being called hours after the incident occurred, about "knowing her rights" with respect to access to Mariana, and about both the boy and the school authorities using knowledge of her "mental disability" to "blow it all into craziness." At the same time the mother recounts having advised Mariana to manage her situation and feelings better and make better choices, but also not to be as manipulative and "make up stuff" to draw attention to her emotional state as a way to distract from the trouble and disruption in which she had become embroiled.

Salvador was a seventeen-year-old of Hispanic background living with his mother, his younger brother, a cousin, and a paying lodger. The family resided in a two-story stucco house in a gated community that was part of a newer suburb. He had a nineteen-year-old half-brother who, like Salvador, had a problem with alcohol abuse and who had recently been sent to prison for holding up a liquor store with a knife. Salvador reported that his first major mental health issues occurred three or four years before he had been hospitalized in another state for what he called "anorexia." He described his eating problems as being driven more by just being out running around and not focusing on eating, which may reflect some detachment or perhaps anxiety/agitation due to unmet self-care needs. He said that he was never trying to lose weight but that he was always out skateboarding and getting high. He said that since moving from California he had had several admissions to CPC, including one for "running away and bad sleep," and another admission in California for self-harm threats because he did not want to live in Albuquerque. Salvador's alcohol problems seemed to be the most serious threat to his stability, and he claimed to have used alcohol to cope with depressive feelings over the years.

> *Salvador:* Uh, I was caught shoplifting at Walmart. And, um, they found alcohol on me and I was intoxicated at the time. And, um, I don't really remember saying this, but I guess when I got to the detention center I told the police that I was trying to hurt myself. They took me to, uh, like, an emergency room for the mental health thing. I woke up there and then in the morning, they took me to CPC. . . . [I've been depressed] since I can remember.

> *Salvador's mother:* Well, I didn't notice too much, until I found out that he was already in the hospital [*laughs*]. He was taking his medication, so I thought he was doing OK, except that he wasn't sleeping and he wasn't doing well at school. And, he was not showing up to his classes, which got him kicked out of school [*laughs*]. But other than that, I really thought he was doing OK with the medication [Zoloft]. He left the house in the middle of the night with his cousin and they went to Walmart, and I guess he decided to get drunk at Walmart. I didn't hear about it till the next morning when my other son told me, and then they told me that the police had taken him, had arrested him from Walmart. Then I started calling the detention center and they told me he wasn't there, and then I didn't find out where he was until like four o'clock, when my friend actually found out from someone she

knows that works there [*small laugh*] that he was in the hospital so that's when I finally found him. . . . It was scary because I know he's been through the depression and the suicide attempts before so I was scared enough to know that the police had taken him. And, well, it's pretty scary when you know [*laughs*]—when you know that your kids have been disappeared, nobody knows where they're at [*laughs*].

Although Salvador acknowledges having been depressed ever since he can remember, he narrates the shoplifting incident that resulted in hospitalization as a discrete event with little context or buildup. He was evidently both intoxicated and disoriented, without recollection that he had acknowledged suicidal intent to the police, and unable to notify his family of what had happened to him, since they ended up having to search for him. Salvador's mother provides a bit more context with respect to his concurrent trouble sleeping and trouble in school, but her overarching sense that otherwise he had been "doing OK" on his medication consolidates the narrative effect of understanding his Walmart episode as an isolated and surprising event. This effect is amplified by her not becoming aware of the event till the next morning and her frightened search to determine his whereabouts, as well as by her nervous and embarrassed laughter while telling the story. It is also of note that a number of others are involved in the narrative, including the cousin who was with Salvador at Walmart but who was not himself arrested, Salvador's brother who told the mother of the arrest, and her friend who had an acquaintance who worked at the hospital.

LAST TRIGGER, LAST STRAW

Families can tolerate a remarkable amount of turmoil and chaos before there is a disruption of equilibrium severe enough to result in hospitalization. Like the first two narratives above, the two that follow involve a critical incident. However, particularly in the parents' versions, these narratives vividly depict situations of cumulative stress that reaches a point of rupture. While we cannot say for certain, it is possible that this quality of the narratives indicates not a difference in the circumstances that surround a precipitating event but a difference in narrative propensity to recognize and articulate a pattern and trajectory both to events and to the overall illness process in which the family is caught up.

We first met Ben, a fifteen-year-old Anglo-American male, when he was living with his adoptive mother, stepfather, stepsister, and several pets, including five dogs, four cats, and two guinea pigs. Ben had lived with his biological mother until he was nine, during which time his life had been unstable, with periods of homelessness in relation to his mother's mental illness, a type of schizophrenia. At the age of nine, he entered the foster care system. At age twelve, after a series of unstable or abusive placements, he began receiving mental health services and was adopted by his current family. During the study, Ben's adoptive mother's ex-husband, a war veteran with post-traumatic stress disorder and depression who was threatening toward Ben, "disowned" him and did not want to see Ben again. Ben was in tenth grade in a Christian school but reported his religion as Satanist. He enjoyed drawing, writing, reading, and spending time with his stepsister and family.

> *Ben:* I was trying to, like, scratch through my skin to get to the vein, like, cut it or something. I took a knife and I tried to slit my wrist [because of] my [adoptive] dad not wanting to be a part of my life, 'cause I split with him and [because] everything that's happened in the past, it's like catching up to me. It was New Year's Day, I was just dealing with a lot of stress and I kind of went overboard. All the stuff from my biological mom to foster homes to getting rejected by adoptions, I'm lost in it . . . the paramedics came and tried to get my pulse and then we went to the doctors to get that all patched up, then back to [the residential facility], and then my mom and stepdad took me to the hospital.

> *Ben's mother:* It was actually a few different things. I think the last trigger point was his adoptive dad, my ex-husband, decided he no longer wanted to be involved and told him pretty much, "Bye!" So that was obviously somewhat traumatic for him. There had been little things leading up to it, but I think that was just a little bit too much. Just immediate depression. . . . New Year's Day he got in trouble for something, I can't remember what it was, he was going to be grounded but he had to sit here so we could see him. He was completely tense and everything was just completely tight and leg shaking and he couldn't pull himself out of it, I don't think he was able to, really. Just a little bit too much and he just kind of calmly got up and walked over and grabbed a kitchen knife and we were both like [*imitates sound of rocket taking off*] across the room, pounced on him . . . they called it superficial so it wasn't real deep or anything but we had a hard time getting it from him. He stayed just completely tense and he was not calmed down and he didn't want me to hold something on it so I had his arm like literally pinned holding tissues on it. I said, "If you can't calm down I am going to have to call the police." And he said, "Do it." And I did [*laughs*]. We had a house full of firemen and paramedics and sheriff's deputies and . . . [*Husband speaks*] The neighbors all flipped out. They were like, "Ooooh!" [*Mother resumes speaking*] And they took him in by ambulance and he spent quite a few hours at the emergency room. By then he was just so physically worn out, he was just like wiped and they said, "Are you OK to take him home?" And we said, "Yeah." And you could see that he was just going to go to sleep. He went

back [to school] the next day and that was our first family [therapy] session. . . . And a little bit after we left, she [the therapist] called and, uh, some of my jewelry and stuff had been gone and we were trying to figure out who did it. Nice, expensive jewelry and his therapist called and said, "Ben has this ring and he says he is giving it to his girlfriend." And I was like, "Really?" So she described it and I was like, "Yeah, that's mine." And he swore up and down that he found it outside by the gate and I was like, "Not buying it." And it just kind of sent him into a pout and he walked out of the therapist's office upset and so we figured, well, and his probation officer was really actively involved and she [also] thought he needs to go back. And she had actually scheduled a court date to force him to go into residential [treatment] and I called her and said, "It's not necessary. We're taking him now" [laughs]. And so we picked him up from school and took him and I sat in the waiting room most of the night and [my husband] drove all the way back here and gathered up clothes, personal care items, drove him all the way back [laughs] and we sat for a few more hours until we finally got him checked in around, um, right around midnight.

Ben's account of his admission is brief but reflective in referring to the cumulative effects of events and stress "catching up to me." Both Ben and his mother agree that the withdrawal of her former partner with whom Ben had a close attachment as adoptive father was in her words a "trigger point" at which in Ben's words he "went overboard." They both mention New Year's Day with the implication that holiday stress played into the suicide attempt. However, it is critical to note in the mother's account that it was not the suicide attempt that led to psychiatric hospital admission, since Ben was allowed to return home after being treated for his self-inflicted wounds in the emergency room. Following his return to school and a therapy session in which his mother's missing jewelry was an issue of discussion, the determination that he had stolen it months before was the disruption of equilibrium that led his parents to take him to the hospital.

Neal was a fifteen-year-old boy who identified as part Hispanic (he also endorsed German, Irish, and Navajo identities). He was in residential treatment at CPC at the time of recruitment. His family (two mothers, two younger brothers, and two younger sisters) lived in Albuquerque, and one of his younger brothers was also in residential treatment during the study. Neal's father underwent a "gender transition"/sex change when he was thirteen or fourteen, and his parents were living together as a gay couple. It was unclear whether or not his father's transition entailed psychological stress for Neal, given that he first went to treatment at the age of six and was admitted to a residential facility at ten or eleven.

From then on, Neal constantly saw psychiatrists and underwent therapy. According to his mothers, problematic behavior had been escalating for a while—Neal had been acting "passive aggressively," fighting with his parents, breaking house rules, accessing pornography at school, stealing, and fighting. After his first discharge, Neal began living at a group home; however, his behavior became unsafe—he stole from cars, tried to run away, and called 1–900 "porno numbers." Eventually Neal was referred to one of the residential facilities in Albuquerque other than CPC, where he tried again to run away and had a destructive episode in which he committed three felonies: criminal damage to property, assault with a deadly weapon, and attempt of suicide. Prior to the current hospitalization, he was again living at home.

> *Neal:* I beat up some kid and I threw some bricks through the school bus windows when they threatened to call the cops on me. I even said, "I'll give you a better reason to call the cops" [*laughs*]. [It was] during track and field and then I was running from some kids that were after me because they couldn't ride the bus home because I just ruined the bus, there was glass everywhere. I said, "Beat me up if you want but I'm going to kill myself afterwards," and so they didn't even beat me up. They looked at me like I was out of my mind and kind of walked away. And then I walked home and didn't tell my parents anything about it. I told them I got kicked out of track and field, nothing about any of that, and then the principal called and told them that I threw bricks through the bus window and that they're going to have to pay for damages. [She] told them what I had said because the kids had apparently reported it to her and that's why they didn't beat me up. So here I am [in the hospital]. . . . [My parents brought me here] and not only that, one of my moms didn't want me to be there anymore, she was going nuts with me there at home.

> *Both parents, who asked for a joint interview:* Well really things have really been escalating for a while. We had a lot of emotional stuff going on here at the house that was getting worse every day. He was becoming very roller coaster like . . . very destructive . . . passive aggressive, bullying [his thirteen-year-old brother] in secret and then sometimes in front of us, and being just unsafe to leave alone. And, he could not be trusted. Every time we would walk out of the door for any reason, if we were only gone for five minutes he would do something insane and screw something up. So we started to do room checks and started finding all of our safety rules being violated. They're not allowed sharps up there and things like that, because [the younger brother] had sliced up the furniture [and] he'll attack you with them so we don't let scissors, and those kind of things be up there yet. We would constantly find them, they were stealing them from the school or something. We found stolen things and we found sharps and items in the room that shouldn't be in there and as we clamped down he began to have more problems at

school and then school clamped down. They reined him in at school [while] we were reining him in here and it just escalated at school where he was in fights all the time and he could not walk down the hallway between class times without getting into a verbal or physical altercation. He had to be escorted between classes and when he went to school he had to sit in the office until school started and someone walked him to class, which is pretty bad for a kid his age, and then the very last thing that happened, the last straw so to speak . . . he threw a rock at a bus window and ran off saying he was going to kill himself. And the thing is that the rock was like the size of somebody's head and he threw it through the front of a moving bus full of people so that it's not just that he was destructive but he was dangerous in the process. And prior to throwing the rock, he got in a fight with an adult at track, got thrown off of track, then went to the office and told them that he wanted his ten dollars back, the fee he paid for track, right now, and they told him to get out of here or else we're gonna call security and he said later that he said, "I'm going to give them a reason to call security," and that's when he threw the rock. And then he started screaming he was going to kill himself and all kinds of other crazy stuff. Then he came home like nothing had happened. The school's right across the street so in the three minutes it took him to walk home he was completely like nothing had happened. They called us like two minutes after he walked in the door and then we found out and we were not surprised. So it was accumulation of all this different stuff, so we took him right down to the hospital, they didn't have a spot for him, we came home, we waited [and on] the weekend was gonna drive him down south to Las Cruces to try to get him in an acute unit there. But we got lucky and got him in here [CPC].

Whereas in Ben's case cumulative stress culminated in a depressive crisis, in Neal's case it was his own escalating emotional instability and aggression that culminated in a crisis of violence. Neal's narrative, as with Mariana's above, focuses on an incident at school, which in his case included attacking another student, being dismissed from the track team, and smashing a school bus window. It appears that his threat of suicide saved him from being beaten by other students in revenge, but landed him in the hospital when they reported the threat to school authorities. Neal's matter-of-fact tone in narration was striking and doubtless indicative of his own sense of being less troubled than others perceived him to be. Unlike the embarrassed laughs of the parents in previous narratives, Neal's laugh was aggressive and defiant. There is substantial agreement between his version and his parents' version of the narrative, including the manner in which Neal came home from school acting as if nothing of grave consequence had happened, beyond his being dismissed from the track team. His parents affirm the escalation of Neal's problematic and dangerous behavior both at home and at school, with the acknowledgment that they were fortunate to succeed in getting him admitted to CPC.

THREE DAYS IN A ROW

Whereas the first two narratives describe a single event that led to hospitalization and thus exhibit the immediacy of a rupture without an evident precursor or even trigger, and the next two describe a relatively long-term cumulative process culminating in a final rupture, the two we are about to consider have in common that the hospitalization is described as the outcome of an event extending over several days. The complexity of these events is due, in part, to the ambiguity of when and whether to resort to hospitalization despite significant disruption of emotional and domestic equilibrium. It is also partly due to the often vexed path to admission, where clinical staff must not only decide on whether to admit but determine whether there is space—a "bed"—to accommodate the potential patient.

Hayley, a notably talkative Anglo-American girl, began participating in the study when she was thirteen years old. She lived with her mother, stepfather, stepsister, and stepbrother in a comfortable bungalow-style house with many plants and several pets, including a dog, a snake, birds, and rodents. By the end of the study both of her stepsiblings were living elsewhere. Hayley had an older biological sister and six stepsiblings from her stepfather's previous relationships. Her biological father had died by suicide three years before we met her, and while alive he was not a significant presence in her life. When Hayley, her mother, and her stepfather were together there was considerable tension and fighting in the house, although they reported enjoying each other's company on a one-on-one basis, and overall Hayley saw her stepfather as an improvement in her home. Hayley had witnessed a traumatizing event a year earlier when she discovered her sister attempting to commit suicide by self-cutting. After the incident, Hayley engaged in self-harm herself, which she said she did out of boredom and because it gave her a sense of relief. When Hayley entered our study, she had been admitted again after her mother had tried to do a body check for self-cutting, and though she did not find anything, a few hours later Hayley began threatening to kill herself.

> *Hayley:* Me and my mom, we got in a fight, and I got really mad, so I kinda snapped and then took more of my medication than I was supposed to. She

just way overreacted, and it was like building up over time and I was pretty mad anyways [with] some people at school. They were just fighting, they're two of my best friends. They're fighting, and it's like I have to choose who my best friend is and it is so hard. It's just like really stressful. . . . [Also, the] day before, her and my stepdad were fighting and, and it made me mad so I just went in my room and threw this thing at my wall, and it put two holes in my wall . . . it was an oatmeal pot, that I forgot to put in the dishwasher, so she [mother] freaked out [about the oatmeal pot], it's really stupid . . . I said, "OK sorry," and then she started going on and on and on and on and on about just, really, unimportant stuff and then I just said stop, and she didn't stop and I just yelled "stop!" And then, I just got mad and then we started to be like arguing. And she wanted to give me a body check because I was in the hospital previously for, um, self-harm and she just wanted to take extra precaution, so that made me really mad, and I went to take a shower in the back house apartment and she just got like pissed off and started invading my privacy so I went overboard and then I said I wanted to kill myself, you know, if I don't get to talk to my sister, and my mom was on all the phones trying to get me a crisis line to talk to but I wasn't gonna talk to somebody that I didn't know. And then I was like, oh, it's time to take my medication, after I told my mom, you know, I want to kill myself and then, she, she just, you know, she's like call 911 and then when the paramedics came, they're just like, evaluating me. When the ambulance came they're just like, did you take more of your medication than you're supposed to and I said yeah, and then, they took me in and here I am. [It was] about ten pills of twenty milligrams of Prozac but it didn't really do anything, just made me really shaky. . . . I really wasn't thinking. I just, kind of acted on impulse. Very angry.

Hayley's mother: I think it'd been leading up to it for about three days, 'cause she had taken three diphenhydramine [antihistamine], which was fifty milligrams, three days before that, but acted like she didn't know any better, and I told her, "No that's like taking six Benadryl, you don't do that." And she'd been real good with the medication up till then. But, I always know when something's goin' on because she has a tendency to take it all out on me, and so she starts getting more hostile with me, and she was doing that for three days, and the day that she ended up taking that Prozac basically from the time she got home it just got worse and worse and then I decided that I'd do a body check. I hadn't done a body check [recently] but I felt like somethin' might be going on. And I didn't see anything [cutting], although [Hayley's sister] says that she thought she saw a cut on her leg. A couple hours later she started telling everybody she wanted to kill herself. I tried calling a bunch of people, but I wasn't really getting the response I wanted, so I finally just called 911. Yeah, it was building up and then the next morning, when I was going over to the hospital to sign papers, my next-door neighbor [whose daughter and Hayley] go to school together and they're friends, was feeling bad because she didn't tell us that Hayley told [her daughter] the night before that she was havin' a real hard time at school. . . .

The reason is because she was very into the "goth," "emo" thing. And basically, I think the two months in the hospital kind of pulled her out of that a little bit, and so her friends weren't taking that very well. So she wasn't being as popular as she was and was having problems with her friends. I think that was part of what was building up. And then I talked to the [school] nurse who said she hadn't been lookin' good for a few days. She saw it comin' too, basically.

Hayley's narrative highlights a struggle not with her illness, but a struggle in the form of a fight with her mother, in the context of a fight between her mother and stepfather, and another fight between two of her school friends. Her mother was aware of Hayley's problems at school but attributed them to her becoming less popular among the "goth and emo"[1] clique after withdrawing from that element of youth culture following her previous two-month inpatient hospitalization. Twice in this three-day period, Hayley had taken too much medication (an antihistamine and Prozac) without a clear indication that either time was an attempt at suicide. It is noteworthy that Hayley emphasized the exacerbation of her state in the argument with her mother over a trivial incident of an unwashed oatmeal pot, which does not figure at all in her mother's account. What they do both recount, from somewhat different experiential stances, is the mother's "body check" to see if Hayley had any scars from self-cutting during what she recognized as a three-day escalation of hostility on Hayley's part. Hayley understood that her mother "just wanted to take extra precaution" because self-harm had been a reason for the previous hospitalization, and her mother indicated Hayley had been "OK with it" at the time. However, while Hayley said "that made me really mad" because it was "invading my privacy so I went overboard and then I said I wanted to kill myself," her mother did not perceive a connection between the body check and Hayley's crisis, saying, "It was a couple hours later. She started telling everybody she wanted to kill herself."

Sherine was a fourteen-year-old girl whose father was Guatemalan and whose mother was Chinese, although she preferred to identify herself simply as "Guatemalan" because she felt it set her apart from others in her community. She was the youngest of five children, and evidently her family, doctors, and Sherine herself agreed that her issues stemmed, in part, from being a "spoiled" youngest child. She had two brothers ages sixteen and thirty-four and two sisters ages thirty-one and thirty-three, and when we met her she lived with her sixteen-year-old brother and biological parents in a dangerous neighborhood located in the South Valley of Albuquerque. Since birth she had moved often due to her parents' employment. Her mother, who said she was on antidepressants because of the stress of dealing with Sherine, also described how the family's constant attention to Sherine had isolated the girl's brother, and said that this had caused her to "hate" Sherine. Sherine's relationship with her older siblings deteriorated over the course of the study. Her hospitalization at CPC was the result of a culmination of incidents that began with Sherine being expelled from her charter school after an incident with her teacher, having already been suspended multiple times for being "completely out of control." Sherine cut herself three days in a row, and was only hospitalized after her mother brought her to the emergency room three days in a row. In the three months following her first hospitalization, she reportedly began doing drugs, engaging in unsafe sexual practices, and being violent with her mother, which led to a second hospitalization. Her third hospitalization came after an attempt to overdose on Prozac when feeling depressed after ingesting ecstasy (MDMA). Sherine's parents traced her malcontentedness to a materialistic orientation, and her father analyzed her problems in terms of depression.

> *Sherine:* I guess I've been depressed for a long time and I've had some anger issues and one day my parents kept telling me I couldn't see certain friends, and I had just been cutting like the last few days because I was just like really, really depressed, like more depressed than I've ever been and then, finally they were just like, we're taking you to the psychiatric emergency room and so I started throwing stuff and just breaking stuff and so my mom like took me to the emergency room and I had already been there before but I went there the next day and they sent me here.

> *Sherine's mother:* She was just out of control, completely out of control and she cut herself three days in a row. Her behavior had deteriorated in the last three months, three to six months and she was just out of control and so I brought her to emergency three times before I could get her admitted. Three days in a row. I took her to the hospital, even though we were one of the first ones there in the middle of the night, people who were heroin addicts would come in on an emergency basis and Sherine would get bumped so basically at one o'clock in the morning after her cutting herself the first time we signed a waiver and went home. The following night we went to UNM psychiatric emergency and they don't have any psychiatrists that treat adolescents there, so it was "Don't cut yourself anymore and behave yourself and go home." The third night we got in there, got another psychiatrist to look at her and he actually said, "You want her to stay?" If I had said no, I guess she would have gone home, and that's basically how she ended up here. I said yes, I need her to be here because I can't see how she can go on. . . . I had told the doctor she almost wore it like a badge of honor, she calls herself "scene" and

I know a lot of their music's about cutting, it's kind of the cool thing and that's the way I had always looked at it, but it was always just like a cut and then wear your little badge of honor, a Band-Aid, but the night before she came in she cut herself so bad, it was [her whole arm] from here to here and it was bleeding everywhere, more serious than we had ever seen . . . so on the third day of emergency she took her blouse off, well she threw up on herself. She was very, very upset and at this point I didn't want to deal with her because we clash and so I don't worry a whole lot when she cuts herself because it's not like suicidal, so I stayed in the living room and [her father] dealt with her and she's very abusive towards me so I can't tell all that went on in there except that, um, that she was probably cussing like she usually does when she's mad, um, breaking things, and I know she was sticking her fingers down her throat to make herself throw up. She took off her blouse and she was yelling, "Please somebody help me, why doesn't anybody care enough to help me?" and [her father] came out of the bedroom and asked me to call the police . . . [*Father speaks*] Before my wife brought her to the hospital she was yelling and screaming, cussing and she would bang her head on the wall and she put a hole in the wall with her head, and then she was trying to look for something to cut herself. She got something and I grabbed it from her and I threw it out and after a while I hug her and she calmed down and she would ask me, "Daddy, what am I going to do, you know, tell me what to do," and I said, "Baby, if I knew what to do you wouldn't be doing this."

Sherine's narrative focuses on intense depression, self-cutting, and angry, violent frustration. She mentions being forbidden from seeing certain friends, which is not mentioned by her mother, who does, however, observe that (like Hayley) she is involved in "scene" or "emo" youth culture, which includes self-cutting as a kind of "badge of honor" (see Csordas and Jenkins 2018). Again, in this case we see an event developing over the course of three days, as well as three nighttime trips to different emergency rooms before successfully getting an admission. The parents' persistence is connected in the narrative with a sense of dedication to helping their daughter. It is likewise evident in a remarkably equanimous recognition of their daughter's desperate struggle, with Sherine's father attempting to comfort her while her mother backed off to avoid conflict until taking her to the hospital once she was sufficiently calm.

IN THE REVOLVING DOOR

The infelicitous metaphor of a revolving door (discussed further in this book's closing remarks) is often invoked to describe a consequence of increasing denial by managed care administrators of extended residential treatment for the troubled youth who most need it. An inpatient treatment period of days or even two to three weeks might barely stabilize a young patient without effectively addressing the core issues of their illness. Once they are discharged, experienced clinicians see it as virtually inevitable that they will return again, or be admitted to another facility, perhaps on a repeated basis. The following pair of narratives exhibits the painful reality of having barely been released from the hospital and being plunged back into circumstances that lead within a short period—four days in both cases—to rehospitalization.

We first met Jacob, an articulate and reflective sixteen-year-old Anglo-American male, when he had been an inpatient for several weeks. Prior to being admitted, Jacob lived with his mother and sister in a stable and secure middle-income neighborhood. His father and mother separated when Jacob was a year old. Although he was not very close to his father, Jacob thought he would be proud to see him working on his anger issues and coping skills. All three members of the family had depression and said this causes tension and drama. When Jacob was two years old, his mother's boyfriend began physically abusing him and his sister until the couple separated. Jacob did not begin speaking until he was three years old, and even then, it was difficult for most people to understand him. The resulting frustration appears to have played a part in the beginning of his anger issues. Jacob was first hospitalized when he was eight years old after an angry outburst during which he tried to run his head through a window. When he was twelve, Jacob was hospitalized for two weeks after an argument with campus security at his school. Four years later he was hospitalized again in three back-to-back periods for outbursts of anger and frustration. Three months prior to the current hospitalization, Jacob's great-grandfather died and this led to his inability to control his depression any longer.

> *Jacob:* I was discharged for four days and I started feeling suicidal again, and cutting my wrists and took 350 milligrams of Benadryl and started drinking alcohol. I'd been feeling a little suicidal for a while. I started cutting myself, and my friends were calling each other names and I just got mad, punched him in the face, threw him down on the ground, kicked him, ran him out of the classroom, calmed down for a little bit, went to the office, blew up there, jumped the fence at school, the cops tackled me and I was threatening to kill myself. . . . I was just telling my cousin the night before that I was cutting myself, 'cause I needed someone to talk to and he told my aunt, my aunt called my mom the next day and told my mom I was cutting myself. And then, later I threw [my friend on the ground] that day, so the therapist told us to come here. . . . My grandpa just died. And I was feelin' bad about how

I didn't love him, like I don't feel like I was that great, compared to other people. I feel like, by my body and stuff, I feel like it doesn't look as good as other people's. [I've been feeling that way] all my life.

Jacob's mother: Well, my grandfather had passed away, and then I got real depressed and had to get on antidepressants, and my daughter and my son are depressed at the moment. And, we are all on antidepressants at this point, but he's been in the hospital previously [twice]. And, I think he has an underlying problem other than the depression—the depression just set it off where he couldn't control it. He's been tested for all sorts of things, and treated for ADHD and bipolar, and, you know I'm not sure exactly.

Standing out against the background of clinical discourse that impinges on the everyday life of a trio, all of whom have been diagnosed with depression, is the radical fact of the recent death of Jacob's great-grandfather, cited by both Jacob and his mother. Given that disruption of everyday life is the norm for this family, they need to have this concrete experiential event to help them account for why this hospitalization is occurring now. Jacob's own account discloses a complex network of affect and embodiment with multiple struggles involving drug and alcohol abuse, self-cutting, suicidality, guilt and bereavement regarding his great-grandfather, poor self-esteem related to negative body image, a string of relevant diagnoses, disrupted family relations and a household atmosphere of depression, and a history of multiple hospitalizations. Yet despite this being a perfect storm of troubled existence that jeopardized his developmental trajectory as much as any of our participants, Jacob reports having friends and being able to attend school when not in the hospital.

We first met Anna, an Anglo-American female, two weeks prior to her turning thirteen years old. Anna's father was unemployed and her mother did not work, and this left the family in a precarious financial situation. She lived in a modest subdivision with her mother, father, and two older siblings. The relationships in the family were "difficult," "fractured," "abusive," and "sometimes supportive," and Anna had witnessed and experienced periodic violent episodes. Anna was the youngest of six children—three boys, three girls. All of the children faced physical, mental, and emotional challenges, such as attention-deficit/hyperactivity disorder (ADHD), lupus, dyslexia, epilepsy, bipolar disorder, paranoid schizophrenia, and rheumatoid arthritis. The three eldest children were from her mother's first marriage. All three of the boys had sexually assaulted all three of the girls. While Anna was certainly sexually assaulted, the extent is unknown due to a contradiction of facts from both Anna and the brother in question. Anna was also reputed to be a compulsive liar, and telling the truth was something she was working on in therapy. Prior to hospitalization, Anna had tried to run away with one of her brothers, who was now homeless; the only family member he kept in contact with was Anna. Nevertheless, during her time in psychiatric care, Anna cited her family as the best part of her life and looked forward to returning home and becoming a good role model for younger children.

Anna: Well, I started running away from my house with my brother because I was having hallucinations and I didn't want to tell anyone because they might lock me up in a mental hospital—like they did. But, yeah, I was having hallucinations and I didn't know they were hallucinations until I was talking to one of my hallucinations and my brother asked who I was talking to and I was like, "I'm talking to this person." And he's like, "No one's there," and it was all weird. I kept running, I wasn't running away because of my parents or anything like that, I was running away from my hallucinations because my hallucinations wouldn't follow me, and I didn't have a place to go so I would just run to my brother. And I knew that I couldn't run to my sister because she would just take me right back home. They thought that I was running away just to run away, that I didn't have a reason. . . . I am mad at my brother [because] he's like, "I don't want to get in trouble for kidnapping." So he made a police report and CYFD [New Mexico Children, Youth and Families Department] came. And he basically sent me to the hospital. Because CYFD had to talk to me and I accidentally said that I am suicidal [which I was] so they took me to the hospital and that's what [started the chain of events that] got me here. I'm pissed at him. Knock him upside the head if I could. . . . So, after about five times of running away, I started cutting at my house, I don't even know why I started cutting, but I knew that I couldn't get a hold of drugs so I just started cutting. So, after about a week of cutting, my mom eventually found out because she is very observant and so they took me to [a hospital] in Albuquerque and I stayed there for four days and then they discharged me because I was doing well. And then I shaved my head and I was high on ecstasy and pot at my house, so my mom did a urine test on me so she had that proof and then took me back to that hospital, but they didn't have any beds. So they took me over to CPC and I stayed there for three weeks and then I got discharged and started snorting pills, Tylenol, ibuprofen, and my mom caught me in the act so she took me to CPC, they didn't have any room. They're like, "She's a hazard," this is basically like a hotel—three weeks. So they sent me here [a residential facility in another town] and I have been here for a month and a half.

Anna's mother: So, she was with those people and [she says her brother] was afraid that he would get picked up for kidnapping her and that he called CYFD and had her picked up. Upon her return, four days later, she was resentful and withdrawn and the CYFD officer and police officer and me were all immediately in complete agreement, Anna needs to be hospitalized. I saw to it that she had a quick nourishing dinner, she went to the bathroom and took her straight to the hospital. Took us many many hours to get her into the hospital because we had to go through ER at one thirty in the morning. She is in there four days and they said, "OK, she's good. She can go home!" She's home four days. She's high on some [drug], I have no idea what, but I know it wasn't pot. I think it must have been some kind of stimulant, possibly an inhalant from what I saw of her equilibrium and her speech and her pinpointed pupils. She started scratching up her left wrist, um, I found her with a very sharp pocketknife. She stayed secluded in her room, she was very withdrawn, very resentful. And she did run off from home once. She said she was going for a jog, that she would be back in thirty minutes. At forty-five minutes we started looking for her, at an hour we called the police. Two hours after that we found her at the park and she gives various stories as to whether she was high on pot or not. We tried to rehospitalize her at the same hospital and again after many, many hours, they said, "No beds. Go home, she'll see a counselor tomorrow." I said, "No, she's not stable enough to keep her at home." They said, "Try and send her to CPC," which I did. She stayed there three weeks, the absolute maximum allowed is two weeks, but there was an insurance hassle. Then she started leveling sex abuse accusations at her seventeen-year-old brother and the insurance finally agreed to keep her at [an out-of-town facility] until August first so that we could get her on Medicaid because then she would be out of the home long enough, Medicaid would consider her a family of one with no income, which would help her get state services.

Like Jacob, Anna lived in a stable, middle-class, Anglo-American suburb, and like him she had an unstable domestic environment, in her case including a blended family with multiple siblings. Her narrative centers on repeated episodes of running away from hallucinations that she claims she did not realize were hallucinations, and an accidental or unintentional admission of suicidal thinking. Her ambiguity about hallucination is perhaps connected to her experience with MDMA and marijuana, given the hallucinogenic properties of both substances. A distinctive tendency to seek stimulation is evident in her acknowledgment that for her, self-cutting was a substitute for these drugs. It is unclear whether her accusation of sexual abuse by her brother, as reported by her mother, was in revenge for him having turned her in for fear of being accused of kidnapping her. With respect to the revolving door of hospitalization, Anna's situation includes not only multiple admissions but a process of moving from one hospital to another, in fact among three hospitals, over what can be understood as a single extended episode. From her mother's narrative it is clear that this is associated both with the availability of beds and with the available insurance coverage.

The revolving-door experience of these young people dramatically underscores the possible negative consequences of abbreviated lengths of hospital stay under the regime of managed care. Their trajectories into and among institutions will be a theme in chapter 5 when we consider their experience of psychiatric treatment.

KILL OR BE KILLED

Insofar as troubled youth survive on the edge of experience, it is unsurprising that death often inhabits their worlds, either as the possibility of suicidality, the trauma of bereavement, or exposure to violent acts and assaults, some of them fatal (e.g., an uncle who was gunned down in the front yard, a parent who attempted suicide). The admission narratives in this section exhibit another form in which death appears, now in the form of a deep ambivalence in the parent-child relationship. In the first instance it is the young person's threat to kill his parents that leads him into the hospital, and in the second it is the youth's fear of being killed by her mother that leads to her inpatient admission.

Scott was a fifteen-year-old boy who self-reported as Anglo/Native American (his mother reported that he was "Anglo"), living at home in a middle-class suburb with his biological mother, stepfather, thirteen-year-old sister, and younger half-siblings (half-sister, three; half-brother, eighteen months). In the past, Scott had lived with his father in Iowa, where he reported being much happier. Scott's mother had a fairly organized narrative of his problems, mentioning a combative relationship with her, a history of uneven discipline with his father, and an extreme interest in anime. She and her son had a contentious relationship, which she attributed to his resentment of her for divorcing his father, and which he attributed to her strictness and unfairness. Scott's extreme interest in anime contributed to the contentiousness—he spent most of his time watching anime, and it was a common interest among most of his friends. Scott's mother said it was taking over his life, and she forbade him to have any anime that she did not approve of. His mother also saw other interests he held as unhealthy obsessions, such as video games, which she felt were gateways into more problematic interests and behaviors. Scott had had mental health care prior to these episodes, due to an ADHD diagnosis, but CPC was his first hospitalization.

> *Scott:* I threatened my parents, that I'd kill them. Which was a really bad remark because I was really angry and I said something out randomly. I usually say something random when I get really angry. They were just really on

my nerves, and because, um, they were taking away my Naruto cards. And they shredded them after a while. I had like, I don't know how many cards I had, but they could have been like three hundred dollars' worth of cards. I was not happy when I found out they were all shredded. They figured it was controlling my life. I think they're wrong. [*Mock dramatically*] They're wrong!

Scott's mother: Before [Scott's stepfather] and I got married, [Scott's stepfather] caught him shoplifting at Walmart. I don't remember what the particular brand was or particular cartoon play cards that he had shoplifted, Pokémon or Digimon or something along those lines. It's anime regardless . . . we haven't had any more issues with that, but he was constantly bringing home cards. Which he wasn't allowed to have. We don't know how he was able to acquire them, but he would have a stack like this. And he would take them everywhere he goes. In fact, even now he's got a folder of anime drawings he's colored, and he'll take that everywhere he goes. He's absolutely obsessed with it. . . . Anime is very violent, to me it encourages violence. It's got scantily clad girls and you can't un-see things, right? So once you poison your mind, that's it. And I don't want him to have this negative worldview that says this sort of thing is OK because, I mean, he's fifteen. He still has maturing to do. If this is OK now, with the scantily clad girls and the violent pictures, what's going to happen when he's twenty-five? So [the admitting incident] was kind of the one that broke the camel's back. He didn't come home after school, so I'm like, "You know what? I just can't deal with this," 'cause it wasn't the first time. And I was so angry, so [my husband] told me to, or suggested rather, to take [Scott's sister] to the movies, and about an hour before we got back from the movie, Scott had apparently called. He was at a friend's house that's three, four miles to the west of us. Our house is on the way to this kid's house from high school. So he didn't stop home. He didn't call until eight o'clock at night. And [my husband] went and got him. So when I got home, they were sitting on the couch, and they were talking, and [my husband] had asked him to empty his pockets, and Scott gave him everything but the anime cards that he wasn't supposed to have. So I came across the room to try to take them from him. That didn't go over well. So it ends up in a wrestling match here on the couch with the three of us. I felt nailed against my arm, but only briefly. It was like you could tell Scott had started, and then he redirected his attention to [my husband] and started scratching him. And he actually did break the skin, and I guess he bit him. It moved from the couch to the door, so he started slamming on the door 'cause [my husband] had already locked it, and did this wrestling move on him and took him to the floor. And Scott just kept screaming at us about how we were ruining his dream of being an anime artist. And we're trying to explain to him that, you know, you got to get through high school, and maybe a little bit of formal training if you want to go anywhere with any kind of career. You know, you got to have something to build on. And, I think at that time he had been failing three of his classes. I can't remember if he told me he wanted to kill himself that night, and I argued that point, and then he told us that he wanted to kill us, or how that went. That was on a Thursday, I believe, and his social worker from school, she meets with him on Mondays. Monday after she had met with Scott she called me because he told her that he wanted to kill us. And he told her how he would do it. He had a plan. And so she called me, she's like, you need to have him assessed.

Scott and his parents agree that his threat to kill them and the violent episode that resulted in his hospitalization are rooted in a conflict over Scott's single-minded absorption in anime art and cards. He claims that he uttered his threat in a fit of anger, which encompassed not only his parents' confiscation but also their destruction of cards with an ostensibly large monetary value, in the context both of a peer network whose shared interests validated his own and of his stated ambition of becoming an anime artist himself. His mother, in contrast, uses telling language such as that Scott was "absolutely obsessed" with the content, including "scantily clad girls and the violent pictures" that inculcated a "negative world view," and implying that his devotion to anime was contributing to his failing three classes in school. Resentment over his parents' divorce and hostility toward both his mother and stepfather are barely below the surface in the violent confrontation following Scott's rebellious after-school visit to a friend without informing them of his whereabouts. The attempt to physically dispossess Scott of contraband Naruto cards resulted in a "wrestling match" with scratching and biting. Despite this massive disruption of equilibrium, it was only the following week that the family initiated the hospital admission process, based on a report from Scott's school social worker that his threat had developed into an actual plan to kill them. The admission required an additional day to overcome bureaucratic obstacles.

Nadine was a seventeen-year-old female, of mixed African American and Anglo-American heritage, living in a ranch-style house in an Albuquerque suburb with her mother, grandmother, and older sister. The house was located in a safe neighborhood where "everyone [was] really close." Nadine's parents divorced when she was six months old. Her father had been diagnosed with bipolar disorder and died of a drug overdose when Nadine was two years old. Nadine discussed how the circumstances of his death precipitated her manic delusions. Both Nadine and her mother understood Nadine's problems to be inherited genetically from her bipolar/substance-abusing father, and this was reinforced by Nadine's use of a "chemical imbalance" trope to describe her problems. Prior to the hospitalization at CPC, Nadine had been at another institution for one week for suicidality. Twice she attempted suicide: once with a knife and the second time overdosing on pills. In the first instance, police escorted her to a local hospital, where she was refused admittance. After the second attempt her mother tried again, but she said Nadine had not taken enough pills to meet admission standards. In the interim between her week at the other institution and her first CPC hospitalization, Nadine claimed that she had an episode of mania precipitated by the antidepressant drug Wellbutrin. The story of Nadine's first CPC hospitalization is quite dramatic—she thought her mother was trying to kill her and called the police. A commitment hearing was held to get Nadine into CPC. Three weeks before our second interview, Nadine was readmitted at CPC for depression and suicidality. She had gone off her medications (lithium and Abilify) a few weeks prior because she thought they were causing her to gain weight. She had also recommenced a previous pattern of bingeing and purging.

> *Nadine:* Um, because I thought my mom was gonna kill me so I called the cops on her a couple times. And then I went to a shelter and then from the shelter they took me to here. I got really paranoid and I thought she was trying to take my money and I thought that she killed my dad. And I just thought she was going to poison me, or she already had poisoned me. And I just got really paranoid . . . for about a week [before I came here to CPC]. I was at [a hospital for an appointment] where my therapist and my psychologist are and she wanted to take me home, but she was getting really angry, so I thought she was going to kill me so I called the cops on her. And then I told the cops that she was going to kill me and that she might be using drugs. They took me to a shelter [and from there] they took me over here. . . . It started with her not wanting to file my W-2 alone and then I thought it was money, and then I thought back that she said they investigated my dad's death. And they said my dad's death was murder. And so I thought maybe my mom did it and that got me thinking that she wants to kill me too. I brought it up to my friend's family and they said that they couldn't really help and I had to do it on my own. . . . [When the police came] I felt like I was kinda getting my mom, getting revenge. She was just calm 'cause she didn't want any problems with the cops. And she talked to them and said that she thought I was bipolar. And she tried to get me to a hospital. . . . [The police took me to the shelter], it was pretty nice and there was a few kids there. I was only there for two days, I think. Or one day. And then I complained of chest pains and went to the hospital over here [UNM]. And then from the ER they took me here [CPC].

> *Nadine's mother:* I thought she was using drugs for like maybe even two weeks before she came to the hospital. And then, um, she started getting worse and worse, and I did not know that she was having hallucinations. I just uh, got to the point where—her thing was dialing 911 and having the police come to wherever she was, and pick her up, and that I was going to kill her, and so I would tell the police, I'm sure she's bipolar—just because she was acting so strangely and so scared. And her face could—almost like it

could blow up to twice the size, and turn beet red, and she started crying and stomping her feet, and telling everyone that I was going to kill her. So that's when I took her to [the hospital where] they could not take her, so then I tried to bring her back home and see exactly what was going on with her, at least trying to keep her home, but she would not stay home, so I had more problems with her calling 911, and then finally she was able to get into—I don't know [some type] of a halfway house for one day. And even there she was so agitated and almost getting ready to try to hurt the other teenagers there, and they could not handle her, so they called me right away that morning and say they had to bring her down to UNM hospital to the emergency room . . . I think I was here twelve or thirteen hours, between her being in the emergency room, and them saying, "Yes, she's having serious mental health problems," to where they finally decided to keep her. Against her will, because she's over the age of fourteen. So, then that's when I found out she was definitely bipolar and hallucinating, and then, uh, Dr. C said she's definitely in the top ten of the most mentally ill people he's ever examined, because she's bipolar, and when she's on the manic high, she's paranoid and schizophrenic. So, uh, she didn't believe he was a doctor, and she thought he was even going to poison her, because then she switched to poison, and at her commitment hearing, she even said that the whole family had slowly been poisoning her. So it was very difficult. Because she is very manipulative and believable, too. And highly intelligent . . . she can really trick people.

Nadine did not hesitate to use the word "paranoid" in her narrative of how she was admitted to the hospital. As is common in delusional thinking, there is a logic based on a false premise: if perhaps her mother had killed her father and was after her money, if she was exhibiting anger when arguing that her daughter should come home, and if she was behaving calmly in the presence of police so as not to arouse their suspicion, then it made sense to Nadine to be taken to a shelter both to protect herself and (as she admits) to get some kind of revenge on her mother. Interestingly, Nadine and her mother each thought the other might be using drugs, and while Nadine described the shelter as a nice place, her mother said that Nadine was agitated and threateningly disruptive in the one day she spent there. Nadine's mother used clinical terms such as "bipolar," "manic," "paranoid," and "schizophrenic," pointedly referring to what she reported as the CPC psychiatrist's comment that her daughter was one of the ten most severely mentally ill people he had encountered.

CLINICAL VOLUNTEERS

Perhaps the most experientially vexing aspect of hospital admission for these youth is their sense of a loss of autonomy and freedom. Thus, it is noteworthy that some of the youth explicitly recount volunteering to enter the hospital. In a state in which no one at least fourteen years of age can be forced into inpatient care, it is critical that these narratives do not merely acknowledge consent or agreement, but attribute initiative to the adolescent patient. Two motives can be inferred from these narratives: frank recognition of a need for help in the form of inpatient treatment, and an attempt to preserve a degree of autonomy in a struggle for personal dignity. A substantial minority (19.1%) of these youth asserted their voluntary submission to hospitalization. Of even greater note, these nine included five of the seven self-identified Native Americans among the youth. While the interview material cannot indisputably confirm a cultural component in this result, the finding is intriguingly suggestive with respect to a connection between an indigenous value of personal dignity and voluntary entrance into therapeutic confinement under the fraught colonial/postcolonial conditions of New Mexico.

Audrey was a fifteen-year-old girl who lived with her mother, her younger sister and brother, and her younger nephew in a small town reputedly without violence and gangs. At the time of our final interview the younger nephew had moved out. Audrey's upbringing was one of the least stable of all the participants. Her mother had been in a gang for decades and did what she described (with a laugh) as some "some really bad shit" until recently having "found Jesus" (pointing to a framed poster on the wall). She presented a challenge to ethnographic empathy within fifteen minutes after the ethnographer (JHJ) arrived at her home. In reporting how many children she had, she said she had "lost" a baby. The ethnographer responded that she was sorry to hear that, and said how difficult that must have been for her. She rejoined by flatly saying that it wasn't really hard since "me and my boyfriend were high on meth for three days and I guess somebody musta rolled over the baby and that was it. So." (Sitting just two feet away on a sofa, with two decades of ethnographic-clinical-personal commitment to "always stay in the room and never flinch," I allowed an ethnographic shiver to pass, hopefully unnoticed.) Audrey's father was in prison most of her life for a number of convictions, including robbery, drugs, and violation of parole, although Audrey expressed wanting to have a relationship with him and wrote letters to him. Audrey seems to have spent much of her childhood worrying about her mother and witnessing profoundly frightening events, including her mother's suicide attempts and recurrent incapacitation related to substance use. Her mother mentioned that

Audrey had been through a great deal as a child, but felt that her mental illness could have stemmed from being "wired wrong." She felt that Audrey didn't have enough motivation to "move on." Audrey seemed to attribute her depression to her maturity level, her upbringing, and the sexual abuse that she both suffered and inflicted upon her cousin. The domestic environment included ongoing psychosocial stressors related to current home instability, with a history of severe to catastrophic recurrent psychosocial stressors. Audrey had previously been in treatment foster care as well as having had an inpatient admission.

Audrey: I had gotten molested by my uncle when I was about nine or ten, I didn't tell nobody, until recently. And I had been acting out sexually with my ten-year-old cousin. My mom's not the one that wanted me to go in here. I thought that I needed help so I put myself in here. [The incident happened] Tuesday of last week. . . . I didn't know that me being molested could act out on my actions? So that's why I told [my mother]—and me and my cousin were caught kissing recently, and I thought I didn't wanna be like that no more so that's why I needed help. And I came here, and after this place I'm going to an all-girls hospital. 'Cause, I feel bad doing that? But, I didn't tell nobody that I got molested because I was like, you know he's *gone,* he won't do it *again,* and it's all gonna go away. But when my mom told me that those [memories] in me, it makes me act out sexually? And I didn't know that so that's why I told my mom. And she did not want to put me in here at all. I thought I don't wanna be like that no more, I wanted to learn why I did that, I wanna get it off my chest.

Audrey's mother: She had always been mean to her sisters and brothers, that's why she went away the first time. Just real defiant. She got help that year, came back, doing OK, we kept doing our counseling and all that. All of us have counselors. And I was here one night and she and my nephew were acting kinda strange, like they wanted me to go to sleep, so I was feeling weird so I dozed off for a minute and then I woke up and I walk in the den, and my nephew comes out of this side, and I said what are you doing in there? And he said, "I was scared!" And I was like, "Well if you're scared you're not gonna be in the dark." And I turned around and Audrey was coming out of the kitchen part of the den, total darkness, you know, and she just started crying and saying, "I can't believe you thought we were doing something. I can't believe you think that about me." . . . I knew something happened. . . . The next morning we were on the way to my brother's house. I told her, "When we get there, your uncle is gonna sit you down and make you tell him what happened. So you're better off tellin' me the truth right now." And so she just came out and told me that they were touching each other and kissing and stuff like that, I thought it was a one-time thing even though we had caught them doing this last year in Albuquerque. . . . Audrey ended up telling the truth about how she was bothering him every day that he was here since we moved here. Which I didn't see none of that. I'm always here, I'm always watching them play, but she said she was bothering him all day long all the time. Tellin' him either you come here and kiss me, and then touch each other, or I'm gonna tell your dad this and that. . . . And I didn't want to put Audrey back in the hospital, so I told her, "Let's think about this, what we wanna do." So the counselor was here. Audrey drags the counselor in her room, and tells her that she's gonna kill herself. The counselor comes out and she's like, "We've gotta go now, there's no other way. Audrey's told me that she wants to hurt herself." She's really so nice, because I didn't have a vehicle, she went with me to CPC. I'm thinking [she wanted to hurt herself] because my brother was mad at her. I wasn't letting her play with the kids at *all*. I stopped it all. If I would have brought her home with me the other day, I was gonna make her feel more like a child molester than anybody . . . so I think [having] her in there is a lot better, and she accepted it a lot better than I thought. Because I promised her, I said, "Audrey, if you do go away, I promise you it's not gonna be more than a month. You're not gonna go into a year this time." I said I just need help getting started on what I'm supposed to do because I'm not a professional, I don't know.

Audrey's narrative exhibits a remarkable candor about her discovery of a connection between having been sexually abused and becoming an abuser. She expresses both guilt and agency in articulations like "I thought that I needed help. . . . I don't wanna be like that no more, I wanted to learn why I did that, I wanna get it off my chest." She welcomes the plan to be placed in an all-girls facility, one that in fact explicitly addresses sexual abuse issues. Her mother acknowledges that everyone in the household has a counselor, and given her own troubles with suicidality and substance abuse it is not entirely surprising that she did not appear to be fully aware of Audrey's sexual transgression even though the other children seemed to know what was going on. Retrospectively she appears to recognize that there was an ongoing pattern insofar as Audrey had already been caught in similar behavior a year earlier, and that she had been otherwise mean to her siblings. Though she does not want Audrey to be hospitalized again, she insightfully, and with some relief, feels that the degree of strict discipline she would have to impose if Audrey remained at home "was gonna make her feel more like a child molester." Her report that Audrey told her counselor privately during a home visit that she was going to kill herself suggests that the threat was itself the mechanism Audrey used to volunteer her own hospital admission.

We first met Kevin, a gregarious and eager Anglo-American male, when he was fifteen years old. His family consisted of his mother, father, and younger brother, who lived in a modest and quiet neighborhood despite describing themselves as living "paycheck to paycheck." The family had just moved into the neighborhood after spending the past three years living with Kevin's verbally abusive grandmother, which was a difficult living environment for the family. By the end of their time in the study, the family lived in a rental house a few blocks away from their previous home. Kevin's illness had been a large source of stress for his parents. When Kevin was diagnosed with ADHD at age five, then hospitalized at age nine, the family was alienated from their numerous relatives in the surrounding area who didn't understand Kevin's illness and were "petrified" to be around him. The nuclear family had begun attending extended family events again in the past few years, and while tension remained, they believed it had made them stronger. Additionally, Kevin's younger brother was being teased at school for his older brother being a "freak" and had thus begun to see a therapist to come to terms with his older brother's illnesses. Kevin's current admission came in the wake of smashing his mother's car windshield, suicidal thoughts, self-cutting, and aggression toward his parents and brother.

Kevin: Um, I was being real suicidal, like, I'd try to cut my wrist and my throat and I was angry and I threatened my mom, my dad, my brother, and I did a lot of other stuff, like I broke my mom's windshield with my golf club and . . . that's probably what—those were strikes one, two, and three, and I was just, I volunteered to go in there. I didn't feel safe around anybody else and I didn't think they felt safe—I know they weren't safe—around me. It was difficult for me, because I thought they didn't understand me and they actually didn't care about me because my brother would get all the good stuff, expensive stuff, and I would just get "congratulations" told to me and get all the out-of-date stuff, and that kinda pissed me off about my life—plus the financial situations, so I just wanted to get it over with. I didn't want to suffer anymore. I just couldn't, but I couldn't do it. I wanted to, it was in my heart to kill myself and in my mind, but I guess, just I didn't want to. I don't know why. One, because I thought it was going to hurt, and I wanted a quick death. And two, I just, I was always thinking of another way, but when I refused to think there was any other way to get through this, or through those issues, I just wanted to kill myself. I look back and it's just stupid. I mean, I've had those little thoughts, but I just push them out of my mind and just think what'll happen, like I can end up somewhere worse than the hospital.

Kevin's mother: Kevin was just in one of his moods Sunday night, and he went to bed, and I guess he had a very vivid nightmare, where he had stuck a lit firework in his mouth and he said he could see his face and head just blow up. And the blood was there, and it was just very real. And he was telling the counselor this. But that Monday morning, he and I sat here, ate breakfast, talked, I congratulated him on the way to school that he got ready on time and what a great job he had done, and [said nothing about the nightmare]. And we had an appointment that same night at five [but] his counselor came out, she goes, "He's not going. We're gonna admit him." And I was in the hallway and I looked at [my husband], and I was like, "What?" She started saying, "He's not safe," and then we walked in the room and he just blew us apart. And he kinda was angry on the way over there. 'Cause he was looking at school cars. But he's looking at cars that are fourteen to fifteen thousand dollars and he wants that for a school car. I said, "Kevin, we can't afford that." So that sent him into one of his triggers. Then he told [the counselor] about his dream, and so she introduced me to Dr. B and she says, "I've been talking to him, and we're just gonna do it." Well then [my husband] and Kevin had some exchanges of words and so she sent [my husband] on his way, and she drove with me and Kevin to the hospital and I admitted Kevin and he was saying, "Oh, you're not strong, you're a weak bitch, you're not gonna admit me, you're not gonna admit me," and I just kept signing the papers and I was crying the whole entire time and I was just signing, and giving them insurance cards, and he just kept berating me. And he goes, "That's OK, I'm just gonna be here a couple days. And then I'm gonna go home." And I said, "This isn't like Club Med, that you decide when you get to come home." And I just kept signing papers, and finally they took him to the cottage and they made me leave because they didn't want me to see—'cause they have to do a body search on him. And that just killed me. I came home to pick up clothes that he needed, and he's on that growth hormone, so we had to get that together. . . . And he did really good the first three days, and they're like, we're gonna have to discharge him, because he's not showing anything that you have explained. And I was like, "Oh my god. I can't believe this." That third day he threw a tantrum, and he just went off on them. And they were like, "Oh my god."

Kevin is quite reflexive in his enumeration of three events that constituted "three strikes" leading to the self-appraisal that led him to enter the hospital voluntarily. He based this on concern for the safety of both himself and others as well as the statement that he "didn't want to suffer anymore." Some of this suffering was based in struggles with his violent behavior, the effects of being short in stature and under treatment with growth hormones, and his unrealistic materialistic expectations. The latter are evident in his comparison between things his brother got that he didn't and his explicit mention of "financial situations," at least in part confirmed by his mother's mentioning that he wanted a $15,000 car for driving to school. Kevin retrospectively describes his suicidality as "stupid," but his mother cites a violently self-destructive nightmare as the opening motif of her narrative of his admission. She also refers to his behavioral volatility in relation to others, with key words including "triggers," "tantrum," and "moods." As with Audrey, the hospital admission occured after a conversation with a counselor; if Kevin in fact volunteered to be admitted it was likely in this conversation, since his mother makes no mention of a voluntary admission. Kevin's internal conflict is expressed in his mother's report of how he taunted her as too weak to follow through with the necessary paperwork, as well as saying that he would probably be there only a couple of days in any case. It is possible that even though he claims to have gone voluntarily into the hospital, he may not have been completely cognizant of all such an admission might involve even though he had been hospitalized once before at a younger age.

NARRATIVE, EXPERIENCE, AND TEMPORALITY

In this chapter we have met a number of troubled young people and devoted considerable attention to the singular event of admission to inpatient psychiatric care as our initial focus in understanding their lived experience. In examining admission narratives, we have seen how language can give access to lived experience, or, to phrase it in terms closer to those of Heidegger, can disclose existence and being-in-the-world. This has given us comparative purchase on the one thing each of them has in common, namely temporary internment in the Children's Psychiatric Center. This hospital is the bottleneck through which all of them have passed and the institution in which they have come to the attention (not always for the first time) of a system of professional care beyond their homes and neighborhoods. From their standpoint, it could be said that they are thrust outward from their familiar, if fraught, private worlds into a complex public world; or, to adopt a literary metaphor, they find themselves plunged down a rabbit hole into a bureaucratic tangle of treatment institutions and insurance providers. Through our analysis we have acquired a concrete initial sense of how these troubled young people describe and narrate their own experience and the manner in which the narrative intersubjectivity of children and parents produces a co-construction of mutual contradictions and confirmations of events and experiences.

Through a close reading of these admission narratives we were able to identify six subtypes. What stands out in retrospect is that, while we derived these six types inductively and not with respect to any a priori categories, taken together they constitute a set of temporal schemas each of which encodes a particular form of agency or lack thereof. *The Precipitating Event* is essentially a moment of spontaneity in the immediate present, and the narrative is concerned neither about what came before nor about what comes after, with little emphasis on agency. The *Last Trigger, Last Straw* narrative portrays a cumulative, escalating temporal sequence and includes some agentive anticipation that hospitalization is a potential outcome of successive events. *Three Days in a Row* expresses a compressed temporal sequence with discrete beginning and end, 1–2–3, a kind of temporal bubble likely characterized by periods of waxing and waning stress, interpersonal tension, and moments of reflection and reconciliation. *In the Revolving Door* describes a longer and cyclical narrative temporality, one that connotes long-term frustration that could undermine hope for the future and that also bespeaks the influence of repeated encounters with the bureaucratized mental health care system. *Kill or Be Killed* invokes a temporality of ultimate finality, looking out into the abyss of death where agency is hypertrophied into an impulse to kill or a struggle for survival in the face of murder. Finally, *Clinical Volunteers* operates within a temporality somewhat closer to the quotidian, one that includes the possibility of deliberateness and deciding; compared to the other types, it expresses enhanced agency, making hospitalization a life choice if not a choice for life. We offer this analysis and the insight it brings about temporality and agency in lived experience with the anticipation that future research may determine that the way such events are narrated can have consequences for the young people's subsequent encounters with the treatment system and perhaps even their clinical and developmental trajectories.

The admission narrative opens a window into lived experience constituted by a delimited account of a specific event co-created in the narrative intersubjectivity of afflicted youth and struggling parent/guardian. Language discloses lived experience, and narrative language discloses it in a particular way that has especially to do with temporality. Philosopher and narrative theorist Paul Ricoeur has written that "time becomes human time to the extent that it is organized after the manner of narrative; narrative, in turn, is meaningful to the extent that it portrays the features of temporal existence" (Ricoeur 1984: 3). The struggles and disruptions that we have portrayed in this chapter define the first and most narrow of three concentric temporal horizons, namely that surrounding the discrete event of admission to the hospital. In chapter 5 we will expand our event horizon to encompass these youth's trajectories through a "career" as adolescent mental patient insofar as we were able to follow it over a two-year period. In chapter 6 we will again expand the horizon to consider the conditions, prospects, possibilities, and hopes for them having a life in the future. To set the stage for this discussion of trajectories of treatment and having a life, in the next chapter we pose the question, essential from both clinical and ethnographic standpoints, of how to define the problems of these young people. How would we define their problems in terms of psychiatric research diagnosis? How would we define their problems in terms of life events and experiences? How do they and their parents define their problems in the context of lived experience—do they engage in a discourse of diagnosis based on psychiatric categories, or do they engage in a nonmedical mode of conceptualizing the problem with their own forms of elaborating, minimizing, explaining, or denying?

CHAPTER 3

Defining the Problem

Ethnography may be the most inductive of all scholarly approaches to human experience. As ethnographers we have an aversion to bringing a priori categories to our research, out of the concern that framing an inquiry in terms of such categories might cause us to miss an important dimension of our interlocutors' experience or, even worse, introduce an ethnocentric bias into our work. Now that we have established a narrative understanding of how the young members of the study cohort came to be in the hospital, our task is to determine, in the broadest possible sense, what is troubling these troubled youth. In this respect we do presume that there is a problem for each of them, and assert that only with a multifaceted inquiry can we achieve the ethnographic validity, clinical research reliability, and existential breadth necessary for adequately describing these problems. Put another way, our presentation synthesizes multiple levels of analysis in order both to *characterize* this group of troubled youth with respect to the range of problems they face and to *illuminate* the subjectivity that is embedded in how they experience and talk about those problems (Jenkins and Barrett 2004; Biehl, Good, and Kleinman 2007; Parish 2008; Martin 2010; Carpenter-Song 2019). Tacking between characterizing and illuminating—between the stories or narratives that we tell about them and the stories or narratives they tell about themselves—is critical for discerning the lived experience of this group of youth. Rather than lives that are largely invisible, the extreme of the extremes, we must show them as lives worthy of careful attention, as lives that matter.

Accordingly, in this chapter our aim is to define the nature of the problems faced by the youth from a series of interrelated standpoints: (1) the moral and economic milieu from which the problems emerge; (2) the clinical-research-based psychiatric diagnostic categories that apply to their struggles; (3) the life experiences the youth have undergone; (4) the etiological concepts articulated by youth and families; (5) the conceptions of illness and normalcy articulated by youth and families; (6) the way the young people discuss their illness and how that may vary over time; and (7) the structured discourse of diagnosis embedded in lived experience. We begin by elaborating some critical contextual features about the social, economic, political, and moral milieu inhabited by these youth.

THE MORAL MILIEU AND PATHOLOGIES OF POVERTY

The intersection of moral milieu and pathologies of poverty (illnesses the social determinants of which are economic and social inequity) is highlighted by a vast and growing corpus of scholarly works from medicine, anthropology, psychiatry, epidemiology, health policy, and allied fields (Farmer 2004b; Patel 2005; Marmot and Wilkinson 2006; Marmot et al. 2008; Good et al. 2011; Macartney 2011; Lende 2012; Lund 2012; Brodwin 2013; Boozary and Shojania 2017; Carpenter-Song 2019). These studies document the ways in which health and well-being are undermined and harmed by structural violence, very much to include the health care system (or the inadequacy thereof) as it affects persons and populations who live under conditions of strain and scarcity. Under such conditions it is abundantly clear that mental illness is a fundamentally social phenomenon. As a matter of lived experience in situations of mental illness, *there can be no such thing as individual pathology* because such situations are intersubjectively constituted and shaped by social relations, economic conditions, and gendered and political status (Jenkins 2015a: 3). In our field site in New Mexico, this social determinacy of mental illness among troubled adolescents was already partially evident in a description by one of the clinicians who contributed to Hendren and Berlin's volume documenting the development of CPC in the 1980s:

> Many of the children have suffered multiple losses, separation, or abandonments from primary caretakers. Severe deprivation and abuse, extended family history of major psychiatric disorders, and family multisubstance abuse are part of these patients' histories. The children present with low frustration tolerance, impulsivity, aggressive outbursts, and poor peer relationships. They are needy, are unable to feel positively about themselves, and have

poor self-esteem. . . . Most have major deficits in ego functions; behavior, rather than speech, is the primary means of communication. These children have little capacity to talk meaningfully about painful internal experiences or interpersonal relationships. (Stearns 1991: 116)

This observation is critical to the intent of this chapter. What differs between Stearns's observations and those of our research team, however, is the degree to which many of our young interlocutors were in fact able to talk meaningfully about their experiences within ethnographic encounters. Although likely in part a function of which patients were referred to the project and which among those chose to participate, the point remains that there are young people, even among the seriously disturbed, who can articulate or reflect on what is happening in their lives.

Anthropological and psychological approaches to adolescence are in accord in noting that cohort effects are developmentally critical (LeVine 2011), and that immediate social conditions are vital to shaping everyday experience. These immediate social conditions define a local moral world, that is, a setting of moral experience that expresses what is most at stake for people in their local networks of relationships in communities (Kleinman 1999, 2006). During the period of our study, managed care for behavioral and mental health in New Mexico was dominated initially by Value Options (2005–9) and then by Optum Health Care (2009–13), both corporations that have been sued by multiple states within the United States for fraud and mismanagement (see chapter 1). This was also the period of the Great Recession in the United States, the economic impact of which led to increasing homelessness and drug use among patients and families treated at CPC. At the time the project began, New Mexico was particularly affected by drug abuse; in 2005 it had the highest rate of deaths due to overdose (27/100,000) in the country, and by 2014 it was second only to West Virginia (though, with the rapid rise of the opioid epidemic in Appalachian and northeastern states, its rank had declined to twelfth by 2016) (CDC 2018). In addition to the persistence over time of significant substance abuse problems, CPC staff had experienced several short-term trends. One was a two-year period of increased suicide rates among Pueblo teenagers living in small, face-to-face communities where a pattern of copycat suicides can easily gain a foothold. Clinicians also reported a year and a half of increased contact with autism patients in need of clinical stabilization, while offering no account of what might have fueled this trend. This is not to mention the roles of a cultural rhetoric of wartime since the terrorist attacks of September 11, 2001, and a resurgent social conservativism in the national discourse. Taken together, these are the social conditions under which the youth lived during the years of continuous data collection (2005–11).

The moral milieu or local moral world surrounding these adolescents is also one in which mental illness is heavily stigmatized, with a mental health system that perpetuates an artificial scarcity of resources. Some families generate violence and abuse from within while others are overwhelmed with strains and constraints from without. Obstacles to development and maturity can provoke the question of what it means to have a life at all. Insofar as Erikson (1963) observed that peer relationships are critical at this age, the following observations about youth culture in New Mexico by a CPC clinician are also relevant to defining the moral milieu:

> It's more and more cool to be cruel. To be cruel to one another. And to present as a hardened person without sympathy for others . . . it's almost like a reality TV thing. I think the media—and almost all the kids have smartphones, rich or poor have the smartphones, and act out a kind of Mean Girl thing. All I can call it is reality TV, which I don't watch and don't approve of. But this very theatrical, dramatic, edgy, high-risk sort of way of living . . . in real time, but none of it face-to-face. All via the smartphone. It's almost as if they're aping the shows they're watching . . . I think it's more the girls than boys but I think the boys are participating in it more now than they did five or six years ago. . . . What we're talking about is more predominant in the larger cities, of which New Mexico doesn't have many, but I think among the Native American kids from the pueblos and from the places around Gallup and Grants there's not as much of the "It's cool to be mean" stuff. Those kids are more preoccupied with drug and alcohol abuse and community problems.

This rendering of adolescent style includes an embrace of anything "high risk," thus potentially fueling the drug epidemic; the same clinician observed that just in the past year CPC had seen an increasing number of younger and younger heroin addicts who had previously also used methamphetamine. Although cannabis remains predominant, and ecstasy and psilocybin are common, the trend was toward methamphetamine, crack cocaine, and heroin. This was accompanied by an increase in sexually transmitted diseases, date rape, and violence between girlfriends and boyfriends, as well as violence against same-sex rivals and authority figures. Overall, says this therapist, "the kids I treat seem to be more and more disheartened, disenchanted, discouraged . . . um, angry. More 'conducty.'"

In these reflections the relation between disordered conduct and psychiatric disorder points directly to the relation between the moral milieu and individual suffering, and the comment about anger points directly to issues we raise in chapter 4. In the continuation of comments from the same therapist, we see the idea of moral poverty introduced as one of the social determinants of the kinds of problems faced by adolescents, especially those who become patients at CPC:

> I think it is a moral poverty. I think it's a loss of the compass. I'm getting— I'm also getting more and more kids who are saying they're atheists. This is also cool. You're smarter if you're atheist. Now most of the kids who say this—because we do ask about your tradition. I ask about ancestry. Kids—a lot of the kids say, "What do you mean ancestry?" The more educated kids know what I'm talking about and I try to engage them in this discussion, just to think about. 'Cause they're struggling with identity and—and—and a lot of them are not very well grounded. They're not rooted in anything. They're almost like a lost generation. And sometimes I can get them to be curious about those things and to begin to build some sense of core meaning in their lives. I had a little boy. Well, not little boy. But a boy who was about sixteen . . . a couple of months ago who was Hispanic and in the course of working with him, he—he made some—and he made some anti-Semitic comments and talked about Nazis and this and that and then he said that his grandfather was a German Jew! But he hadn't put this together with his comments! And it was really important because he didn't like himself very much . . . so it was important to the therapy to talk about this. And this is a kid who is intelligent enough and self-aware enough to be able to begin to talk about these things, you know. Who are you?

While there is certainly a moral component to the experience of troubled adolescents, and while they most certainly inhabit a local moral world, there is also a possibility that the clinician's reading of contemporary youth culture might be substantially shaped by a predominant exposure to the struggles of an inpatient clientele. Any analysis of "pathology" and "moral poverty" must be pursued in broadening circles from the individual to peers, family, treatment system, and society at large—it is such a comprehensive view that in part protects moral analysis from moralism.

DIAGNOSIS AND DISTRESS

Given that these are youth who find themselves imbricated in the formal system of psychiatric care, we must come to terms with how their problems can be defined as psychiatric disorder in the terms of research clinical diagnosis. Above, we outlined our methodological position regarding the need to cast a broad net by beginning with the general category of "problem," with full awareness that anthropologists are generally wary about categories of psychiatric disorder as repositories of ethno-centrism and ethnopsychology. Indeed, the successive iterations of the *Diagnostic and Statistical Manual of Mental Disorders* (DSM) and the *International Classification of Diseases* (ICD) are not progressively more accurate approximations of an objective system of disease entities, but reflections both of changes in how mental illness is conceptualized and of shifting epidemiological patterns of affliction. Thus, it is "far more fashionable in anthropology to criticize or even ridicule psychia-try's construction of diagnostic categories than to suggest a research agenda formulated in terms of them" (Good 1992: 181).

Our approach to the ethnographic use of psychiatric diagnostic cat-egories is in accord with that proposed by Good (1992: 187) insofar as productive interdisciplinary collaboration requires submission of these categories and their criteria to systematic cross-cultural investigation. In this study, as in other large-scale studies we have conducted (Karno et al. 1987; Jenkins and Karno 1992; Jenkins 1996, 1997; Storck et al. 2000; Hollifield et al. 2001, 2006; Jenkins et al. 2005; Csordas et al. 2008, 2010), diagnostic categories serve as a "useful starting point for cross-cultural comparison by identifying constellations of symptoms that tend to 'go together' by virtue of neurobiology, social etiology, and the structure of subjective experience" (Jenkins 2015a: 22). In anthro-pological analyses, diagnostic categories can never be an end point. They require scrutiny, particularly given the long-standing recognition within psychiatry itself of substantial heterogeneity in any given diag-nostic category (Bleuler 1950 [1911]). Of great concern also is the core issue of cultural validity for diagnostic practice and therapeutic inter-vention (Kleinman 1988a; Kaiser et al. 2019a, b; Shohet 2018; Leocata 2018; Leocata, Patel, and Kleinman, in review). As in others of our studies, in the present work we use empirical research diagnostic data both to inform the anthropological critique of diagnostic categories and to inform our understanding of the cultural patterning of subjectivity. That such patterning is demonstrably uneven, partial, and overlapping within and across categories is an observation upon which cultural anthropologists, clinical psychologists, psychiatrists, and neuroscien-tists would readily agree. In sum, our critical stance is to recognize that psychiatric nosologies are cultural artifacts insofar as they reflect the cultural and historical contexts in which they are developed, but that at the same time they can offer a descriptively useful if limited etic frame-work for cross-cultural comparison of psychic affliction in psychiatric anthropology, cultural psychiatry, and global mental health research.

With these considerations in mind, we turn to the results of our psychiatric diagnostic interview, the KID-SCID. As detailed in the appendix, the KID-SCID is a research assessment administered by a clinician with rigorous training in its use to determine psychiatric diagnosis according to research-reliable criteria. To "meet research criteria for" any disorder a high threshold number of symptoms, duration, and severity must be present, along with significant problems in functioning. A great many of our cases met subthreshold (moderate degrees) research criteria for certain diagnoses while meeting full criteria for others. This observation is germane to the familiar clinical reality of "comorbidity" or concurrently present disorders. However, since a comprehensive presentation and discussion of the full SCID profiles that would incorporate subthreshold diagnoses for the forty-seven adolescent participants could constitute a book unto itself, we restrict ourselves here to SCID diagnostic results meeting full criteria for *DSM-IV* disorders.

Results for the most common disorders identified are summarized in table 4. Overall for the cohort, major depression/dysthymia (persistent depression) was the most common diagnosis (57.4%), followed by generalized anxiety or panic disorder (40.4%) and substance abuse or dependence (38.3%). Somewhat less frequent were oppositional defiant disorder (ODD) or conduct disorder (27.7%), post-traumatic stress disorder (PTSD) (27.7%), and attention-deficit/hyperactivity disorder (ADHD) (27.7%). Rates of psychotic disorders (21.3%) and of bipolar disorder/cyclothymia (14.9%) were both relatively high for this age group. Compared with other diagnoses, eating disorders ranked lower (10.6%).

With respect to comorbidity, it is important to note that the mean number of diagnoses in table 4 for these young persons is 2.7. This indicates that most youth "made criteria" for more than two types of disorder. The co-occurrence of depression and anxiety (the most frequently observed disorders in this study) has been noted among youth in numerous other studies. Shelli Avenevoli and colleagues (2008) provide an extensive review of work utilizing epidemiological and survey data, concluding that depression and anxiety disorders are "the most common concurrent conditions in youth, with median prevalence estimates of more than 39 percent anxiety among youth with depression and almost 17 percent depression among children and adolescents with anxiety disorders" (2008: 15).

Table 4 also reveals the salience of sex/gender differences for several diagnostic categories. Bearing in mind that sex and gender should not be conflated, as commonly occurs in the social and health sciences (cf.

TABLE 4 SCID PSYCHIATRIC RESEARCH DIAGNOSES OF ADOLESCENT PARTICIPANTS BY GENDER

	Major depression/ dysthymia	Anxiety/ panic disorder	Substance abuse/ dependence	ODD/ conduct disorder	ADHD	PTSD	Psychotic disorder	Bipolar disorder/ cyclothymia	Eating disorder	Mean number of diagnoses per participant
Female (n = 22)	18 (81.8%)	12 (54.5%)	8 (36.4%)	5 (22.7%)	5 (22.7%)	8 (36.4%)	4 (18.2%)	4 (18.2%)	4 (18.2%)	3.1
Male (n = 25)	9 (36.0%)	7 (28.0%)	10 (40.0%)	8 (32.0%)	8 (32.0%)	5 (20.0%)	6 (24.0%)	3 (12.0%)	1 (4.0%)	2.3
Total (N = 47)	27 (57.4%)	19 (40.4%)	18 (38.3%)	13 (27.7%)	13 (27.7%)	13 (27.7%)	10 (21.3%)	7 (14.9%)	5 (10.6%)	2.7

Nasser, Walders, and Jenkins 2002), and that both concepts encompass phenomena existing on a continuum, the study participants all identified as either male or female. Although our ethnographic and clinical research in no way constitutes an epidemiological study, it is nonetheless striking that depression—the most common diagnosis for the cohort overall—is much more common among females (81.8%) than among males (36%). In accord with epidemiological findings from adult studies of depression, in this study girls are more than twice as likely as boys to be living with depression. The greater frequency among the girls likewise applies to anxiety/panic disorder (54.5% and 28% respectively), PTSD (36.4% and 20% respectively), and eating disorders (18.2% and 4% respectively). For boys, we observed higher frequencies of ODD/conduct disorder (32% and 22.7% respectively), ADHD (32% and 18.2% respectively), and psychotic disorders (24% and 18.2% respectively). Of interest is that frequencies of substance abuse/dependence among girls and boys are fairly similar (36.4% and 40% respectively). Finally, the mean number of psychiatric diagnoses is higher for girls than for boys (3.1 and 2.3 respectively). The range for the total number of comorbid SCID diagnoses is 1–6, wherein the highest number (6) applied to two girls, with only one boy being close (with 5).

We can compare the interviewer-generated results obtained from the KID-SCID with adolescents' own self-perceptions of their problems and distress using data from the Achenbach Youth Self-Report profiles, which we were able to generate for a substantial proportion of the participants ($N = 35$). Affective disorders are most prominent in both KID-SCID and Achenbach results, but across the *DSM*-oriented Achenbach categories a dramatically higher proportion of youth report a borderline/clinical level of distress than is evident in the KID-SCID results (e.g., 83% for affective disorders vs. 59.6% in the KID-SCID). This is likely due to the rigor of the SCID method, which entails a high threshold to meet clinical research diagnostic criteria. Nevertheless, it is noteworthy that the youth themselves report such substantial distress. On the parallel Achenbach Child Behavior Checklist their parents largely agree, with the exception that parents report even higher levels of affective distress for their children than do the children themselves. This is in contrast with a comparison group of nonpatient adolescents we recruited from public schools who have been neither diagnosed nor treated for any emotional problems, who reported a higher level of distress than did their parents. Although we cannot pursue this comparison here, it suggests that recognizing a problem as an illness may amplify family members' perceptions of suffering, whereas a presumption that there are no problems diminishes their awareness of distress that adolescents may be experiencing. Finally, on the Achenbach checklist parents do not appear to notice significant differences between boys and girls, though among the youth themselves girls appear to report an incrementally higher level of symptoms than their male peers.

LIFE EVENTS AND EXPERIENCE

The process of coming to have a life requires developing a sense of identity and morality. With reference to the age range of twelve to eighteen, precisely the ages of our study participants, Erikson (1963) identified the most characteristic psychic conflict as that of identity versus role confusion. This conflict can be especially vexing when mental illness, disorganized family relationships, trouble with peers and school, and a complex treatment system militate against the secure consolidation of identity (cf. Jenkins 2015a for gender identity confusion). From the standpoint of developmental psychology, we might address this issue in terms of a typology of adolescent modes of dealing with the identity crisis (Marcia 1980) or modes of autobiographical coherence (Habermas and Block 2000). However, from an ethnographic standpoint we are concerned with the structure and coherence of a lifeworld where mental illness in social and interpersonal context poses a significant challenge to personal integrity, identity, and well-being. In the ethnographic context and in relation to our earlier discussion of the moral milieu, the development of identity and morality go hand in hand. In this respect the best point of contact between psychology and anthropology is Carol Gilligan's (1977, 1982) observation that morality is not necessarily a matter of abstract principles in hypothetical decontextualized situations. She uses as a case in point the relative degree to which girls and women do not operate according to abstract principles but rather are guided by context, care, and compassion. Gilligan's feminist ethics of care come close to our concern with equity and social justice in the local moral world inhabited by troubled adolescents.

While we have affirmed the value of formal psychiatric research diagnosis, recognizing the centrality of developing identity and morality in coming to have a life requires us to focus on formative life experiences as a parallel and complementary way of characterizing the problems of troubled youth. The diagnostic categories of psychiatric disorder we discussed above and present in table 4 impose a highly particular construction of experience. As descriptors of the existential realities of peoples' lives, the nature of their affliction, and the problems they are struggling with, psychiatric diagnoses invariably present a partial and two-dimensional picture. In previous research using data from the Navajo Healing Project, we demonstrated precisely how SCID interviews and ethnographic interviews approach experience from standpoints that generate complementary data (Csordas et al. 2010). In the same vein, for an understanding of salient problems in the adolescents' lived experience, we have prepared table 5, which summarizes a set of problematic life experiences derived from our ethnographic data in a form parallel to the way table 4 summarizes the psychiatric research diagnostic data. We explicitly choose "problematic life experiences" as opposed to the commonly used "adverse childhood events" (CDC 2018) because the latter term typically refers to events that befall children, whereas our categories include not only things that happen to them but things they do themselves. That is, an adolescent can be physically or sexually abused but also may be the perpetrator of violent and abusive acts—both are problematic life experiences. The complementarity of the diagnostic and the ethnographic also allows us to productively blur the boundary between cause and consequence in the relation of illness and experience. One cannot (and should not) say without detailed case studies that a disorder causes or facilitates a problematic experience or, on the contrary, that a problematic experience (whether the child is an active agent or a passive victim) causes an illness.

Table 5 shows that overall, violent behavior is the most characteristic feature of the youth's life experience, evident among 74.5 percent of the cohort. This fact will be critical to our discussion in chapter 4, where we address anger as a deep-seated problem for a substantial proportion of the youth. Yet, since anger is reported by a relatively smaller proportion of 57 percent, it cannot account for the totality of violent behavior. The second most common among problematic life experiences is suicide attempts, at a rate of 68.1 percent; while often associated with depression, this rate is higher than the 57.4 percent of youth with a SCID diagnosis of major depression or dysthymia; while suicide may be common in depression, not all who are suicidal meet the criteria for a depressive disorder. Next most common is police involvement or legal trouble (66.0%), followed by bereavement (59.6%). Among forms of self-destructive behavior, drug and/or alcohol abuse is a common issue (59.6%), as is self-cutting (57.4%). It is common for the adolescents (46.8%) to have experienced physical abuse, and nearly a third (31.9%) have been sexually abused.

TABLE 5 PROBLEMATIC LIFE EXPERIENCES OF ADOLESCENT PARTICIPANTS BY GENDER

	Perpetrator of violent acts	Suicide attempt/ preoccupation	Police/legal trouble	Bereavement	Drugs/ alcohol	Self-cutting	Has been physically abused	Has been sexually abused	Mean number of life experiences per participant
Female (n = 22)	16 (72.7%)	18 (81.8%)	11 (50.0%)	14 (63.6%)	15 (68.2%)	17 (77.3%)	11 (50.0%)	10 (45.5%)	5.1
Male (n = 25)	19 (76.0%)	14 (56.0%)	20 (80.0%)	14 (56.0%)	13 (52.0%)	10 (40.0%)	11 (44.0%)	5 (20.0%)	4.2
Total (N = 47)	35 (74.5%)	32 (68.1%)	31 (66.0%)	28 (59.6%)	28 (59.6%)	27 (57.4%)	22 (46.8%)	15 (31.9%)	4.6

Aside from these high rates for each of the problematic life experiences we documented, it is critical to observe that almost all of these youth had experiences in multiple categories, with a mean of 4.6 overall (4.2 for boys and 5.1 for girls). Comparing across genders for particular experiences, the proportion of girls and boys who have perpetrated violence is remarkably close (72.7% and 76% respectively). Boys are far more likely to have had encounters with the police or legal system (80% and 50% respectively). Girls are more likely to have had experiences in all the other categories, with the largest gender differences being in suicide attempts (81.8% and 56% respectively), self-cutting (77.3% and 40% respectively), and having undergone sexual abuse (45% and 20% respectively). Girls also have more experience with drug and alcohol abuse (68.2% and 52% respectively), while there are smaller gender differences in bereavement (63.6% and 56% respectively) and with having undergone physical abuse (50% and 44% respectively).

The interpretive consequences of simultaneously entertaining psychiatric diagnosis and problematic life experience as approaches to characterizing participants become vivid when we juxtapose tables 4 and 5. However, these two ways of defining problems do not directly map onto one another, and may indeed be thought of as orthogonal to one another. Moreover, as we have already suggested, it would be too simplistic to say either that the illness causes the events or that the events cause the illness. Ethnographically, the manner in which the problematic experiences shape the lifeworld of troubled adolescents and are negotiated by them is of paramount importance. In fact, from the ethnographic standpoint, being subject to a diagnosis and undergoing treatment themselves constitute a category of life experience alongside these others, regardless of the descriptive or clinical value of the diagnostic categories per se.

A final point to repeat about problematic life experience as we have documented it is that some of the categories have to do with things that the children have done themselves and some have to do with things that have been done to them or that happened to them. This is less a matter of activity and passivity than of the "vexed" agency we observed in the consideration of hospital admission narratives in chapter 2. If it is too much to suggest that they are like leaves blown in the wind of events, it is certainly relevant to understand their agency as stymied in such a way as to subvert development and biographical coherence or, as we have said, the process of coming to have a life. The structural violence of poverty persisting over generations, family instability that ensues from such conditions, a mental health care system that when responsive remains without adequate resources, and conditions of psychological affliction that color a world of distress to which they know no alternative, all conspire to define their lives.

DIAGNOSIS AND LIFE EVENTS: GENDER AND DEPRESSION AS DEVELOPMENTAL ILLUSTRATION

Although we cannot speak further to all of the SCID psychiatric diagnostic disorders reported, we will briefly examine the differences observed between girls and boys for depression in relation to life events and experiences. Here we must grapple with the major issues from the extensive literature on sex differences for depression in relation to epidemiological, biological, psychological, cultural, and social structural factors and processes. While the application of adult models to children and adolescents cannot be presumed a priori in the absence of sufficient empirical data for youth nationally and globally, Avenevoli and colleagues (2008: 7) provide an extensive review suggesting that "child and adolescent studies collectively support the downward extension of adult criteria." Three decades ago, psychologist Susan Nolen-Hoeksema (1990) documented depression as more common among women than men by roughly a 2:1 ratio. This finding has been replicated in many epidemiological studies as summarized by Kessler (2003). Avenevoli and colleagues (2008) interpret these epidemiological data for adolescence as due in part to an earlier age of onset (around age thirteen). They argue for a multifactorial approach to variance in which biological-developmental processes emerging at puberty (along with menstruation and endocrinological changes) are conceived to interact with environmentally provoking experiences.

A summary of research by leading scholars suggests that there is a biological embedding of experience in the sense that life experiences can modify biological processes to affect health and well-being (Aristizabal et al. 2019). They note a fundamental and consistently recurring problem in neuroscience of conflating correlation with causation. Thus, while epigenetic mechanisms such as DNA methylation are suggestive, they do not demonstrate biological etiology or "underlying mechanisms" with respect to stress-related disorders. Aristizabal and colleagues call for a nuanced approach to relationships among genome, epigenome, and gene expression to include factors of tissue or cell type, age, temporal aspects of experience, sex, and DNA sequence (2019: 1). Regarding mental health in humans, they call in the same article for additional evidence to define the biological embedding of experience.[1]

In the earliest formulation of sex differences and depression, Nolen-Hoeksema (1990) proposed a multifactorial analysis to include psychological, social, and biological processes. At the psychological level, she identified distinctions of cognitive style wherein women were more prone to "ruminative" thinking and men to "distractive" activities. Our data do not show such clear distinctions between girls and boys, and this might be due to developmental differences in age. However, social structural and cultural forces of adversity and possibility mark the lives of our young interlocutors in such a way that we can grasp the situated standpoints of experiential epistemologies (Harding 1991, 2015) that define their lived experience.

Take, for illustration, Taciana (we introduced her in chapter 1 pp. 1–6 and will see her again in chapter 5 pp. 185–90), who presented as "depressed." Taciana is left to wonder *why* it is that she is "the one" to be repeatedly raped. She agonizes over how in the world it can be that so frequently it is her. Her situation of gendered precarity is a powerful example of a social-structural arrangement that produces depression. An article entitled "The Global Burden of Rape" (Koss, Heise, and Russo 1994) foregrounds that which is rarely foregrounded in the dominant discourse on the "global burden of disease." Koss and colleagues identify commonplace cultural presumptions worldwide that rape is a rare event perpetrated by typically unknown and "unbalanced" assailants, and that it is more a matter for criminal justice than a violation of bodily integrity with serious long-term consequences for psychological, physical, and social health (1994: 509–10).

Yet in global perspective, Irina Anderson (2017: 1) summarizes estimates of worldwide rape prevalence of "21–25 percent in industrialized nations, increasing to 42–90 percent in nonindustrialized ones." While anyone can be raped, globally women and girls are disproportionately raped more frequently, and there are no known risk factors for rape except the perpetrator being male. Summarizing results from available studies, Koss and colleagues find that "consistent are cross-national findings on the typical victims and perpetrators of rape. . . . The majority of perpetrators are people known to the victim, and a substantial subset of victims are very young girls. Across diverse continents and hemispheres, between one and two thirds of the victims are 15 years and younger" (1994: 518). These researchers observe that rape is culturally normative across a variety of context-specific settings or relationships (acquaintance, date, marital, punitive, weapon of war, ceremonial ritual). They note that rape therefore creates an enormous global health burden on societies, with broad health consequences that are bodily and sociocultural. Sexual abuse and violence against girls have been recognized as prominent factors in social theories of gender differences in depression (Nolen-Hoeksema 1995). Taciana is not alone.

More broadly, the majority of researchers agree that exposure to adverse social and economic conditions affects mental health status across a spectrum of serious mental disorders, across countries worldwide, and across the life span (Kessler et al. 2010). Both rigorous epidemiological and close clinical-ethnographic research have demonstrated that for adult women living in communities with particular interlocking sets of adverse conditions (poverty and unemployment, maternal burden of child care, lack of social support, and the cultural devaluation of women), precise predictions can be made for depression. Without discounting individual suffering, this research suggests that the diagnosis of depression is more apt for particular social *situations* rather than *persons* (Fields 1960; Brown and Harris 1978). These situations have temporal resonance over the full course of the life span, and certainly for the developmental trajectories of adolescents in our study cohort.

LIVED EXPERIENCE IN FAMILY CONCEPTIONS OF THE PROBLEM

As much as we have already done to define the problems of the study cohort, we have barely scratched the surface. This is because we have not yet examined the conceptions of the problem articulated by youth and their families over the time of their participation in the project. We must take a step back from the presupposition of psychopathology or even problematic life events to a fully engaged ethnographic sensibility that begins again with the query of whether our interlocutors recognize a problem in the first place, even in the context of their engagement with the treatment system. From this starting point we recognize that in any society, including our own, the understanding of what is normal and abnormal, or healthy and pathological, is culturally constituted (Benedict 1934). Whether an explicit distinction between normal and abnormal is culturally available cannot be taken for granted. Neither can we take for granted how people determine what is normal or abnormal in a particular case, or how they determine when and whether a therapeutic intervention is called for. Nor can we presume that in a particular social setting the distinction between normal and pathological is a categorical one (you're either normal or you're not) as opposed to being understood as a continuum (you can be more or less normal) (Canguilhem 1989; Sullivan 1953; Jenkins 2015a). The significance of this observation goes to the existential and methodological consequences of the shifting and ambiguous threshold between normal and abnormal.

In our ethnographic setting, the question of what counts as normal and how to talk about a particular adolescent in relation to what counts as normal played a significant role in how people conceived of what was wrong. In this respect, what we will call a *problematic of normalcy* was explicitly observable in twenty (43%) of the cases. However, the idea of the normal appears in a variety of ways. Not all conceptions of normalcy are as clear-cut as one girl's avowal that with her bipolar disorder, "it can be just all of the sudden really high up or really down low like just not normal, and I'll stay like that for a longer period of time than most people do when they're like that." One grandmother referred behaviorally to her grandson's abnormal and perseverative response to situations. A mother referred etiologically to brain abnormalities in her son. One youth commented that having a diagnosis of mental illness means never having a normal life, while her mother commented that she was not a normal child even when she was very young. Similarly, another girl disagreed with her diagnosis of premenstrual dysphoric disorder because she thought it normal to be emotional during a menstrual period, while her mother recalled that the girl had abnormal behavior as a baby. One mother disagreed that her son had bipolar disorder but indicated he was not normal either, having had mental health issues since he was a baby. Three mothers said it was important for their child to have accurate diagnosis and appropriate treatment/medication in order to have a normal childhood or normal life or to act normal.

Beyond the observation of how people conceptualize and talk about normality, we can also discern a tendency toward normalization of diagnosis and distress. Compelling in this respect is the following statement by a young girl:

> The way things are now is they're not normal and I think people should be allowed to make their own mistakes, which really isn't possible for me because I have the mental disorder hanging over my head. So normal people make mistakes, and I make a mistake and they call me crazy, they say screwed up . . . because I would make a decision and people would be saying, "Oh, you made this decision because you were manic, you made this decision because you were crazy." I want to be a normal person that makes bad decisions occasionally but that also makes good decisions too. I just want to be normal and I don't think that's possible. I mean, now that I'm off of my medication, it makes me think, well, did I go through all this for nothing because I don't feel bipolar, I don't see it, and honestly, a lot of people never have.

Such normalizing statements are often made with reference to adolescence as a developmental stage, with a cultural assumption that it is normal for the teenage years to be fraught and filled with angst. Several young people commented that they had no more anger or aggression than a normal kid, that mood swings are part of being a normal teenager, that the therapists "say I'm a pretty normal teenager," that an intermittent explosive disorder is just part of the teenager stage, that all teenage boys get into fights, that mood swings are part of being a normal teenager, or that hallucinations are a normal part of life (a young woman made this last statement without any indication that she was aware of the recent "voice hearers" movement). Several mothers made similar remarks: that her son has moody and normal days like everyone, that her daughter's fatigue and depression had declined to a normal level for a teenager, that her son's oppositional defiance is just part of being a teenager, that her son was dealing with regular teenage stuff, or that her daughter's problems had less to do with her diagnosis of bipolar disorder and were more "teenage related and PTSD related." Perhaps summarizing the ambiguous and contested nature of normality, a father referring to his son said, "For the longest time he wanted to be normal. And I told him, 'Normal? What is normal?' It could be, of course you can't explain, but I think if he can get his hallucinations under control, get his thought processes clear, then he'll be OK."

A final example of the problematic of normalcy illustrates both its cultural complexity and the concordance between parent and child conceptions of the problem. In her first interview, one girl who reported being diagnosed with schizophrenia and bipolar disorder said she thought that her problem is a disorder because "it doesn't go away. It doesn't really come and go with situations; it's just always there." In her second interview she rejected the bipolar diagnosis on the grounds that

> I am sure there is something else wrong with me, but I am not a normal bipolar, not like some days I am manic some days I'm not. It's like my mom said, this [whole] month I am usually manic. . . . I think, in a way, everyone is bipolar to some degree. I just notice a lot of people have down times and they have up times and it's just how everyone is. It's the cycle of life and it's not a disorder, it's just normal.

Here the girl's reference to "normal bipolar" evidently has the sense of "typical bipolar." Moreover, she explains that because she has a new boyfriend and more positive friends, she no longer has the same issues, an explanation that indicates a conception of the problem heavily influenced by circumstances rather than the presence of a disorder. Her mother mentioned a diagnosis of bipolar but not schizophrenia and, in her first interview, framed her daughter's problems in terms of adolescence and maturity. She said, "You're not dealing with, you know, a regular sixteen-year-old. Does she have more than bipolar? Sometimes I wonder. . . . I don't know if she'll ever be able to be on her own."

At the time of her second interview this mother, like her daughter, doubted the diagnosis of bipolar, but unlike her daughter she suspected it was a personality disorder. Moreover,

> I think there is something else going on with her. I think they are not treating her completely. I think there is something missing. I think that once we figure out the piece of the pie that is missing, and get it fixed or find out what it is, and switch the medication to go with that, we may have a whole new child on our hands.

By the third interview, the mother still thought there might be more going on than had been diagnosed, but commented that for the most part her daughter needs to know how to manage her bipolar disorder and stay on medications. This situation points directly to the unstable threshold between normal and abnormal in participants' experience, and even when a problem is formulated in psychiatric terms, the possibility remains of negotiating and renegotiating meanings. Indeed, how is someone supposed to know from a subjective standpoint whether they are off the norm or how far from the norm they are? Evidently, being hospitalized and placed in treatment are not in themselves adequate. Not only is it not always self-evident that one is not normal, but it does not appear that one can always say for certain that one is suffering, especially if one's life is the same, by and large, as it has always been.

Considering the problematic of normalcy takes us another step closer to lived experience in our characterization of young people's problems. The psychiatric research diagnoses we present in table 4, based on the KID-SCID, are valuable background data but are not the same as how the youth struggle with normalcy or talk about diagnoses they are given in clinical encounters. The problematic life experiences we present in table 5 do not tell us whether they consider their experiences as extraordinary or how they relate those experiences to why they are in the hospital. Thus, when—in order to avoid ethnocentric (or, as it were, clinic-centric) bias or presupposition—we asked interlocutors broadly about how they conceive of their "problems," we had to be prepared for any number of types of responses, including references to disorders (e.g., bipolar), symptoms (e.g., paranoia), behaviors (e.g., fighting), relationships (e.g., rejection), emotions (e.g., anger), or no problem at all.

In order to identify patterns among conceptions of the problem that would be both ethnographically and clinically relevant, we categorized responses as recognizing no problems, only psychiatric problems, only nonpsychiatric problems, or a mixture of psychiatric and nonpsychiatric problems. We made this categorization across all three ethnographic interviews in order to gauge consistency and/or change over time. Only one youth consistently denied having a problem across the initial and two follow-up interviews. Those who reported only psychiatric problems accounted for 17 percent of the adolescents, and those who reported only nonpsychiatric problems accounted for another 17 percent. The remaining 64 percent of youth showed a variety of mixed patterns. Some of these were patterns of change in a specific direction: three moved from conceptualizing their problems as nonpsychiatric to conceptualizing them as psychiatric, mostly in terms of coming to understand or grow comfortable with what the diagnoses meant; ten moved from psychiatric to nonpsychiatric while not necessarily repudiating their diagnoses, and likely because a period of time had elapsed since their hospitalization; and two moved from having problems to having no problems, primarily in the sense of feeling that their problems had been ameliorated. Complicating these shifts over time in how adolescents described their problems and related to diagnoses, only five consistently indicated they had a single problem, while all the rest described multiple problems.

The single youth who denied anything was wrong repeated in multiple interviews that he does not have any problems and that the diagnoses are made up. He said that his problems started when he went to another adolescent psychiatric hospital where he "started going mad" and attained "my own level of madness." He reported coming to CPC because he got depressed after his grandparents died. However, he did not believe he was mentally unstable at all ("nothing is wrong with me") and, due to bad experiences with doctors, did not seem to value diagnosis and treatment. He explained how sickness is taught to people and it is all in their heads, and he expressed belief that he can control all of his issues. His mother said the problems started when her son was molested, mentioning that he hallucinates, hears voices, and thinks he has split personalities. She was very concerned that he would commit suicide. She reported that the doctors diagnosed him as schizoaffective, and in a later interview said that although she "kind of agrees" with this diagnosis, it has all gotten much better. She commented that he is a very

smart and advanced kid and that she does not think he is bipolar anymore but is depressed. Questioning the very idea of diagnosing as she
discussed how each person is unique, she still concluded that depression
is real and probably hereditary. This unique situation may be one in
which the severity of the problem prevents the problem from being
seen, and in which the boy's conceptualization is tied to his mother's
apparent ambivalence about his diagnostic status and about whether
his condition has improved.

We now turn to examine the conceptualizations of several youth who
explicitly and consistently defined their problems in psychiatric terms,
several who expressed ambivalence and ambiguity with respect to psychiatric diagnosis, and several whose positions shifted over the course
of their participation.

Endorsing Psychiatric Diagnosis

Robbie, a seventeen-year-old Pueblo Indian boy, said right away in his
first interview that he has schizophrenia and Asperger's, adding that
doctors used an MRI to confirm paranoia-schizophrenia, and specifying
that his problems are getting worse and worse. He distinguished explicitly between physical and emotional distress, the former manifest in
migraines and "killer headaches" and the latter in a ruminative process
in which thoughts play over and over. The combination of these two
distresses constituted his problem and made him oversensitive, causing
"episodes." He said that the schizophrenia developed after abuse by his
mother, the absence of his dad, and bad treatment by siblings, and that
because this all happened while he was just a child, his brain development was impaired. In his second interview he acknowledged that at
first, he did not like the idea of having a psychiatric diagnosis, but then
as he thought about it more and observed himself and others, he came
to conclude that it was true. In his third interview he seemed to find
much comfort in the psychiatric diagnoses, and reported having spent a
considerable amount of time trying to understand them through
research. He was able to talk with his psychiatrist about research on
Asperger's and how to move forward. He believed that his problems had
gotten much better with education and making the effort to understand.
His grandmother explained that he was first diagnosed after the school
psychologist saw him pacing and muttering to himself and that he subsequently had an episode in which he threw a chair at a wall near a
bully. She consistently noted the difference between how "normal peo-

ple" handle things and how her grandson is abnormal in his perseverative worrying in response to stressors.

Also fitting this model is Quincy, a twelve-year-old Anglo boy who said that he came to CPC for depression (being alone in his room and crying) and anger (throwing things, punching things, yelling, and cutting himself). He said that one therapist actually gave him the right diagnosis, which included depression, anxiety, and bipolar disorder. Bipolar disorder to him was mood swings (switching from being happy to sad and depressed) that came from genetics, as his mom, grandma, and great-grandmother all have bipolar disorder. In his second interview he reported feeling relieved to be diagnosed with bipolar disorder and that things were much better since being on the right medication. He said he still got angry but did not get depressed anymore. By the time of his third interview, he had been readmitted to CPC once and was currently in foster care. He still agreed with his diagnoses, which now included depression, anxiety, ADHD, attention deficit disorder (ADD), and hypomanic disorder. He had not thought about the latter diagnosis much, but continued to avow that taking his medication made him better and that his bipolar disorder was inherited from his family. His mother's account was strongly concordant, and in her first and second interviews she reported being happy when he was diagnosed with bipolar disorder, saying she knew that he had it before he was diagnosed. He also had been diagnosed with ADHD at age two and a half, and she reported working hard to figure out what therapy, parenting methods, and medication he should be given. She even attended conferences about ADHD and got her bachelor's degree in a field related to psychology. In her third interview, the mother discussed her own experiences being bipolar and how her diagnosis and treatment came about, talking about the similarities between her son's and her own mental illnesses. She very much agreed with the psychiatric/psychological conception of her illness and thought that she and her son were alike and that he would get accustomed to the need to be medicated his entire life in order to control his behaviors and live normally. She also mentioned that her son may have been sexually and physically abused when he was younger than ten.

Neal is another young man who described his problem explicitly as Asperger's syndrome because of "having troubles with social cues" and depression caused by "everything I am going through." A fifteen-year-old Hispanic youth with mixed Anglo and Native American ethnic background, Neal was diagnosed with attention deficit disorder but did not think he had that disorder because "I'm a loner and don't need much attention." He also thought he was born with autism because his mother bled throughout her pregnancy and that the condition may have been made worse by injections he had received containing mercury. In his second interview he de-emphasized Asperger's as a relatively minor issue while noting that "they say my main problem would be anger and depression and impulsivity, three main problems. I'm very impulsive." In his third interview there was very little discussion of his problems, and he simply mentioned that his issues were anger and depression. In general, he accepted the psychiatric diagnoses while understanding that he must be the one to make progress toward getting better. His parents said that he has been seeing a psychiatrist since he was two years old and has had many diagnoses, including sensory integration disorder, dysthymia, Asperger's, autism, ADHD, and narcissistic personality disorder. They seemed to agree with these, and his mother explained how Asperger's is different from depression or bipolar in that it is a neurobiological brain disorder. Thus, "the way that it presents is different and so nobody can ever really keep him long because he doesn't have that acuity, what he has is he's annoying, he has no social skills, he's different." In their second interview, Neal's parents expressed that his symptoms and levels of mental health issues make Asperger's an insufficient diagnosis, that there is something more than just Asperger's. In their third interview, the parents explicitly discussed the helpfulness of diagnoses. They said that their son too often relies on the benefits of his disorder (as an excuse to justify behavior) and instead "he needs to accept the fact that he has a disorder and he needs to be willing to work positives and negatives." They also talked about how Asperger's is no easier to deal with than autism, since "with nonverbal autism people help you along the way. With Asperger's, people just see him as a kid that is screwing up."

Christopher, a fourteen-year-old Anglo boy, was hospitalized after trying to commit suicide. Chris said that what bothers him most are his bad sexual behavior, physical aggression, and depression. He reported that the doctors have said he has psychosis, PTSD, and possibly bipolar disorder, agreeing that these "pretty much describe me." He considered his problem a psychological one that has to do with his thoughts and emotions. He did not believe that his problem is genetic, but he did consider it his personal responsibility and thought that he should have used his coping tools better to control his anger. In his second interview he reported that his main problems were anger, behavior management, depression, psychosis, family issues, and sexual aggression, adding that his anger, psychosis, and depression had gotten worse while his family issues, behavior management, and anxiety had gotten better. He accepted the concept that his brain chemistry is "different" and he needs medications to balance it. He said that his diagnoses were currently PTSD and schizoaffective disorder and again agreed that "I think they kind of explain my issues." In his third interview it seemed that he viewed psychosis as the main problem. He talked about what he does when he is in a psychotic episode (fighting, self-harm) and about how the psychiatrist and therapists have helped him to recognize signs of psychosis and develop coping strategies to handle it. It bothered him that the doctors said that because of his psychosis he will never be able to live on his own. He articulated the ambition to be a psychiatrist one day, and it was obvious that he endorsed these diagnoses and engaged in therapy.

His stepfather believed that Chris's main problem is his thought processes (confusion and hallucinations) and reported the diagnoses as bipolar disorder/schizoaffective bipolar disorder with psychotic episodes. He indicated that medical science does not know much about the brain, and that moreover the boy's grandparents were both addicts and that it is hard to follow the family line to see if his issues are genetic. He reported a history of abuse by Chris's biological father, which he thought may have contributed to the problem. In his second interview the stepfather discussed how his son's current psychiatric diagnosis was good because it is treatable but worried that he could be diagnosed with "schizophrenic bipolar disorder" because that would be much worse. In his final interview he predicted that his stepson's future problems will be psychosis and delusions and that he will need to fight to keep these in control his entire life. He distinguished between whether the problems originated in old "bad behaviors" or from his diagnosis. If they were from his diagnosis, they consisted of "more psychosis, manic behaviors, head banging, punching walls, violent and sexual thoughts, and verbalizing those to staff and peers." If they were bad behaviors, they were more habitual, as when recently he stopped going to school and purposefully dropped his level within the hospital school "from 3 to 1 because everybody was making fun of him and he wanted to be like everyone else." In this respect the stepfather accepts the diagnosis but does not think it accounts for all the problems.

Diagnostic Ambivalence

Among those who acknowledged problems without consistently endorsing psychiatric or diagnostic terms, Andrew was a twelve-year-old Anglo boy who in his first interview said simply that medication helped but that he was unclear how it helped. In his second interview he said that he had learned to control his "full anger," but did not clearly describe how he did that and stated that he did not use the coping skills learned at the hospital because they were stupid. At the time of his third interview, having been readmitted to CPC because he choked his brother, he conceptualized his problem as that he fights with his brother a lot. Being at the hospital helped because he was able to talk, learn coping skills, and get medications, but when the topic of diagnoses was brought up, he referred to his mother and was silent. For her part, she said that her son was very aggressive; he would fight, threaten, interrupt. She thought there were a lot of factors that caused her son to have psychiatric problems, including heredity and his father being on drugs. When he was diagnosed as bipolar, she was confused, having no idea what bipolar was or if her son had mixed diagnoses. She thought he was "schizophrenic," but because of his age he couldn't be diagnosed, and she considered this was wrong because it makes the parents suffer. She wished that the psychiatrists would "actually diagnose" her kids, four of whom were in treatment, feeling that clinicians are reluctant to diagnose children: "Diagnose them. Do it. Get them under control and give us a chance of life." In general, she trusted psychiatric diagnoses and medication and advocated for her son to receive higher medication dosages and more diagnoses, as she considered this the only chance he had at getting better, being safe, and having a life.

Jess, a fifteen-year-old Hispanic girl who had been hospitalized multiple times for seizures, depression, and hallucinations that resulted in suicide attempts or overdoses, said that her depression is influenced by stressful family events (death of her father and uncle), family sickness (grandma and mother), and income struggles. She explained how she had to "do a lot more around the house" because her mother did not do enough. When asked if this was caused by her mother's depression, her response was "Uh, she's just lazy." She considered her hallucinations a normal part of her life, her epilepsy a problem in her brain, and her depression an emotional problem outside her brain. In her second interview she said she did not think she needed therapy anymore because she had been doing much better and she had not been having anger problems. She said that her depression was much better, although she had just cut herself. She continued thinking that her hallucinations were not a problem and said that she felt comfortable about them. In her final interview she said her main diagnosis was for depression but that she disliked diagnoses. "[It's] not a big deal for me. I know what is wrong with me. I don't need to have a specific label on it." She was no longer hallucinating and said her depression was better. Her mother said the main problem was not just one thing, and that her daughter's depression and epilepsy came as a package. "I don't say one more than the other because one month we're struggling with her anxieties and stuff like that, then the other month we're suffering with her thyroid or with her lupus, so it's everything." She said the girl had been diagnosed with depression, anxiety, and bipolar, but not PTSD. She did not consider the hallucinations medical, but thought they were just imaginary friends. The mother herself had a history of severe mental illness, but unlike other parents with a history of mental illness she seemed unfamiliar with or unaccepting of psychiatric diagnoses. During her second interview the mother denied that her daughter actually heard voices, saying she made this up for attention. She rejected the idea of an overarching mental health problem because Jess underwent a series of tests to determine whether she was "schizophrenic" and depressed and came out fine except in the test for short-term memory. She said the girl might have some anxiety, eating problems, and attention problems but these would not be considered mental. In her final interview the mother reported that more recent tests suggested that if she were eighteen, she would be diagnosed with a personality disorder. Her mother recalled that Jess had been diagnosed for depression, bipolar disorder, and schizoaffective disorder, agreeing that she had depression and might be bipolar but indicating that the overarching issue was her daughter's seizures.

Michael, a fourteen-year-old Anglo boy who had been suicidal, reported that doctors had told him he had paranoia, claustrophobia, and bipolar disorder but referred to the diagnoses from a "they" perspective: "They told me . . ."; "They thought. . . ." Yet he was on medication because he did think something was working. He said that his mom had attempted suicide also. He reported that his problem was just dealing with people and being around them all the time. In his second interview, when we asked what his most recent diagnosis was, he responded, "I don't really know, I didn't even talk to them about me like that." He said that he was taking medication for anxiety and so he was getting much less nervous and was less paranoid. He did not necessarily attribute the change to his medication, but attributed it to thinking more. His mother and grandmother reported that he had been diagnosed with paranoia, anger management issues, severe depression, and most recently bipolar disorder. Michael's mother was very afraid that he might be diagnosed with bipolar/schizophrenia because she knew a girl who had that and she had "many issues." She said that depression runs in the family and that she was currently taking medication for it herself. She thought that her daughters might have contributed to Michael's paranoia. In her second interview the mother recalled that her son had mental health issues since he was a baby and required brain surgery because his soft spot closed up. Doctors at the time told her that he may have issues in adolescence of being antisocial and anxious. She stated that she started noticing changes that confirmed the doctors' predictions, and that his mental health issues had increased since he had gotten older. She said that currently "he's antisocial, he's bipolar, he's got some antisocial anxiety, there's a few other things, but like I said a lot of it goes back to the brain" and being exposed to her own suicidal depression when he was eleven. By the third interview she disagreed that her son is bipolar. She said, "He doesn't have mood swings, he doesn't have these highs and lows. He will have some real lows, but that has to do with the anger problem that he has." Michael's mother and grandmother agreed that he was not normal because he did not exhibit the social skills that average seventeen-year-olds have and he had issues with bonding. They attributed these social anxiety and anger issues to his brain surgery at three months and to physical abuse by his mother's boyfriend.

Scott was a fifteen-year-old Anglo/Native American boy who said he was diagnosed a "psycho" by a doctor and that offended him very much. "Yeah, I wasn't a psycho. I'm not a psycho at all." At points, he said, he had problems with rage and anger, but he offered no examples. In his second interview he said that the doctors had not given him a psychiatric diagnosis for his anger and that his main issue was not seeing his girlfriend. His mother said he had been diagnosed with pervasive developmental disorder (PDD), ODD, ADHD, and childhood schizophrenia. Twice she said she agreed with schizophrenia because she was most familiar with this disease and it made sense with respect to her son's symptoms, particularly hearing voices. She was not sure about PDD, mainly because she did not know much about it. In her second interview she enumerated obsessive-compulsive disorder (OCD), ODD, PDD, schizophrenia, and psychotic disorder. She said that at first, she completely agreed with the diagnosis of schizophrenia, but now she thought he actually might have OCD. She expressed frustration with modern medicine because the doctors could not give her answers about what was wrong with Scott. She wanted a diagnosis because "I need to know how to deal with this, you know is it anything specific that has a generally specific set of symptoms that I can learn and deal with." A diagnosis would help her deal with her son's problem by providing her with a standard set of symptoms related to the disorder. She also thought that diet could influence behavior, saying that at her house they only eat homemade food but after two weeks at his father's house Scott returned in problematic condition, probably because of his diet there. In her third interview his mother reported that he had been diagnosed with an early stage of schizophrenia or a general psychotic disorder. His younger sister, present during the interview, reported that in conjunction with his involvement with anime, he claimed to be possessed by a "fox demon" and was unsuccessfully trying to get control of himself again. She also said that he called himself a "hell praiser," which she assumed was a Satan worshipper.

Shifts over Time

A number of the youth had conceptualizations of their problem that dramatically shifted across the course of their participation. Katie, a sixteen-year-old girl of mixed Anglo and Hispanic heritage, said multiple times in her first interview that "I am bipolar," which she described as "like where you have ups and downs, and manics and depressives, and does all kinds of funky things to your brain." Subsequently she decided that the bipolar diagnosis was wrong and that the medications were causing her to act out. She said she was not currently on medications and claimed to be feeling much better, saying, "Now that I'm off of my medication, it makes me think, well, did I go through all this for nothing because I don't feel bipolar, I don't see it, and honestly, a lot of people never have." Her mother in her first interview reported having been convinced by her daughter's doctor to have her evaluated for bipolar disorder but said that she was unsure whether the girl "is lying, is acting bipolar, or if she is acting true." Katie's mother was ambivalent about accepting a bipolar diagnosis for herself and thought that the way she was raised and being a single parent caused her own mood swings. In her second interview she indicated that doctors had imposed the diagnosis in order to push medication and that Depo-Provera had helped her daughter by diminishing her PMS. By the third interview Katie had run away from home for a second time and her mother emphasized that she was a manipulative liar, concluding that medicating without figuring out the real problem and labeling her with a psychiatric disorder were both ineffective. In this instance both the dramatic shift away from a psychiatric conception of the problem and the concordance between mother and daughter are noteworthy.

In his first interview Nielsen, a fifteen-year-old Anglo boy, said that he had ADD, ADHD, bipolar, mania, and chronic depression. It was obvious that he knew what these disorders are and how they are different from each other. He clearly understood his diagnoses but did not think they really made any difference in his life. He considered his problems genetic because his dad had higher levels of ADD, ADHD, depression, and bipolar and his mom was also diagnosed with mental disorders. He also thought an explanation for his mental disorder might be a chemical imbalance in his brain. By the second interview he thought that his problem was that he would listen only to his dad, but his dad did not attempt to control him. When asked what he thought about previous psychiatric diagnoses, he responded by saying that none of them made sense to him except maybe the ADHD diagnosis. He is among the group of normalizing youth we identified above, and regarding the disorder he said that "it might be I just don't see any signs of it. Nope. Well, um mood swings, yeah, but those must be normal for a teenager." There is a dramatic change in the conception of the problem between these two interviews, such that he recognized the relevance of psychiatric diagnoses in the second interview but no longer identified his problems as related to a mental illness or as psychiatric. In their first interview, his mother and father reported that the father had been diagnosed with bipolar disorder for over twenty years and worked in advocacy as a bipolar disorder survivor. During most of the interview, his father was explaining bipolar disorder and educating Nielsen's mother and the interviewer about the different types and levels of bipolar disorder. The mother believed completely that her son had bipolar disorder and that he was born with it in the same way people are born with diabetes or other chronic diseases. Nielsen's mother and aunt were strongly in favor of diagnosing people with bipolar and not being weak about the need to label people. In the second interview his father reported that Nielsen was recently diagnosed with PTSD because his mother was engaging in irresponsible behavior when the boy was around, like smoking crack. The father thought he agreed with the diagnosis of PTSD.

John was a fourteen-year-old Hispanic boy who said in his first interview that he was diagnosed with PTSD and bipolar disorder. He believed he had these because the medication helped. At points in the second interview, he said that he did not have a problem. He had received therapy in the past for his anger, his smoking, and to formulate his relapse plan, but claimed that since he had therapy he no longer did those things. At other points, he said that arguing was his problem. In his third interview he explained how he was very anxious and worried about everything (his family, himself, his clothes). He also said that he was very paranoid about what people were thinking, and stated that the doctors were now thinking his ticks and behaviors were a product of his anxiety rather than

ADHD. Yet overall he felt like he controlled his anger better, though he experienced bad mood swings every two weeks. Thus, the conception of his problem changed dramatically in each interview: (1) has PTSD and bipolar disorder, (2) no problem, (3) the problem is mainly anxiety. His grandmother believed he had behavioral problems that consisted of anger. She agreed with his diagnoses of ADHD, severe depression, and bipolar disorder, and in fact was advised by her sister when her grandson was seven to get him checked for ADHD. His grandmother had read up about the disorders and said that "he fits right into bipolar." In her second interview the grandmother noted that Nielsen had been having problems with fighting other kids, adding that he was depressed and had ADHD and bipolar disorder. She thought he was bipolar because of how he would break things constantly and destroy things. She maintained her adherence to bipolar in her third interview because he would get into a bad temper. She had read about it and it made sense for him. She observed that the doctors wanted to change his diagnosis to anxiety and PTSD because of his mother's death, but she disagreed because the boy had problems long before his mother's death. She was unsure about other psychiatric diagnoses because he didn't fit into those either.

THE DISCOURSE OF DIAGNOSIS

Regardless of whether they endorsed psychiatric categories, expressed ambivalence about them, or shifted their position over time, there is one critical feature common to how youth and parents/guardians conceptualize their problems. We have discovered that embedded within their accounts is what we will call a distinctive *discourse of diagnosis*. This discourse is a function of the nosological system that reaches beyond the clinical domain and colonizes the everyday language and lifeworld of families. It is not an artifact of the interview process—the frequent concordance between adolescent and parent/guardian discussion of problems suggests that they are talked about in families and in therapeutic encounters, not just in response to ethnographic interrogation. Distinct from the research diagnosis we derived from the KID-SCID and reported above, the diagnoses and explanations these youth receive from clinicians who treat them may vary from one clinical setting to another and from one time to another. What we must attend to is the manner in which patients, families, and mental health care professionals take up the clinical discourse of diagnostic categories in a way that is consequential for their lived experience of illness. To be precise, we must recognize that psychiatric categories can be deployed as rhetorical weapons, metaphorical containers, sources of emotional relief, opportunities for blame, epithets to throw, therapeutic tools, and points of reference (Jenkins 2015a). We attribute this insight to having taken the methodological step away from labeled and entified categories of disorder to the broader question of conceptions of the problem. This move allows us to identify a field of discourse characterized by a distinct *discursive structure* and within which diagnostic terms can be understood in their function as *discursive operators*. Following this line of interpretation entails a particular theoretical claim about the relationship between language and experience, and elaborating that claim is the aim of this concluding section.

Understanding the discourse of diagnosis embedded within how these young people and their parents/guardians talk about their problems begins with recognizing the instability and "diagnostic fluidity" (Nissen and Risor 2018) of terms designating psychiatric disorder as they are used and circulated in speech. This instability and fluidity are present both with respect to the nosological systems themselves and to the manner in which they are deployed in both clinical and everyday speech. The nosological systems are inherently unstable in two ways. First, the fact that categories of psychiatric disorder in *DSM* and *ICD* do not precisely correspond is already evidence that they can only be approximations of the real and do not describe discrete pathological entities. Second, as we noted earlier in this chapter, the periodic revision of the classifications cannot be said to result in successively more accurate descriptions of pathological reality, but instead reflect both changing epidemiological profiles of mental illness and the rethinking of categories influenced by diagnostic trends as well as cultural styles, fashions, and fads.

Research and clinical diagnoses differ as well. The KID-SCID instrument that we used is administered by a trained clinician but is based on a single interview, and generates diagnoses that are standardized for research purposes. Clinical diagnoses may be generated over the course of several encounters and also may be revised over time or differ from one mental health care provider and treatment setting to another. It is critical to note that with reference to the *DSM* the SCID covers only Axis I disorders, whereas there is no limit on clinical diagnoses. Indeed, in the process of doing the KID-SCID interviews, the SWYEPT child psychiatrist and clinical psychologist recorded adolescents' report of symptoms for a number of diagnoses not identified by the KID-SCID. These included four instances of Asperger's disorder, three of learning disorders/disabilities, five of nonpsychiatric medical conditions (including epilepsy/lupus/thyroid, diabetes, mononucleosis, asthma/allergies, and craniosynostosis), two of reactive attachment disorder, and one of PDD.

There were also ten instances in which personality factors (Axis II of the *DSM* nosology) were invoked in a variety of ways. Generally, Axis II diagnoses are applied to this age group with reluctance in clinical practice in light of developmental changes. Three of these were reports of a clinical diagnosis of borderline, narcissistic, and "bipolar and/or a personality diagnosis." Four were reports by mothers, who made statements including that she suspected her child has "histrionic personality disorder"; that her child had a "personality disorder"; that based on recent tests, if she were eighteen her daughter "would be diagnosed" with a personality disorder; and that a therapist friend had suggested the girl had borderline personality disorder with problems that "seemed to combine" medical, personality, and abuse factors. In three instances, reference to personality was more general: one girl said that people misinterpret her good mood as a bad mood "but this is my normal personality"; a mother said that bad behavior and aggression "are her personality"; another mother said that her daughter is "a good kid with a good personality."

We must reiterate that it was not part of our protocol to report to participants the results of the KID-SCID research diagnostic interview, and the diagnoses they reported and discussed with us came from their clinical encounters and hospital experience. When we explicitly compared research and clinical diagnoses for each young person, there was typically overlap in the enumeration of disorders—recall that in 94 percent of young people the KID-SCID showed more than one and as many as six disorders—but there were no instances in which the results corresponded precisely. Thus, it is the self-reported (by patient and parent) clinical diagnoses that are in question in identifying the discourse of diagnosis as an element of the lived experience of dealing with and making sense of problems. To the extent that this discourse is deployed in daily life and clinical encounters, it works to transform the flow of experience into a structured subjectivity and intersubjectivity. Let us look more closely at how this comes about.

Discursive Structure

Having considered the variety of ways in which adolescents and their parents/guardians articulate conceptions of the problem, we can describe the use of psychiatric labels and diagnostic terms as a coherent discourse of diagnosis structured in the following way. The first level of this structure is how they understand the diagnosis, particularly with reference to whether their understanding conforms to the psychiatric definition. The second level, regardless of how they understand it, is whether the person agrees or disagrees with the diagnosis they cite. Third is whether or not they find a diagnosis useful or helpful to account for or deal with their problems. Fourth is whether or not they are actively engaged in the discourse of diagnosis as evidenced by how they circulate diagnostic terms through their utterances. This structure is depicted in figure 8, along with brief interview excerpts exemplifying the alternative positions at each level. We can also briefly elaborate some of the nuance at each of these levels, as follows.

Understanding: From an ethnographic standpoint, the issue is not *whether* people understand diagnoses in a canonical, authoritative sense, but *how* they understand it in ways that are experientially and pragmatically consequential. Consider one boy who reported that an MRI had been used to diagnose his paranoia-schizophrenia, and another who disagreed with his diagnosis of ADD because "I'm a loner. I don't need much attention" (figure 8). Although both statements seem eccentric, the first boy in fact was otherwise quite well informed about the disorders of schizophrenia and Asperger's with which he identified, although schizophrenia did not figure in his SCID diagnostic profile. The second boy understood his own Asperger's in terms of having trouble with social cues and had a complex understanding of the relation between depression and anger, even while misunderstanding ADD. The example of understanding we give in figure 8 indicates awareness of celebrities who also have bipolar disorder and how "racing thoughts" distinguish this girl from "normal" people. Two mothers commented that bipolar disorder was a common diagnosis, but one did so in the context of the disorder having been explained by clinicians while the other spoke from a critical stance and thought that bipolar is *too* commonly diagnosed. A number of participants indicated that they had engaged in their own research about particular diagnoses. This included an adolescent who researched Asperger's and two who researched bipolar disorder, as well as a mother who looked into schizophrenia, two who researched bipolar disorder, and one who sought information on antidepressant drugs.

Agreeing: It is critical in identifying a discourse of diagnosis that clinical determinations were not necessarily accepted at face value on medical or psychiatric authority but agreed or disagreed with—17 percent of adolescents made explicit statements either agreeing or disagreeing with a diagnosis. The example of disagreement in figure 8 is from a

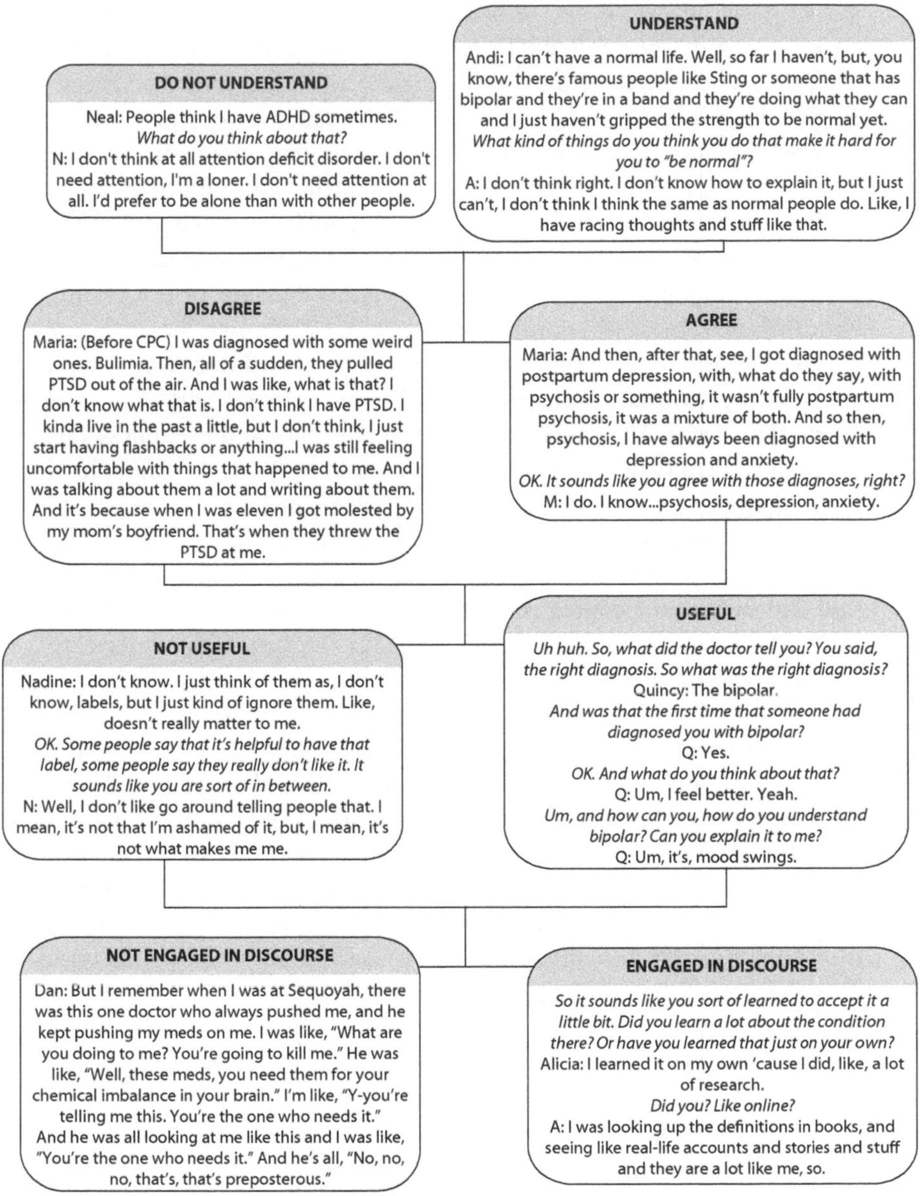

DO NOT UNDERSTAND

Neal: People think I have ADHD sometimes.
What do you think about that?
N: I don't think at all attention deficit disorder. I don't need attention, I'm a loner. I don't need attention at all. I'd prefer to be alone than with other people.

UNDERSTAND

Andi: I can't have a normal life. Well, so far I haven't, but, you know, there's famous people like Sting or someone that has bipolar and they're in a band and they're doing what they can and I just haven't gripped the strength to be normal yet.
What kind of things do you think you do that make it hard for you to "be normal"?
A: I don't think right. I don't know how to explain it, but I just can't, I don't think I think the same as normal people do. Like, I have racing thoughts and stuff like that.

DISAGREE

Maria: (Before CPC) I was diagnosed with some weird ones. Bulimia. Then, all of a sudden, they pulled PTSD out of the air. And I was like, what is that? I don't know what that is. I don't think I have PTSD. I kinda live in the past a little, but I don't think, I just start having flashbacks or anything...I was still feeling uncomfortable with things that happened to me. And I was talking about them a lot and writing about them. And it's because when I was eleven I got molested by my mom's boyfriend. That's when they threw the PTSD at me.

AGREE

Maria: And then, after that, see, I got diagnosed with postpartum depression, with, what do they say, with psychosis or something, it wasn't fully postpartum psychosis, it was a mixture of both. And so then, psychosis, I have always been diagnosed with depression and anxiety.
OK. It sounds like you agree with those diagnoses, right?
M: I do. I know...psychosis, depression, anxiety.

NOT USEFUL

Nadine: I don't know. I just think of them as, I don't know, labels, but I just kind of ignore them. Like, doesn't really matter to me.
OK. Some people say that it's helpful to have that label, some people say they really don't like it. It sounds like you are sort of in between.
N: Well, I don't like go around telling people that. I mean, it's not that I'm ashamed of it, but, I mean, it's not what makes me me.

USEFUL

Uh huh. So, what did the doctor tell you? You said, the right diagnosis. So what was the right diagnosis?
Quincy: The bipolar.
And was that the first time that someone had diagnosed you with bipolar?
Q: Yes.
OK. And what do you think about that?
Q: Um, I feel better. Yeah.
Um, and how can you, how do you understand bipolar? Can you explain it to me?
Q: Um, it's, mood swings.

NOT ENGAGED IN DISCOURSE

Dan: But I remember when I was at Sequoyah, there was this one doctor who always pushed me, and he kept pushing my meds on me. I was like, "What are you doing to me? You're going to kill me." He was like, "Well, these meds, you need them for your chemical imbalance in your brain." I'm like, "Y-you're telling me this. You're the one who needs it." And he was all looking at me like this and I was like, "You're the one who needs it." And he's all, "No, no, no, that's, that's preposterous."

ENGAGED IN DISCOURSE

So it sounds like you sort of learned to accept it a little bit. Did you learn a lot about the condition there? Or have you learned that just on your own?
Alicia: I learned it on my own 'cause I did, like, a lot of research.
Did you? Like online?
A: I was looking up the definitions in books, and seeing like real-life accounts and stories and stuff and they are a lot like me, so.

FIGURE 8. Adolescent discourse of diagnosis: a structural model.

girl who not only disagreed with PTSD because she did not have flash-backs, but said "they pulled PTSD out of the air" and "threw the PTSD at me." The example of agreement is from the same girl, who recognized herself as delusional and accepted the simultaneous presence of depression, anxiety, and psychosis. Several participants expressed the importance of having the right diagnosis, but this importance could be in the form of either satisfaction with a diagnosis or a feeling that the correct diagnosis had not yet been identified. Others recognized the legitimacy of diagnoses in principle, while either agreeing or disagreeing with the correctness or continued adequacy of their own diagnosis, or agreeing with one diagnosis they had been given and disagreeing with another. Three of the youth rejected their diagnoses outright.

Finding useful: The degree of perceived relevance and usefulness varied even when a diagnosis was not disputed. In figure 8, the example of not finding diagnoses useful is from a girl who claimed to "ignore them" because it "doesn't really matter to me" and moreover "it's not what makes me." The boy who provides the example of diagnosis as useful said that because of finding the right diagnosis "I feel better," and now he could better account for his "mood swings." Again, with reference to the methodological importance of asking about problems in the broadest sense, three young people conceived their problem independently of their disorder, and two stated that the disorder was under control and hence not a problem. One youth acknowledged the diagnosis while not considering his problems to be medical; one was quite familiar with and agreed with the diagnoses without caring much because they had been repeatedly revised and new diagnoses introduced over time; one avowed not understanding the diagnosis and losing interest. Several referred to the manner in which diagnosis could be used as an "excuse," as with one adolescent who said he had done so in order "to not control a problem" and another who did so to "pull back from society." Two mothers invoked diagnoses as excuses used by their teenager in this same sense, while a father said that his child "too often relies on the benefits of the disorder." A grandmother said that her daughter used her own mental illness as an excuse not to take care of her kids, which contributed to the adolescent grandchild's mental health issues.

Engaging the discourse: A person can understand their diagnosis, agree with it, and find it useful, but still may or may not actively engage in talking about it or accepting its consequences. Our example in figure 8 of not engaging is from a boy who rejected the diagnosis, rejected the idea of a "chemical imbalance" in his brain, rejected the need for medication, and was confrontational with his doctor about it. The example of someone who was engaged is a girl who was not only "looking up the definitions" but seeking out "real-life accounts and stories." Indeed, one youth was described as an "expert on the diagnosis" and fluent in discussing its relevance. Yet fluency in the discourse of diagnosis could be accompanied by thinking of the diagnostic process as inadequate. One mother was particularly articulate in this respect:

> I've been looking stuff up and everything and, yeah, he is a schizophrenic. And that's a big problem because I guess our society or the FDA or whoever, whoever has control of all these diagnoses and everything, they won't diagnose kids with things that they normally see in older people. 'Cause they say, like the schizophrenia starts at, like, college age and everything. I think that's not right. You know, if they have all the signs and everything, their mind developed or not, if they have all the signs, diagnose them, give 'em the medication that they need and everything, instead of making the family suffer with them all those years until they can diagnose them and give them the medication that's gonna control that disease and everything. Sonia, she has other personalities and everything, but they can't diagnose her with multiple personalities because of her age. And I'm like, "She has it. Diagnose her. Get her what she needs." Like that, she could have a chance of having a normal childhood. Yeah, it's rare to see any of these diseases, mental diseases and everything in these kids and everything, this age and everything, but my kids have it. Diagnose them. Do it. Get them under control and give us a chance of life. But, that's why when they said do I want to do this study and everything, I'm like, "Well, what is it gonna do," and they're like, "Well it can help in the hospital situation and everything." And I'm like, "Well why are you guys just doing it for the, the adolescents and everything. Do it for, for all age groups."

In this case being engaged in the discourse of diagnosis includes a plea for more adequate diagnosis that is part of a critique of diagnostic process and conventions.

Figure 8 shows how the discourse of diagnosis is structured, drawing on the entire cohort of youth who participated in the study to provide particularly vivid examples for each component of the model. The model can also map how individuals talk about diagnosis. In principle, for example, someone might understand the diagnosis, agree with it, yet find it not useful and not be engaged in diagnostic discourse; any number of permutations is possible. The next two figures show examples of individual discourses of diagnosis that are, for the most part, self-consistent in accepting or rejecting diagnostic conventions and categories as relevant to their own situations.

Figure 9 shows how Kevin not only expressed understanding but felt that not knowing his diagnosis exacerbated his problems. He explicitly

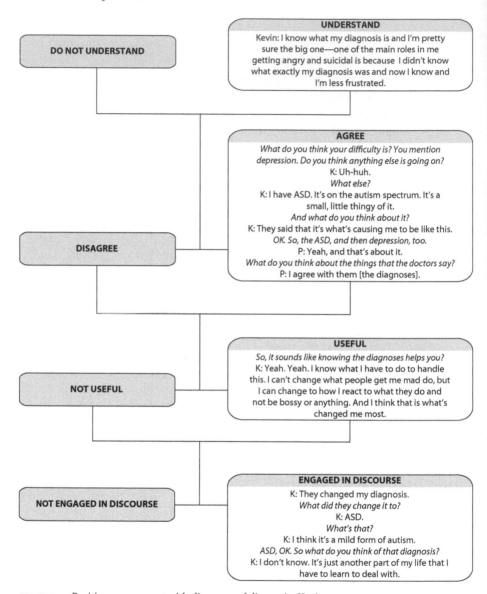

UNDERSTAND

Kevin: I know what my diagnosis is and I'm pretty sure the big one—one of the main roles in me getting angry and suicidal is because I didn't know what exactly my diagnosis was and now I know and I'm less frustrated.

DO NOT UNDERSTAND

AGREE

What do you think your difficulty is? You mention depression. Do you think anything else is going on?
K: Uh-huh.
What else?
K: I have ASD. It's on the autism spectrum. It's a small, little thingy of it.
And what do you think about it?
K: They said that it's what's causing me to be like this.
OK. So, the ASD, and then depression, too.
P: Yeah, and that's about it.
What do you think about the things that the doctors say?
P: I agree with them [the diagnoses].

DISAGREE

USEFUL

So, it sounds like knowing the diagnoses helps you?
K: Yeah. Yeah. I know what I have to do to handle this. I can't change what people get me mad do, but I can change to how I react to what they do and not be bossy or anything. And I think that is what's changed me most.

NOT USEFUL

ENGAGED IN DISCOURSE

K: They changed my diagnosis.
What did they change it to?
K: ASD.
What's that?
K: I think it's a mild form of autism.
ASD, OK. So what do you think of that diagnosis?
K: I don't know. It's just another part of my life that I have to learn to deal with.

NOT ENGAGED IN DISCOURSE

FIGURE 9. Positive engagement with discourse of diagnosis: Kevin.

agreed with the diagnoses of depression and autism spectrum disorder, and found them useful in helping him know what to do to handle his situation. He actively engaged in diagnostic discourse about the consequences of adding a new diagnosis that defines "another part of my life that I have to learn to deal with." As shown in figure 10, Sherine demon-

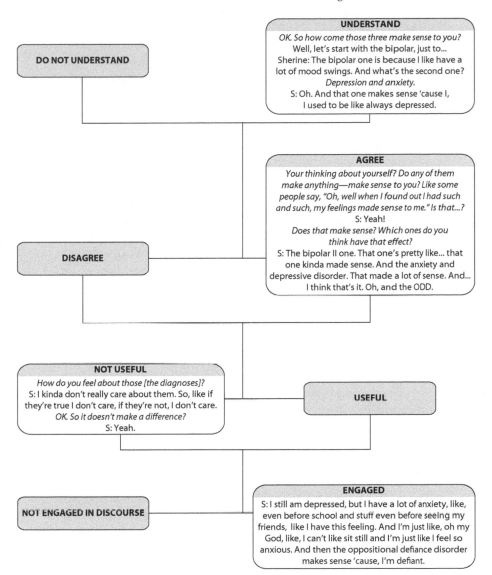

DO NOT UNDERSTAND

UNDERSTAND
OK. So how come those three make sense to you?
Well, let's start with the bipolar, just to...
Sherine: The bipolar one is because I like have a
lot of mood swings. *And what's the second one?*
Depression and anxiety.
S: Oh. And that one makes sense 'cause I,
I used to be like always depressed.

DISAGREE

AGREE
Your thinking about yourself? Do any of them
make anything—make sense to you? Like some
people say, "Oh, well when I found out I had such
and such, my feelings made sense to me." Is that...?
S: Yeah!
Does that make sense? Which ones do you
think have that effect?
S: The bipolar II one. That one's pretty like... that
one kinda made sense. And the anxiety and
depressive disorder. That made a lot of sense. And...
I think that's it. Oh, and the ODD.

NOT USEFUL
How do you feel about those [the diagnoses]?
S: I kinda don't really care about them. So, like if
they're true I don't care, if they're not, I don't care.
OK. So it doesn't make a difference?
S: Yeah.

USEFUL

NOT ENGAGED IN DISCOURSE

ENGAGED
S: I still am depressed, but I have a lot of anxiety, like,
even before school and stuff even before seeing my
friends, like I have this feeling. And I'm just like, oh my
God, like, I can't like sit still and I'm just like I feel so
anxious. And then the oppositional defiance disorder
makes sense 'cause, I'm defiant.

FIGURE 10. Negative engagement with discourse of diagnosis: Sherine.

strated her understanding of bipolar disorder, depression, and anxiety in terms of her moods. She agreed with the diagnoses because they "made sense" and even added, as an afterthought, her diagnosis of ODD. Yet she indicated that the diagnoses are not useful by expressing her indifference and saying, "I kinda don't really care about them." In spite of this, she engaged in a discourse of diagnosis insofar as she referred her descriptions of lived experience back to the diagnostic categories in expressions like "I have this feeling," "I can't sit still," and "I'm defiant."

Our final two figures outline a dramatic change in the discourse of diagnosis articulated by the same adolescent at two different moments of her participation in the project. Alicia (figure 11), a Native American girl diagnosed with bipolar disorder on her first hospitalization, did not like that diagnosis and did not think it applied to her "because I have reasons why I get upset." This rationale suggests that she did not understand the clinical sense of the diagnosis. She disagreed with the diagnosis of bipolar "because I'm not." She felt that neither bipolar nor any other diagnosis would be useful, that her issue was "just emotional problems," and that the only thing she needed was to "just be by myself." By the time of her second interview Alicia had undergone a significant transformation, reflected in a radically new way of talking about diagnosis (figure 12). She now understood the diagnosis as describing the "reason why I am here." She agreed with the diagnosis of bipolar, saying that she was not ashamed of it and that "I'm not trying to deny anything." She also found it useful in the sense that "I'm a little bit more aware of how they treat people with disorders." She was engaged with the discourse to the degree that she "looked up some bipolar stuff" and became determined to "do something about it."

Alicia's situation is worth pursuing a bit further, not only because of the dramatic transformation of her attitude toward diagnosis, but also because it shows the kind of resources available to her and because it is a rich example of how the discourse of diagnosis can be deployed in a family's process of defining the problem. Alicia's mother was herself a social worker who reported that she and her two sisters as well as her son were all diagnosed with bipolar disorder. This mother's own explanation was biological and genetic, while her sisters rejected the diagnosis and argued instead that the adolescent was possessed by evil spirits or was the victim of witchcraft. They had a Native American ceremony performed to "pull out the evil spirits," during which the patient was covered in sheep's fat and ashes. In her first interview Alicia rejected not only the psychiatric diagnosis of bipolar disorder but also the indigenous diagnosis of spirit possession, saying that her problems were purely emotional (not medical) and would get better if she was left alone. As we have seen, in a subsequent interview she endorsed the bipolar diagnosis. In the interview it was clear that this transformation was based on the acceptance she experienced at the hospital in being able to talk openly about her experience, on her overcoming being

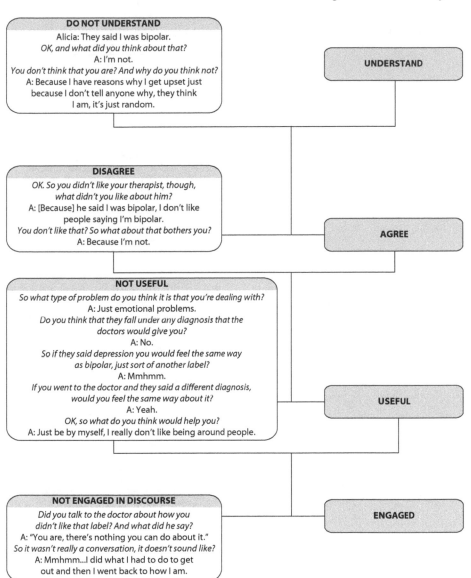

DO NOT UNDERSTAND

Alicia: They said I was bipolar.
OK, and what did you think about that?
A: I'm not.
You don't think that you are? And why do you think not?
A: Because I have reasons why I get upset just
because I don't tell anyone why, they think
I am, it's just random.

UNDERSTAND

DISAGREE

*OK. So you didn't like your therapist, though,
what didn't you like about him?*
A: [Because] he said I was bipolar, I don't like
people saying I'm bipolar.
You don't like that? So what about that bothers you?
A: Because I'm not.

AGREE

NOT USEFUL

So what type of problem do you think it is that you're dealing with?
A: Just emotional problems.
*Do you think that they fall under any diagnosis that the
doctors would give you?*
A: No.
*So if they said depression you would feel the same way
as bipolar, just sort of another label?*
A: Mmhmm.
*If you went to the doctor and they said a different diagnosis,
would you feel the same way about it?*
A: Yeah.
OK, so what do you think would help you?
A: Just be by myself, I really don't like being around people.

USEFUL

NOT ENGAGED IN DISCOURSE

*Did you talk to the doctor about how you
didn't like that label? And what did he say?*
A: "You are, there's nothing you can do about it."
So it wasn't really a conversation, it doesn't sound like?
A: Mmhmm...I did what I had to do to get
out and then I went back to how I am.

ENGAGED

FIGURE 11. Negative engagement with discourse of diagnosis at first interview: Alicia.

ashamed of the label because the diagnosis helped her, and on the research she conducted on the disorder on her own initiative.

Doing her own research on bipolar disorder was crucial for this girl not feeling ashamed of her disorder and being able to understand her problem better. This went along with a decrease in perceived stigma and

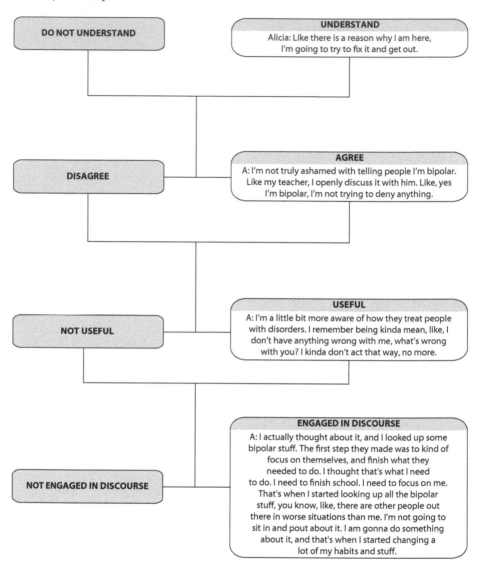

DO NOT UNDERSTAND

UNDERSTAND
Alicia: Like there is a reason why I am here,
I'm going to try to fix it and get out.

DISAGREE

AGREE
A: I'm not truly ashamed with telling people I'm bipolar.
Like my teacher, I openly discuss it with him. Like, yes
I'm bipolar, I'm not trying to deny anything.

NOT USEFUL

USEFUL
A: I'm a little bit more aware of how they treat people
with disorders. I remember being kinda mean, like, I
don't have anything wrong with me, what's wrong
with you? I kinda don't act that way, no more.

NOT ENGAGED IN DISCOURSE

ENGAGED IN DISCOURSE
A: I actually thought about it, and I looked up some
bipolar stuff. The first step they made was to kind of
focus on themselves, and finish what they
needed to do. I thought that's what I need
to do. I need to finish school. I need to focus on me.
That's when I started looking up all the bipolar
stuff, you know, like, there are other people out
there in worse situations than me. I'm not going to
sit in and pout about it. I am gonna do something
about it, and that's when I started changing a
lot of my habits and stuff.

FIGURE 12. Positive engagement with discourse of diagnosis at second interview: Alicia.

surprise about how supportive people were when she told them of her condition. During her third interview she continued to agree with the diagnosis of bipolar disorder, saying multiple times that "I am bipolar" and commenting with respect to a recent emotional event that "I relapsed." She said she had identified the signs for when she was starting to get depressed or manic and would let her family and friends know what was happening. According to her, the main problem that remained was learning to control her feelings and moods. Her mother acknowledged having already thought at the time of our first interview that Alicia had bipolar disorder, mainly based on their family history. She said that her daughter's active denial that she is bipolar had made treatment harder, and that because of the disorder she could not really control her anger or prevent herself from getting upset. In a follow-up interview she appeared not to have been updated on her daughter's shift to accepting the bipolar diagnosis. Perhaps the two did not talk about this topic specifically, or perhaps the adolescent was trying to please the interviewer by engaging in the discourse of diagnosis.

Discursive Operators

Having outlined the structure of the discourse of diagnosis and given a number of examples, we want to address how it is possible for this discourse to be deployed and circulated in everyday life for these youth and their families. At the most general level, this is a question of how diagnostic terms function as *discursive operators* in people's talk about their problems. This is a phrase that requires some elaboration of the sense in which we are using it. The concept of discursive operator is most often associated with the literary critic Roland Barthes in his analysis of how historians write, and in particular how history is constituted as a genre. He argues that historical discourse is founded in a "referential illusion" in which "the historian claims to let the referent speak for itself" (Barthes 1986 [1967]: 132); the referents are "existents" and "occurrents" understood as "beings, entities, and their predicates" (133). Historical discourse is actually an "*imaginary* elaboration" (138) of these supposedly real referents internal to language itself, such that "fact never has any but a linguistic existence (as the term of discourse), yet everything happens as if this linguistic discourse were merely a pure and simple 'copy' of *another* existence, situated in an extra-structural field, the 'real'" (138). The discourse is an imaginary elaboration because "the 'real' is never anything but an unformulated signified, sheltered behind the apparent omnipotence of the referent" (139). In this sense the referent is a discursive operator allowing narrative structure to become "both sign and proof of reality" (141). Recognizing and refraining from operation has the consequential outcome that "the sign of History is henceforth not so much *the real* as *the intelligible*" (141). If we accept that diagnostic terms function as discursive operators, and we equate Barthes's "real" with our understanding of "lived experience," we disagree that this experience can be discounted as merely an "unformulated signified." This is because, unlike Barthes, we are not dealing with a scholarly discourse in the form of historical texts, but of a spoken, intersubjective discourse that is articulated *within* lived experience.

A step toward moving the idea of discursive operators from the domain of text to that of lived experience has been taken from the standpoint of sociology by Jean-Michel Berthelot (1995), who has identified the "body" as a complex referent that functions explicitly as a discursive operator. In this formulation the intelligible does not completely efface the real, but there is the possibility of a relationship between the semantic and the pragmatic within the discursive function. Thus, "what is essential is not the nature of the body considered as language but the meaning (semantic) and the efficacy (pragmatic) of the statements that are made through it" (1995: 19). The meaning and efficacy that Berthelot refers to have to be understood as exerting a rhetorical influence on lived experience, not merely performing the function of signifying the unformulated into an "as if" reality. Here there is a conceptual slippage between the term "body" and the lived body, each acting as an instrument rather than an object. In fact, the role of body as a discursive operator is to guarantee the integration of polarities "between objectivism and subjectivism, structures and actors, functions and meanings" (1995: 20). We suggest that diagnostic terms work as discursive operators in a way similar to how Berthelot sees the term "body" working, insofar as

> a knowledge discourse capable of generating precise objects can arise in a meaning situation characterized by the insertion of the referent in question in one or more given practical discourses. . . . More precisely, the referent—here, the body—no longer functions as an object of knowledge, but, via its linguistic sign, as an instrument for constructing a discourse. It is this role that we suggest could be designated by the term discursive operator and which we analyze as the manifestation and the effect of a given discursive regime. (1995: 21–22)

The role as discursive operator that Berthelot sees for the term "body" is precisely the role we suggest is played by each diagnostic term in the "practical discourse" of diagnosis among our young patients, their parents, and mental health professionals. In our case the discursive regime is that established by the nosology of biomedical psychiatry, and each diagnostic term is "an instrument for constructing a discourse." In this analysis, the shift from understanding the diagnostic term as designating an object of knowledge (a diagnostic entity) to recognizing it as an instrument for constructing a discourse (of diagnosis) dissolves the boundary between language and experience, or between the intelligible and the real, hence making possible our attempt to understand this aspect of the experience of troubled young people.

Adapting the term "discursive operator" from these authors required us to reinterpret a concept that exists primarily within the textually inscribed discourses of academic history and sociology. A move toward being able to recognize a discourse enacted and performed in the life-world is present in James Boon's (1972) anthropological elaboration of the notion "cultural operator." In this view, culture is a form of discourse only a step removed from the academic discourse we have just discussed, and the examples Boon deploys of an opera (*La Traviata*) and a form of drama (Javanese *ludruk*) can readily be understood as being within textual discursive traditions. For Boon, culture "pertains to operations which render complex human phenomena communicable. Any set of human phenomena . . . can be *described*, although not necessarily exhaustively, as a juncture of analytically separable orders of elements" (1972: 227), and "a cultural operator can be defined as a succinct and orderly conjunction of elements from what appears to the analyzer, to the actors, or to both, as diverse orders" (230). Referring to Boas's comments on the tricks that memory may play in generating what we now call life history data, he writes that "with a concept like 'cultural operators' in mind, rather than placing hopes in 'reliable factual data,' one welcomes any such 'tricks that memory plays' as clues to differential ways in which significant items from ongoing experiences are selected and ordered in retrospect" (238). This retrospective selection and ordering may reinstate the distinction between real and intelligible. "Yet, whether repeated, contraried, or subversively 'forgotten,' the conjunction remains an ordering principle behind the universe-of-concerns, an operator which steers the recognition, the surprise, the discomfort, the joy, the dismay of those affected, at least temporarily" (240).

The manner in which the diagnostic term as discursive operator serves as an "orderly conjunction of elements" that steers immediate experience is precisely why we have brought to bear this notion derived from structuralist and post-structuralist thinking in an account that emphasizes the lived experience of troubled youth and how people make sense of their problems. From a theoretical standpoint, this analysis describes exactly what we have already seen in the way the term "bipolar disorder" worked in Alicia's discourse of diagnosis. The relevant ethnographic question is not what the correct diagnosis is but the way diagnosis plays a role in how people conduct their lives and negotiate their lived experience. The diagnostic term as discursive operator is not just a recursive feature of discourse circulating within a hermetic field of textuality, but a conjunction of elements of experience circulating through the lifeworld in spoken form. Entrained by the rhetorical operation of terms identifying disorders, the discourse of diagnosis becomes embedded in the lived experience of those who come under its sway and ramifies through their subjectivity as both a tool for sense-making and a form of clinical authoritativeness.

This conclusion advances our discussion in chapter 2 about the relation of language and experience, and the role of narrative intersubjectivity. It returns to the problem created by the post-structuralist unmooring of discourse from the real, rendering the intelligible world as analogous to the text and being-in-the-world as experientially unstable or even inaccessible to the human sciences.[2] But if the discursive operator interrelates cultural orders while linking language and experience, what cultural orders are interrelated by the diagnostic term in the case of the youth who participated in our research? Foremost are the clinical tradition articulated in formal nosologies, the discourse of diagnosis itself, and the lifeworld in which people discuss their problems, struggle over their meaning, and strive to overcome them. The interrelation among these orders is relevant at two levels. First is the relation between the formal nosology and the discourse of diagnosis as we have described it. The key contrast here is between the diagnostic term as a *definitive label* that enacts an authoritative clinical rhetoric of reality and identity ("I am bipolar," "She has PTSD") and the term as a *discursive operator* that enacts a circulating cultural rhetoric of intelligibility and indeterminacy ("They threw the diagnosis at me," "That describes me pretty well"). The second level is the relation between the discourse of diagnosis itself and the lifeworld into the fabric of which that discourse is woven through everyday thought, talk, and action. Regardless of whether the discourse of diagnosis is relevant in any discreet moment of experience or social interaction, it is most certainly sedimented into the lifeworld of this cohort of troubled youth in varying degrees as a relatively perduring element of subjectivity. This is the subjectivity that can be inferred, for example, from the difference between a young person who articulates no diagnosis and another who endorses one; between someone who carries a single diagnosis and one with a repertoire of multiple diagnoses; and between a person who has multiple diagnoses all at once and one who accumulates them over time or whose diagnosis is repeatedly revised.

Within this form of discourse, utterance of the diagnostic term has the consequential result of establishing a claim to the real. Yet the very indeterminacy and complexity of the modes of "defining the problem" we have described in this chapter make it clear that defining the relation between the real and the intelligible is indeed a problem. In the terms we have laid out in this section, we can understand a diagnostic category in its function of operator as analogous to Barthes's literary referent, Berthelot's sociological body, and Boon's anthropological site of conjunction among cultural orders. The critical point is that an ethnography of the kind we are presenting reinserts the intelligible into the lifeworld, phenomenologically as real as it gets. Identification of diagnostic terms as discursive operators allows us to recognize the relation between language and experience as perceptually concrete yet indeterminate, because if language constitutes the sinews of human existence, experience constitutes its flesh.

CHAPTER 4

Angry Boy, Angry Girl

Anger is the single most prominent emotional phenomenon in the lived experience of these troubled youth. It is specifically cited by twenty-seven (or 57.4%) of our interlocutors as a major experiential theme and an explicit problem. Because of this prominence, anger plays a pivotal role in our account, indeed warranting its own chapter. Moreover, anger stands out because it crosscuts the categories of diagnoses and life experience we introduced in chapter 3, simultaneously understandable as a symptom of mental illness and an emotional response to the frustrations of illness, a condition that must be contained and an expectable reaction to extraordinary conditions of family instability or social precarity. Finally, anger is a human phenomenon subject to cultural variation in expression and experience, and hence how it appears is of anthropological import for a situated understanding of the struggle for well-being.

We can consolidate the latter point by beginning with two widely known anthropological instances of anger in cultural context. The first is Jean Briggs's (1970) book *Never in Anger,* which claims that, from a very early age, the Inuit are instilled with an aversion not only to expressing anger but also to experiencing it. This is quite understandable in a small-scale society of requisite intimacy, where slamming the (metaphorical) igloo door and stalking off into a frigid Arctic night is conducive neither to cultural nor to personal survival. The second is Renato Rosaldo's (2003) "Grief and a Headhunter's Rage," in which, following his own experience of bereavement, the anthropologist comes to empathetically grasp how among the Ilongot bereavement incites a rage that can be appropriately assuaged only by violently taking the head of another person. Both are accounts of unfamiliar yet eminently intelligible instances of the meaning of anger in highly particularized cultural contexts. The moral valence of anger in the Inuit case is generally that it is wrong, negatively sanctioned at least in the sense that it is socially dangerous. The moral valence of anger in the Ilongot case is that in certain circumstances it is not only right, but entails an obligation to act in a certain way.

The anger that we outline in this chapter is radically different and poses a different kind of challenge to ethnographic understanding. This is because among our interlocutors, biographical coherence, personal identity, consistency of social environment, and stability of life trajectory are urgently at stake in a manner virtually inconceivable among the Inuit or Ilongot. Anger is not only an unstable category in the face of interpretation, but a destabilizing force in the social milieu of such persons. Anger, like conditions of mental illness, requires interpretation along a continuum rather than in terms of dichotomous categories (such as "normal" and "abnormal"). The continuous relation between emotion and mental disorder in cultural context can be seen, for example, in anger or hostility among Mexican and Anglo-American families living with schizophrenia, or in "engaged depression" and somatic experience of heat (*calor*) among Salvadoran women refugees (Jenkins 2015a). While this approach does not discount the value of diagnostic interpretation from a clinical standpoint, it takes a step backward to problematize the distinction between normal and abnormal by situating emotion, in the present case anger, in the lifeworld and lived experience of these youth and their families.

Hence, our focus is on the following question: What is the meaning of anger in the lived experience of the adolescent psychiatric inpatients with whom we have been working? By invoking the concept of meaning, we emphasize that we are concerned as deeply with how anger is interpreted by youth and their families as we are with its social production, consequences, and prognostic implications. By invoking the concept of lived experience, we emphasize the immediacy of anger in everyday life as those who are afflicted recount it. We address this question by presenting concrete accounts of the experience of anger and its place in the configuration of family relationships. From this standpoint, and given the amount of space available to us, we want to introduce you to one angry boy and one angry girl, first summarizing their circumstances and then allowing them to speak for themselves. Our presentation will trace the young people's perspectives as they were expressed at three points across the slightly more than one year during which we followed them. We will conclude with some general comments on understanding anger as a moral emotion.

AN ANGRY BOY

We met Michael when he was fourteen years old and in ninth grade at his local public high school, and he participated in the research over a sixteen-month period. He was a large-statured, eccentric, and eager-to-please young man who saw himself as good at drawing and enjoyed reading "chapter books," since he read at about a twelfth-grade level. He was interested in looking at the stars, thought he might want to work with NASA when he grows up, and liked to walk dogs and ride bikes. His mother reported that Michael had been in special education after he began failing in middle school. She noted that he had trouble with peer relationships, and that he did not get along well with his younger siblings, though in general he got along well with adults. He had a girlfriend for three months at the beginning of the study, but they broke up. However, at the time of our final interview, he had gotten a new girlfriend just the day before. Michael lived in a low-income neighborhood outside Albuquerque with his mother, who was receiving unemployment assistance through a housing subsidy, two younger sisters (ages nine and ten), and a brother (age seven). All the siblings have different biological fathers. During part of the study, Michael lived with his maternal grandmother in a well-kept, quiet part of Albuquerque so he could attend an alternative school, and possibly also to get away from a neighborhood bully who, Michael's mother said, is psychotic.

Michael indicated that things had started to "get tough" for him at about age ten or eleven. He said, "It was just my anger, my doctor says I have a lot of PTSD," and "The only reason for my anger is I need to distract myself." Some of his aggressive repertoire appeared to have developed to serve a protective role within the family and for himself, in the context of being the eldest sibling in a household with serial and unstable male adult presence. However, his anger clearly had become amplified to a maladaptive level of impulsivity and aggression. He also reported being molested in a foster home sometime in the last several years. He seemed aware of his own stresses and responses to stress and to be more cognizant than many of his peers of what it was he needed to do.

Michael had received outpatient psychiatric treatment since he was five years old and in kindergarten, diagnosed at the time with ADHD, for which he was prescribed medication. Since that time, he had six inpatient hospitalizations for episodes of explosive anger and was diagnosed with ODD and PTSD. These diagnoses were confirmed with the KID-SCID, though our project psychiatrist suggested the relevance of ruling out features of Asperger's, a specific learning disability, and intermittent explosive disorder (IED). With additional information from Michael's mother he was inclined to add bipolar II disorder (hypomanic), as a possibility. At the beginning of his participation in the study Michael was taking 700–1,000 mg of Seroquel, which our project psychiatrist noted was a particularly high dose for a boy who did not appear to exhibit psychotic symptoms, and had also at some point been on Risperdal. He reported feeling less angry while taking medication but did not like the side effects, especially a dramatic weight gain that he would eventually lose as he hit a growth spurt. He also said he would have anger outbursts every day if it weren't for the Seroquel. His mother, on the other hand, took a more critical view. Constant changes to his medications likely contributed to her negative stance toward professional psychiatry, even though she noticed positive changes in his behavior.

The hospitalization during which we encountered Michael was his sixth since age ten and occurred in the wake of a physical fight with his sister for what Michael himself described as "dumb reasons." Michael's mother called the police, who offered either to arrest him or take him for psychiatric hospitalization, and she chose the latter. During the sixteen months that our research team followed him, Michael had another explosive episode during which, according to his mother, he threatened to kill both her and himself. His mother called the police, and he was readmitted for a three-week hospitalization followed by placement in treatment foster care for a six-month period. These arrangements were also presented to Michael as an alternative to going to jail. Asked what he thought of his hospitalization, he said he was there for his "anger, mostly my anger, I have big, erratic blow-ups. I go from flat-line to straight up." He had been in counseling before this, but his mother reported that it did not work because Michael was not fully participating in it. After this hospitalization and subsequent treatment foster care, he continued outpatient therapy. At that time, it appeared that Michael began to be more engaged with his counseling, partly from a growing awareness of the legal repercussions of his actions.

Michael's biological father has been very peripherally involved, and the extreme tension between him and Michael's mother has been a source of provocation for Michael, who would like to be in closer contact with him. Following their separation, Michael's mother had a series of live-in male partners. One of these men, the biological father of Michael's younger brother, lived with the family from 1998 to 2005. Michael recalled that "for seven years, I thought I loved him as my father." Michael was unwavering in his conviction that his problems started with the "trauma" inflicted upon him and his sisters by their stepfather. The main focus of his interviews was the physical, sexual, emotional, and verbal abuse committed by this man against everyone in the family except the youngest, who was his own son. What is clear is that he emotionally and verbally abused Michael's mother and, on a few occasions, physically abused her as well. It was crushing to Michael to have his sisters divulge that for a period of approximately four years (from when he was nine until he was twelve or thirteen), his stepfather had sexually abused them while their mother worked long and late shifts. Moreover, his stepfather was a severe disciplinarian who beat Michael and possibly sexually abused him as well. He handcuffed Michael to his bed to allow for opportunities to abuse his sisters without his interference. Michael reported struggling with the handcuffs, breaking some of the bars on his bed frame, which led the stepfather to cuff him to one of the thicker and sturdier bars instead.

Their mother began to notice something was awry when she would come home and the children would act out against her, which she later attributed to them not being able to take out their own aggression against the stepfather because it would not be safe. When his older sister finally told him about the abuse, Michael threatened to tell their mother himself if she did not do so, refusing to keep such a terrible secret. In the wake of that telling, Michael's mother got a restraining order against the stepfather, who was later arrested and held in custody pending a trial that happened during the course of the study and particularly preoccupied Michael at the time we met him. During the criminal trial we were able to catch glimpses of how the stepfather continued to negatively affect the family. Michael said,

> And I told mom if he ever comes near [my sisters], she's gonna have to call the cops to come restrain me, because—because I will beat him up so bad. And mom says, my mom says, don't do that, just call the cops. . . . I'm glad that he's going to jail but if he doesn't get put to jail time he might come after us, then I'll settle it . . . and maybe it takes fighting to solve a problem, but

Gandhi used to solve problems without violence . . . sometimes it does take violence to solve a problem.

In the end, the stepfather was convicted, sentenced to nine years in jail, and incarcerated.

In his initial ethnographic interview, Michael reflected on the ambiguity of his diagnostic status and its relation to his current situation:

> It's been the anger all the time. They don't know what's wrong, they haven't—they said I have a little bit of that, a little bit of this. They haven't properly diagnosed me yet. I have been trying every ADHD drug known today, and they still can't quite figure out what I am. They say I have a little bit of PTSD. They say that I have a little bit of everything. [PTSD makes sense because of] the stress that's gotten me like this. Stress from the [court] case, because I'm gonna have to get up on that stand and so [are my sisters], and they're only nine and ten. I'm not gonna be even in the same room while they're doing theirs. When they come out, when I'm up on the stand, that's when I think I'll crack.

In this passage Michael evidently associates PTSD with the stress he experiences in the immediate moment, without reference to his lifelong problems or even to the past trauma inflicted by his stepfather, though he appears to understand that potential re-traumatization is what leads responsible adults to fear that he could "crack" on the witness stand.

In her first interview, Michael's mother also expressed an opinion on his diagnostic status, and on what may truly be wrong with him:

> I think there's more than, more than just the PTSD goin' on. I seriously would like a brain scan. I would like to see if there is any abnormalities. He's never had a brain scan. I would love to see if there was any abnormalities in his brain, 'cause I think there is. I seriously think that there is an abnormal in his brain that is causing all this. Because you can't just shut that part of your brain off. I've tried to do things that were against right and wrong, and against common sense, and I can't. It's hard for me. It's like I have to force myself to try to do it, so why is that part of his brain shuttin' off. He has, he has no, you know, it's just—I would love to see a scan of his brain though.

Michael's mother invokes an ethical argument for favoring what in her view is a distinction between a neurological problem of brain abnormality and an emotional problem of stress. The actions against right and wrong to which she refers are evidently those committed by Michael in his anger, and since, in her view, no one with a normal brain would do such things—she says that she has tried to do unethical things and can't make herself do them—there must be something physically wrong. It does not appear particularly relevant to her whether the abnormality might be genetic, congenital, or traumatic in origin.

This narrative raises questions about the relations among *empathy, morality, mental illness,* and the *brain.* While neither parents nor teens often discussed their problems in relation to the brain (chapter 3), when such interpretations were mentioned it was in terms of everyday discourse derived in part from media representations of the brain as the primary site of mental illness and violence. Whereas in the past, problems of mental illness or violent behavior would typically be talked about in relation to experience—often familial, and sometimes in a psychodynamic vein—Michael's mother expressed frustration with what she perceived as clinical "misdiagnoses, left and right," saying that the doctors had overlooked what, in her strong view, was the obvious need "to take a look at his brain." She did not empathically interpret her son's lapses in "common sense" and his capacity for "knowing right from wrong" in light of his physical beatings and psychological abuse at the hands of one of her former live-in boyfriends, nor did she consider her son's anger within a psychological context of preoccupation and fear that the assailant might soon be released from prison. While neuroscientists might agree that dysregulation of certain areas of the brain could affect emotion and behavior, popular understandings of such processes are not rooted in research-based knowledge. Parallel to cultural notions of a mental illness as a "chemical imbalance" (Jenkins 2015a), notions of the brain are remarkably imprecise, making them ideal symbolic matter for the "work of culture" (Obeyesekere 1990), particularly with respect to both self-making (Martin 2010) and other-making.

By the time of his second interview, Michael was able to reflect on how the hospital experience had helped him: "They kept giving me feedback every single day, like when every time I tried to get a level, they said 'no,' but they liked that I kept trying and trying and trying, you know, stopping. Because most of all, you know, I was getting angry, taking things too seriously. [That is,] explode when they might be talking to somebody else." In this remark he was referring to an incident in which he could not get someone's attention because they were in another conversation, and "taking things too seriously" was an element of self-critique in recognizing his explosive response as disproportionate. It is evident that Michael was engaged and trying to control his anger, specifically in a way defined by the inpatient context in which lapses were measured by failure to attain a higher "level" in a behavioral evaluation system linked to when and whether one could be discharged.

At the time of her final interview, Michael's mother reflected on the relative efficacy of inpatient hospitalization and treatment foster care, qualifying her judgment that the latter is more efficacious with recognition that he may not have had sufficient time in the hospital:

[Hospital was less effective] because they only had him in there six months. They only do up to six months. I think that in kids with multitudes [of problems] like Michael, you can't just do six months and be done with it. It's one of those things where that's their rule. They can't do the treatment in six months, then, and that's fine. And I understand. They have some kids in there that go longer, depending. At any time, I can take him back if those issues ever arise. He doesn't threaten to hit me. He doesn't threaten to kill me. He gets angry, and he yells. But he doesn't hit. So to me, it's half of one, a dozen of the other, um, but I think hospitals are not . . . I don't know. Maybe that's why so many people *don't* get better. [They could do more, like] giving people medication and keeping parents informed, because I don't think parents are informed enough. And we're not doctors. We're not clinical people. We don't know the drugs, you know. We didn't go to school for that, we're relying on you guys to help us figure out what we need to do, and to inform us, and I don't think doctors are taking that time. They don't have the human skill part of it, you know? Like back in the olden days, they'd make house calls, and they would keep their patients informed. And now it's gotten more clinical where they don't take the time to, to put that human part into it.

While she is ostensibly comparing inpatient and treatment foster care settings with respect to length of care, she also includes the home setting precisely because Michael's anger does not entail violence, in the absence of which having him at home is no better or worse for his improvement than having him away in treatment. In her view this is especially the case insofar as hospital treatment lacks a human touch. Finally, she commented on his recent behavior:

I can say some of it's the medication. But really, it's Michael. He doesn't want to change. Michael is hell bent on doing what you don't want him to do. I mean he made it to a point of doing it. I mean, he still does it. He *knows* that he's not supposed to do something, and he'll still do it anyways. 'Cause he doesn't think.

Here she is returning to her ethical argument of more than a year earlier, but without invoking brain abnormality and instead invoking personal motivation to change. It is unclear whether this is a contradiction or an evolution of her earlier stance based on everyday interaction since Michael's return home.

As for Michael, at his third and last interview the effects of the trauma endured and remained intimately connected with his anger. We asked whether he felt as though he had acquired enough tools in treatment to calm himself down, and his response was as follows:

> Not enough. It's never going to be enough. [What helps most to calm down is] just being with my family, knowing that I'm not the only one who's going through the thing. Because at foster care, I was the only one going through this. They were going through similar stuff, but not like—one of my foster brothers didn't like his mother, and I don't know how you can hate your mother. He doesn't understand that without her going through labor you wouldn't be on this earth. He said his dad made him, but doesn't matter. He came through the mother. [What calms me down is] either me, Mom, [my mother's current boyfriend], or just me using my coping skills. And maybe talking to social workers. Because I may be mad for a couple days, and out with my social worker and therapist that may kinda settle. I consider myself, because my social worker said that I'm, that I, I use the term I'm like a volcano. I hold everything in, and then I blow it out. I stopped holding things in, and my therapist said that I need to kind of find a way to puncture it and let my anger out slowly rather than letting it out in just one big . . . because then that would do some serious damage to my family, and I might be in jail. And that's not where I want to go. . . . [But I've had flashback dreams.] It's not me . . . in it. It's me looking at it. From, like, the perspective of me looking at it [from above while he's beating me]. And there was a period of time where my mom saw broken bars. She never wondered why. She wondered why are so many bars on this bed broken, and I told her, and that's why. And I've never been able to break those bars. I don't know. I was trying, and I just do that.

Michael's metaphor of himself as a volcano evidently played a role in conversations he had with his social worker and therapist in attempting to manage his anger. He is reflective in talking about how being with his family and using coping skills learned in treatment help him control the anger, as well as about damaging his family and going to jail as consequences of not controlling it. He also, however, returns to the trauma of being handcuffed to the bars of a bed frame and having to break them to get free, and to their presence as a sign of trouble that his mother at first did not notice.

In contrast to his mother's views, Michael framed his struggle not so much in terms of pathological abnormality versus motivation to improve as in terms of the particular challenge of letting go versus holding on to his anger:

> It's, my mom wants me to let it go. It's like I'm not letting it go. And then my mom thinks I'm not letting it go. Personally, I'm trying to, but it's kinda more harder than she seems [to think]. I know something has happened to her in the past. I don't want to say. But for me, it's different because it's more physical—I don't know. My sisters were molested, and I was abused. You can't really compare the two. Mine was worse in the abuse, but it hurt their mind. So it hurt me, like, way worse. They didn't get none of that physical trauma that I had. I had [a] high [level] of that. But they have high [levels] of

mental hurt from him . . . that's one thing, that's the main thing that's holding me back, is that I don't want to let go of this thing. Because it's done so much for me in protecting me. Before I used to be skinny and stuff. Then all of a sudden, I got huge. And it's like . . . the fat people get skinnier, but the skinny, skinny people get taller and bigger. That's how I figure. That day may come when I need it, and if I don't have it then, then I'll have to revert to something that I don't like to do—use weapons, because I don't like using weapons in fights. Yeah, my therapist explained to me: "You've been in trauma for a whole life, so we're always in that defense mode, and we won't let go of that one thing." And I've been trying to. But my old social worker at school, I told him about one of the dreams I had. He said, "If you can in the dream, if you're standing over the sink, reach in there and grab that belt, and take it away, and throw it away if you can." And I've been trying that, but it's been unsuccessful. Because in dreams you can do anything you want outside reality. I've been trying to do that, but I can't really, it's like my hand goes through it.

Michael strains to compare the relative damage of physical abuse and sexual abuse as different kinds of harm, to body and mind. He does not understand his sisters' molestation as violent in the same way as the physical violence he experienced, and hence he says he was hurt worse. His main struggle with letting go of his anger is that it protects him and he may need it in the future as an alternative to using weapons. Michael's emotional response to the absence of protection by his mother for himself and his sisters in the face of life-threatening abuse was the creation of a self-system in which anger is readily and reliably available. More tender emotions of fear and trembling, and even grief over how alone in the world he is when it comes to his own protection, are camouflaged by barefaced and dramatic displays of anger. Perhaps discovering he could break the bars of his bed frame revealed a power within himself of which he had been unaware and that he feels the need to preserve. Perhaps he feels that his unexpected growth spurt reinforces the legitimacy of this power by making him more capable of utilizing it. The struggle is evident in the poignant failure of his attempt to follow the social worker's suggestion to intervene in his own dreams to grab the belt used by his stepfather to beat him.

By the end of our study, Michael's mother had a live-in boyfriend who worked full time as a truck driver and who was a relatively stable influence. She gave him credit for having repaired numerous holes Michael had punched in the sheetrock walls of his bedroom, so that one could not tell they were ever damaged. Yet without the capacity for self-control of anger, the social determinant of Michael's life was the revolving door of the hospital, foster home, and family home. Michael fully recognized this yet remained deeply conflicted: angry blowups had cost him his freedom and residential stability, but "letting go" of anger left him empty-handed and undefended. He knew he "needed" the anger as protection against endangerment. Moreover, anger in his case (and in the cases of many other youth in this study), must be understood not only as psychological protection, but also as unyielding moral protest against the structural violence that formed the conditions of his life. To be sure, this position is at once constructive and destructive. It is dangerous yet vital for a sense of the right to life and for solidity of purpose. In this vein, Michael had also done far more than to devise an elaborate self-system of anger. His interests in astronomy and scientific discoveries, along with involvement in romantic relationships, helped to protect an estimable if fraught capacity for development, resilience, and even idealism. That he crafted these under conditions of psychic trauma and adversity is extraordinary. Both he and his mother credited CPC as the best care they received, as invaluable therapeutic support. Yet they and the dedicated clinical staff knew that there is and should be so much more.

AN ANGRY GIRL

Natalie was a friendly teenager, Hispanic in ethnic background, of average height and somewhat higher-than-average weight, with an eyebrow piercing, a lip piercing, and a bar through the top of her ear, as well as a tattoo on her wrist. Comfortable in sweats and a hoodie sweatshirt with black sneakers, or jeans and t-shirt, she was sixteen years old and a rising high school junior when she joined the project, and she participated over a thirteen-month period. She was in a home-based Christian school program, and explained that this was a result of being "kicked out [of public school] for learning my student's rights." Apparently, this involved lodging a grievance against one of her teachers by going over the head of the principal to the superintendent. Natalie described persistent difficulty with the public school system, including problems getting along with teachers and feeling there were some teachers who picked on students and treated them unfairly, and having herself been a bully in elementary school. Natalie reported that she began having difficulties as a child and had been in and out of counseling for many years. While she was not sure of the exact age at which she started counseling, she said that she was "pretty young." She reported that her mother told her she used to get really angry and bang her head against walls and against concrete when she was young. She then laughed and said, "That's why I have a big forehead."

She was not expansive in discussing issues like medication and mental illness but seemed generally thoughtful and inquisitive. During the Achenbach Youth Self-Report questionnaires, Natalie said that she would prefer to have the questions read aloud to her, as she had some difficulty understanding big words. She asked for clarification on several items, including needing to know the meanings of "inattentive," "self-conscious," "timid," and "stubborn." She mostly answered questions with little commentary, though she occasionally expanded on her thoughts. She had great difficulty generating things that were good about herself and was only able to say that she liked her eyes. When asked about friendships, she said she was going to try to go out less with her friends because this got her into trouble, and that she did not really like getting close to people. She also said that while she knows she is loved, at times it did not feel that way to her and it was hard for her to believe this.

Natalie lived with her mother, twenty-year-old brother, and fourteen-year-old sister in a town of about fourteen thousand people in northern New Mexico. Their neighborhood of public housing, locally known as "the projects," reputedly has several crack houses, a methamphetamine lab, and what Natalie's mother referred to as a whorehouse nearby. The entry to their house was dark and the house a bit warm, with only one swamp cooler languidly running. It was very tidy and neatly organized, yet everything was worn and felt dirty. The carpets were old and stained. The furniture was shabby and jumbled, the couch covered in a pink fleece blanket, and the kitchen table covered in an old plastic table cloth. A shelf near the kitchen was lined with lava lamps and crosses.

Natalie and her two siblings all have different fathers, and there had never been a consistent father figure in Natalie's life. Her mother appeared not to have had many boyfriends since having left the gang life after discovering she was pregnant with her eldest child. Natalie had no contact with her biological father, who lived in the same town but reportedly denied paternity on the grounds that "I don't make whores and bitches" and who had threatened to kill the mother and all her children "if that bitch is mine." The child services agency had partial custody of Natalie in order to provide her mother with transportation to visit her in the hospital, since she expressed significant anxiety about driving. The agency representative had observed sufficient fighting in the home to determine that her mother was abusive and neglectful, and the mother herself reported that they had wanted to take her younger daughter away when they took Natalie to CPC.

Her mother was obese, with health problems including anxiety, depression, and high blood pressure. She was a heavy smoker and was without most of her teeth due to previous cocaine use during her gang period. The mother and daughter were close to the point of emotional enmeshment, considering one another as best friends, and acting simultaneously like siblings, playmates, friends, mother/daughter, and daughter/mother. Natalie was exceedingly concerned with the state of her mother's health. At the same time, her mother claimed that her own health was impaired by Natalie's explosive anger, insofar as she could not "physically take her shit" but could not get away from Natalie because of her own physical problems. She expressed resentment that Natalie received more benefits than the other members of the home, pointing out that her room was painted pink even though they weren't allowed to paint the interior of their government-owned house, and that Natalie had a tattoo (which no one else in the family had), piercings, and a cell phone. Her mother also disapproved of Natalie's marijuana smoking and complained that she acted "like a volcano" when she was high, imitating a stoned Natalie by contorting her face and putting a water bottle in front of her face to mimic the proximity of Natalie's face to hers during these times. She continued by imitating Natalie's crude and provocative language: "What the fuck are you lookin' at? What's your fucking problem?" She concluded that she was afraid someone would be killed in the house. In fact, Natalie appeared to be the healthiest member of her family, with the burden of attending to the others' needs, since her brother was labeled psychotic and her sister autistic, and the family income consisted entirely of disability payments. Her anger in this context seemed to be more healthy than dysfunctional, except that she was violent. She got "upset and explosive" when communication with family members was strained. Natalie's mother said that she tried to get away and go to her room but that Natalie would follow her and kick down the door and "keep getting in my face."

Natalie listed her diagnoses as bipolar disorder, IED, and possibly ADHD, and she had been treated for these on an outpatient basis. She described bipolar as "crazy" and "weird," while with IED "I'm just like a walking volcano. I could be happy one minute and then, like, I'm just a different person. And I basically black out. Practically anything [can get me mad]." She also indicated significant anxiety about eating in front of others, though she said her second-best friend after her mother was "food" because she loved to eat. Her mother attributed her problems to associating with the wrong friends, whom she referred to as violent, but also indicated that Natalie's problems may have been with her from birth. Natalie said that she had been in a car accident with friends a year prior to her interviews, reporting that since then "I can't do a lot of things that I was able to do." Her therapist at CPC reported that she had a mood disorder and ODD. Her research diagnoses by the KID-SCID included recurrent major depressive disorder in partial remission, PTSD in partial remission, ADHD, brief psychotic disorder, separation anxiety disorder, alcohol abuse, and cocaine dependence in sustained full remission. Medications she was taking included Concerta and Seroquel, along with calcium for bone density and Depo-Provera for severe menstrual pain, and she had previous experience with Lamictal and Lexapro.

The hospitalization during which we encountered Natalie was her fourth since age twelve. Natalie reported that just prior to being admitted she was having difficulty with her brother and that her "meds hadn't been adjusted." At one point she stabbed his hand with a pen, commenting that sometimes she "acts without stopping to think." She reported that the worst she had felt in the past year was just prior to her admission, saying that she would "get mad and explode at people." The incident that led to her admission was a severe fight with her brother, during which he admitted he "beat the shit out of her," hitting her harder than ever before and burning her with a cigarette as she fell on the floor and hit her head on the refrigerator. He then called the police. After some discussion about her injuries and her safety, an ambulance took her to an emergency room and from there to the psychiatric hospital in Albuquerque. When we first interviewed her in the hospital she described her situation as follows:

> Well, I was basically holding in most of my anger, 'cause I thought that my mom wouldn't be able to, you know, be willing to talk to me about it, I was holding it in and I was going out with my friends a lot, well, not, you know, like that [i.e., sexually] but [laughs]. But I'd stay out with them for like a long time. And my mom would call me and be like, "You know, you gotta start coming home," and I'd be like, "OK," and I wouldn't go back. And every time I'd go back to my house, I'd feel like, angry, 'cause I didn't want to be there. It's part of the teenager stage but it was like, weird. . . . [What's helpful here at CPC is] me learning how to use coping skills. 'Cause, you know, I think I'm ready to go back home too, and it's just, I gotta learn how to use 'em. And it's been working a lot. . . . I'm excited [about going home] but then in a way, I don't really want to leave here, 'cause I got so attached to it, you know? Because it's going to be a lot different: I'm going to have

more responsibilities out there than in here, but I think I can deal with it. You know, I actually came this time to get myself help 'cause other times I go, you know, like when I went to H Center I was like, "Yeah, you know, blah, blah, whatever, I'm not going to get help." So I was there basically for five months for not doing my treatment goals, and over here it's only been a month and I'll be here like a month and eleven or something days and I'm leaving 'cause I'll have done a lot better.

Particularly compelling in this reflection is Natalie's comment that "it's part of the teenager stage but it was like, weird." As we saw in chapter 3, there is a tendency among some parents and youth to normalize what is in fact an extraordinary condition by appealing to typical adolescent behavior (albeit exaggerated), but in this instance the young person also conveys the sense that her behavior and situation were not just exaggerated, but weird. She expresses attachment to the hospital environment as well as some apprehension and ambivalence about returning home, where she will be faced with responsibilities. She compares her positive and efficacious engagement in treatment with a previous hospitalization in another facility where she resisted help. Also of note is her engagement in the therapeutic discourse and putting "coping skills" into play. As we will see in chapter 5, our interlocutors exhibited a wide range of attitudes toward coping skills and their value, and virtually all of them had been exposed to the concept at some point in their patient trajectory.

At her second interview, no longer an inpatient, Natalie was reflective about the effectiveness of her hospital treatment and her worries about her family:

I was more, I was more . . . very controllable about myself when I got out. Because when I was up there the most thing that I'd worry about every day— this would also keep me from helping to learn some coping skills—I got worried about my mom. She's not in very good condition. I'd be up there, you know, every night praying because she's all I have. Her and my brother and my sister. My grandma's not worth a shit. I'm sorry, but she's not. She's a total "B" [laughs]. So, you know, if something would happen to my mom, my brother and sister are all I have. So, you know, that's what would worry me the most up there. That's why I'd mainly want to come home, but I liked it up there. I kinda didn't want to leave. I'm getting attached to everyone over there. . . . [Now I'm not in treatment], I'm doing my own therapy. I'm being my own therapist.

Natalie's mother, who was present and participating in her interviews at home, indicated having been hurt by her attachment to the hospital environment, reporting that when Natalie said she would miss it and wished she could stay longer, "that really broke my heart. I was like,

'Do you want me to have a taxi turn around and take you back or what?'" Now, however, she was pleased that although Natalie was acting as her own therapist,

> she talks to me too. Yeah, she has a problem, and to me, they're little problems, but to her, they're these humongous things. And we worked together at 'em, you know. I tell her if we can't work together at 'em, then let's talk to somebody together. And I tell her, you know, I've been there, I've gone through that feeling before, and this is what I did, or this is what stupid thing I did, and I tell her the truth.

Natalie was consistent in taking medications but considered them secondary to her own efforts to control her anger and serve as her own therapist:

> They [medications] help out a little. But it's mostly, I am trying to, like, you know, control my anger and stuff. Because it's not only medication that's going to help you. You also need to help yourself at the other stuff too. I've learned that the hard way. . . . When I started getting really bad and stuff, and then I start getting sent to treatment. And I mean treatment, they're not helping you. You gotta help yourself. They don't help you. You know what I mean? They can't change your life and all this and that. . . . Lately I've noticed that it's been a lot better that I am, you know, really don't even have to use coping skills. No, I just, like, blow it off. But it still is kind of hard just letting things go. Still really hard. Trying not to punch people when I'm mad. That's the hardest part, but when I look at it, I am like, "Why do I want to hurt them?" If I'm the one that's pissed off, and I'm the one that's cranky. And they're just sitting here innocent, and I'm here. . . . I'd yell at my mom for no reason. I'd wake up in the mornings, and I used to be real bad.

Despite learning how to help herself, Natalie still finds it "hard just letting things go," but she also has developed a self-reflective questioning of why she would want to hurt others with her anger "for no reason."

Her final interview showed Natalie continuing to control her anger and deploy her coping skills. She said,

> I had my little moments, but I've learned how to, I have learned pretty much to control them since I was up there in CPC and sometimes I use my coping skills, sometimes I don't. Like taking time out and just going to my room and just stay in there. Smoke a cigarette or something. Listening to music, something mellow, not something that's going to rile me up. That wouldn't be pretty.

She also more strongly endorsed the value of medication, saying, "I don't really know why, but it's like, if I don't take them, if I accidentally skip a day or something, my mood just like, totally changes. [I start] getting more angry. Aggravated and more like, urrrrr. . . ." Also, at the final interview, her mother noted that the levels of Natalie's medications had been changed because she had been getting "cranky," though the new dosing appeared to exacerbate obsessive-compulsive behavior. "She is more calm, you know, but still, when she starts getting busy with doing things, she doesn't want to stop, she just keeps on going. And then she says, 'I swear, if I find anything on the carpet I'm gonna be fucking pissed.' And I'm like, there is always gonna be something on the carpet. Always."

Natalie's relationship to her mother recalls the kind of relationship described by Garcia (2010) elsewhere in northern New Mexico that is so close and enmeshed as to include sharing and passing on heroin addiction as a means of mother-daughter bonding. In this instance a balance of intimacy, alienation, autonomy, and care within a family in which each individual had limitations that contributed to a precarious domestic environment created the conditions of dysfunctional anger. Her story during the course of treatment is one of struggle over learning to control her anger. The hospital was a positive environment for Natalie: she referred to it as a "vacation from home" that was a place of respite from the volatile and chaotic family milieu and the stress of her mother's health problems. She claimed it helped her learn coping skills to control her anger, which, following discharge, she wanted do without the assistance of therapy, though she continued to take medications. At the end of her participation in the project Natalie's mother continued to be ill, now having been diagnosed with fibromyalgia and being in chronic pain, with Natalie helping on a daily basis. Natalie had graduated high school through a home study program, was volunteering at a veterinary clinic, and was planning to attend community college to become a mechanic.

ANGRY SITUATIONS

Having looked closely at the circumstances and experiences of one boy and one girl, our next task is to descriptively characterize the range of anger experience across all the participating youth. Psychologists have attempted to identify categories of anger among adolescent males within school settings (Furlong and Smith 1998) and specific factors contributing to anger-provoking incidents among male and female adolescents in inpatient settings (Swaffer and Hollin 1997). For our study cohort, in a fundamental sense we are dealing not just with angry youth but with angry situations in which anger is simultaneously a feature of embodied disorders and lived experience. Accordingly, we must address the question of what kind of problem anger is for these youth. It is not necessarily an illness or a symptom of illness, though it can be cited as the reason for being hospitalized. Thus, we have heard that a youth was hospitalized "for my anger issues" or because of "depression, anxiety, and anger." We heard similar statements from guardians/parents as well. In only one instance did a young person express enjoyment of hurting others, and in the case of Michael we saw that anger was explicitly a strength and mode of self-protection. The attribution of anger to personality was not particularly pronounced even when it was acknowledged that the youth had been angry since they were little. Several said explicitly that they were "not an angry person" by nature, though the occasional metaphorical self-description of being like a volcano or an animal suggests the role of anger as an identity-defining feature. In some cases, anger seemed to be a permanent state and in others it was expected to be temporary; "coping skills" could be used either to control anger or to eliminate it. Medication could be understood as intended to manage either an illness or the anger, and the effect of going off medication was recognized as increasing susceptibility to anger.

Only a case-by-case analysis could completely account for the multiple dimensions of diversity among the situations of anger we encountered. With respect to who they were angry at, it could be parents and/or siblings, teachers and/or peers at school, staff and/or peers in the hospital—but it was almost never at themselves. Any of these people might be experienced as the cause of anger, or they could be simply the target of anger. As for why the youth were angry, there might be a specific cause or none that could be identified, and the youth might become angry about "little things" or about "everything"—though, as we will discuss below, there is virtually always a moral/ethical component to anger, insofar as some real or perceived injustice can be cited in any particular instance. Variation is also evident in the intensity of anger, and how angry a young person becomes can range between full-blown rage and seething irritability; but it was noteworthy that the word "hate" was mentioned only twice across all our interviews, and one of those was an expression of self-hatred. Anger is sometimes expressed by violence; some may direct that violence only against others while some may direct it only against objects, and self-harm is seldom explicitly described as associated with anger toward oneself. Finally, there is variation in temporality, in three respects. First, anger could erupt spontaneously or emerge in a way that a parent, for example, could see it coming in their child's eyes or face. Second, there was considerable variation in how often episodes of anger occurred and how long they lasted, and increases or decreases along this temporal dimension were sometimes cited as concrete evidence of exacerbation or improvement of anger. Third, in some instances parents observed the onset of angry or aggressive behavior at a young age, and in other cases anger emerged at a later age, when the child seemed to depart from a more or less normal mode of behavior and begin a decline that was more or less rapid.

Across these dimensions of variation, there is a distinct vocabulary of anger that we have extracted from the discourse of our interlocutors and their families. We are not concerned so much with differences between terms used by the youth and their parents, or across ethnic groups and diagnostic categories, or across specific instances of anger. What is of more interest is the lexicon presented in box 1 as evidence for the existence of a culturally patterned discourse of anger characterized by the regular recurrence of specific terms. Most striking is the set of recurrent terms used to describe events of anger, all of which emphasize their intensity. The vocabulary also indicates particular attention to the onset of these events, insofar as they are clearly rupturing the emotional fabric of everyday life. Not to be downplayed is the constellation of emotions associated with these events that go well beyond simple reference to being angry or mad and include recognition by youth and their parents that the events can be extremely complex emotionally. Moreover, the events are behaviorally as well as emotionally complex, including a repertoire of actions that are both expressive and violent. What we describe as phases of anger include a variety of temporal modulations and modulations of intensity within the events. Finally, we recorded several descriptions of the events that are explicitly metaphorical, including the most common one comparing the angry youth to a volcano in eruption.

Across the range of angry situations in which these youth come to be embroiled, to what degree are they articulate about what they are doing and what is happening to them? Are there modes of expressivity through which they convey a sense of their own anger as lived experience? In fact, we have identified two such modes: narration and self-observation. The first includes accounts of angry events and situations, while the second includes reflections on the kind of person she/he is and the nature of his/her anger. One of the clearest cases of a youth who offered both narration and self-observation was Neal, a fifteen-year-old boy of mixed Hispanic, German, Irish, and Navajo ethnicity whose diagnostic picture from the KID-SCID included Asperger's syndrome and recurrent major

Box 1 Vocabulary of Anger

Events of anger: blowup/blowout (10), outburst (8), episode (6), fit (5), tantrum (4), meltdown (3), rage (2), rant, tirade, explosion, freak-out attack, state

Onset of events: be triggered (4), get set off, flip off/out (2), freak out, lose it, snap, go ballistic, go off the wall, go over the edge, go up in flames,* come unglued,* get out of control, get out of hand, get tweaky, act outlandish, act out of proportion

Emotions accompanying the events: angry, mad, defiant, upset, out of sorts, cranky, violent, agitated, stubborn, frustrated, stressed, pissed off, hate, depressed, anxious, sad

Actions within events: threaten, sneer, grimace, yell, scream, hit, hurt, punch, throw, kick, beat the shit out of, be physical, be aggressive

Phases of anger: black out (2),** building up, letting out, carrying anger,*** triggering, holding in, letting go, walking away, getting control, coping

Metaphors of anger: like a walking volcano (3), like an animal, beet red

Note: Numbers in parentheses following a term indicate how many respondents used that term; the other terms were each used by one respondent.
* One father's idea of a "type A personality"
** No subsequent memory of what one did
*** Grammatically analogous to "bearing a grudge"

depression/dysthymia (we have met Neal in chapter 2 pp.59–62 and chapter 3 pp. 105–06). The following is his narration of an angry situation /event that occurred in one of the treatment facilities he had been in:

> I got arrested at [a treatment facility] for destruction of property, assault with a deadly weapon, which was a really large cable the size of a baseball bat, and disorderly conduct. I got two fire extinguishers—the first one I used in the hall and sprayed the whole unit down with it so they had to pull the fire alarm, because it was like nobody could breathe. And then I poured cooking oil and broke the window, and took the shards and put them all over the floor with cooking oil. That way, it will be slippery and cutty. And then I just started trashing the kitchen there. Just trashing it, tearing everything apart. Ahm . . . tried to hang myself to get them to come in. They came in and they were slipping all over the place and we were wrestling in the glass. And a lot of them got cut up. Most of them had really severe lung problems after that, they call it some sort of a "dustemonia" or some shit, something I mean. And it was just a really bad experience. The cop restrained me, I was covered in all kinds of cooking oil, and cuts all over me, from the glass. The cops arrested me, they came in with armed Tasers. Because I was dangerous, you know. I was. And they were ready to Tase me in a second. You know the Taser gun, when it

shoots out a little needle, like, zzzzzzz, you know, has a wire attached to it. Yeah, they had that pointed at me the whole time while they were coughing and talking to me, they had Tasers pointed at me. [It happened because] staff were blaming me for getting a guy fired. I was held down in the middle of the room, I was trying to bite one of the staff, while I was in a restraint. He punched me in the face and said try to bite me again. So that's what happened to that [guy because I] reported it. You know? So the staff were all pissed off at me because I got him fired. But he got his own ass fired for punching me in the face and if he didn't punch me in the face, they wouldn't have fired him. You know? So that was a really bad experience, but . . . I guess I'm getting better treatment here [at another treatment facility].

Perhaps most notable about this narration is its matter-of-factness, a relatively cool account of creating chaos that could have been either a calculated and orchestrated episode of vengeance or a highly rageful and inflamed event of acting out. Neal repeats that it was a "really bad experience," and that a police officer had to restrain him because "I was dangerous."

Elaborated self-description and observation rather than narration appear in the following account compiled from parts of two other interviews. Recall from chapter 2 that Neal's father had undergone a sex change operation and his parents were living together as lesbian females, a situation contributing to difficulties with peers at school who were aware of it and also contributing to domestic tension, on which Neal is commenting at the beginning of these self-observations:

[The home situation is deteriorating because of] the fact that I cause so much trouble in school and at home. I pick fights with my parents and I instigate fights with other people at school. I don't even realize that most of the time. I'm just stubborn, so if somebody says you got to do this and I'm in a bad mood and I'm saying, "You know what, I'm doing it in my way, you can go screw yourself if you don't want it that way," is basically what I say with my actions, I don't say it with my words, and that's only if I'm having a bad—if I woke up on the wrong side of the bed. . . . I ran away from a group home that I was at and so they put me back in CPC and CPC put me here. I was getting very unsafe at the group home, tearing a lot of things apart, getting all tweaky, I mean like one of the medications I was on was tweaking with my head. And since I've gotten off of it, um, I haven't been as tweaky, [feeling] the need to tear everything apart, literally, I would tear everything apart, but since then I haven't done anything like that. I was running away and stealing from cars. I got caught out of the house several times. I got caught doing a bunch of stupid stuff. . . . [Now for anger and depression] I'm using coping skills such as deep breathing, arts and crafts, 'cause I love art and reading and writing, those are the things that I use. And when it gets really bad I punch walls or punch out windows. When I get overwhelmingly angry and nothing else works I need to hit something now and let my adrenaline flow. There is no one thing [that makes me angry], it's just the way people go about it, or the way they say it, or the way they do it, anything meant to antagonize me or my family, especially my family. I'm having an argument with you, don't bring my family into it, that's just degrading and makes me think they're lower than dirt and they have no reason to not get their asses beat. [People say] I have two moms, they bring that up a lot. I wish I hadn't shared it with one person and then he went, turned around and betrayed me and told everybody in the fucking unit [here at the hospital. I'm tired] about the fact that I have two moms, tired of it. It's depressing simply because I can't share anything with anybody without them judging me because of my parents. [It's been that way for] years. . . . They [doctors and therapists] say my main problem would be anger and depression and impulsivity. Three main problems. I'm very impulsive. I do things without thinking, or sometimes I think them through and just do it regardless.

Here we see a significantly different expressive mode, more reflective and also more vulnerable and intimate. Neal identifies his behavior and also the fact that he's often not aware of it in the moment. He labels a certain type of violence associated with medication while in a group home as "tweaky," a term often associated with methamphetamine use. He includes among his coping skills punching holes in the wall, though for most therapists that would be recognized as needing the application of a coping skill rather than itself being one. He acknowledges the primacy of his family situation as a provocation to his anger, and identifies impulsivity as a key trait, even explicitly associating it with his Asperger's condition.

The ability to narrate and self-observe is not to be taken for granted, given a tendency among professionals and laypeople alike to presume the inarticulateness both of teenagers and of those afflicted with serious mental illness. As we have already observed repeatedly, at stake is the possibility of having a life—biographical coherence and experience. This is not to say that there is no experience if it cannot be expressed or narrativized, as for example has been argued by Desjarlais (1997) among homeless, often psychotic, mentally ill people. There are certainly instances in which self-observation is present but at a minimal level of elaboration. For example, Alex was a thirteen-year-old Hispanic boy with a complex diagnostic picture including psychosis, whose core self-observation was differentiation of what he called "full anger" and "full-full anger." These were forms of very "powerful anger" that he sometimes referred to as happening by provocation and other times said that he "used." Alex claimed to know how to control his full anger but not his full-full anger, saying "I get super angry, and I used to can't control it in the past, now I know how to control it. I lower it little by little.

When I get mad at my real dad then I punch him." At first Alex said that he had a secret for controlling full anger, then that he used "coping skills" like taking a walk or thinking about his family. He had recurrent dreams in which he used his full anger to kill his real father, a dream that he expected to become real, because the father had tried to kill him when he was a baby. For Alex, "full anger" was a condensed symbol of emotion that was intense, problematic, requiring control, and implicitly valuable in allowing him to extract revenge and kill his father.

HOLES IN THE WALL

At the conclusion of our work at CPC, we made a presentation to the clinical staff summarizing what we had accomplished. We capped our discussion with a statement about how striking the theme of anger was and asked for their comments. The very first was "There is a lot to be angry about in today's world, um, so maybe it is a healthy sign." This comment offers a clue to understanding anger as a moral emotion, but the clinicians had more insights to offer as well. One invoked the distinction between internalized anger that is episodic in its expression and externalized anger that is temperamental and chronic, observing that the younger children tend to exhibit the more episodic form, while by adolescence anger tends to settle into a more habitual pattern. The younger children, including those below our cutoff age of twelve, are "almost like raw nerves when it comes to anger, irrespective of the diagnoses they have." Another clinician distinguished between the emotion of anger and its expression, observing that "for many of our [especially younger] patients it is lack of internal controls . . . coping skills, or the ability to put it together what's going on, it manifests as anger . . . and they act on the dictates of their impulses." In other circumstances the expression of anger is instrumental, political, performative, or manipulative, "like in juvenile detention you will have patients who will display rage-like behaviors but often they are actually enjoying putting on the entire show," perhaps to intimidate or frighten a target individual.

Clinicians thought that in the home environment, anger is "a kind of a function of the family communication," a behavioral style as much as an emotion, learned from a family member for whom it is "the only way they can express themselves and how they get their needs met." Perhaps "within the family everyone gets angry and that's just how they get things done," or it is "the standard way of managing conflict or of managing any sort of situation," such that it becomes the family "language" or the "common currency that the economy of the family is played out in." Anger can thus be, all at once, "a style of illness, a way of life, a way of thinking" that is passed on through families as well as gangs, and may be produced and reproduced under conditions of structural violence. According to some clinicians, this is distinct from bipolar, psychotic, or normal anger in that it involves a "hostile posture like you have been cheated, that life has been completely unfair to you and the only way you can try to redress matters is at least implicitly through violence, toughness, you know, the perpetual badass type." Some may become angry seeking pleasure or reinforcement, others because their expectation that a desire will be met is frustrated. There may be a sense of insult, injury, or injustice that leads to a retaliatory anger. "Some kids learn that other people will do what they want when they get really angry," or that they can storm off to their room and no one will bother them because they are in a rage. As these clinicians talked, it became clear that anger is an umbrella category that includes variations and subtypes, and indeed, as one remarked, "it is almost like anger is too broad of a term, like Eskimos with snow."

These clinicians were talking from the standpoint of their experience with psychiatric inpatients, but in a sense they were in the process of generating a comprehensive theory of anger, relevant to what they considered normal as well as pathological anger. With this in mind, let us consider the possible phenomenological variations[1] in emotional tone of a domestic environment qualified by chronic, episodic, and violent anger, where by "qualified" we mean endowed with a certain quality or valence. If we adopt the metaphor of emotional lightness and heaviness, the first variant is the household where the constant expression of anger, or the persistent possibility for expression of anger, creates a milieu that is heavy, intense, harsh, and on edge. The second variant is that in which, between episodes of disruptive anger, the environment returns to a relative lightness, stability, equilibrium, and perhaps even harmony tinged with sweetness. In the periods of relative calm, family members become vulnerable in a repeated and cyclical way, ever again hurt by the outbreak of violent rage. Contributing to this situation is the frequent tendency of the young person, within a day or even within an hour, to "act like nothing had happened." The presumption of a return to normalcy and the desperation of family members for some degree of equilibrium can be quite compelling. This must certainly have a temporal component that further qualifies the domestic emotional tone, insofar as angry outbursts are "like an everyday occurrence" in some cases, while in others the outbursts may occur every other week. There is no reason to conclude, however, that increasing frequency

necessarily results in the consistently heavy and harsh type of environment, since it is possible for family members to cycle between violence
and vulnerability on relatively short periodicities.

Both types of environment could exhibit tendencies toward normalizing anger or taking it for granted. Crossing a threshold between irritability and anger marks the onset of a crisis that continues through to its
resolution or to a breaking point constituted by a call for intervention by
police or the health care system. In some families a parent can "see it in
her face" or sense the growing inner turmoil of a child, and in other cases
it appears to "come out of the blue." In some families both parents and
children can pinpoint triggering events and reasons, either profoundly
consequential or relatively trivial, while other families report expressions
of anger over "the smallest thing" or "for no reason at all." Normalization is most evident and problematic when people say that the anger is
typical adolescent behavior or "growing pains," while not being certain
of where the boundary of such allegedly typical behavior lies. Such normalizing statements appear to be less an attempt to excuse than to
account for the behavior. Acknowledging that violent rage is "mixed"
with typical behavior may only serve to enhance tolerance while exacerbating frustration and confusion, even in the rare instance where a young
person has the insight to characterize their own behavior as like that of
other kids, only carried to an extreme. What is at issue in each case is the
threshold of this extreme. Perhaps there are two thresholds: the surpassing of one defines emotional damage, and the surpassing of the other
defines a breaking point that demands outside intervention. Although it
may seem contradictory, at first, to describe circumstances characterized
by sudden ruptures in terms of thresholds, it is most accurate to say that
the experience of damage or the resort to intervention occurs in surpassing a threshold of tolerance and endurance that may fluctuate from time
to time, from mood to mood, with the severity of affliction, with the
persons involved, and with what is at stake. In fact this is no surprise, in
that even parents with children who are not severely distressed occasionally find themselves declaring "That's the last straw" in exasperation,
only to be surprised at how many straws actually remain.

ANGER AS A MORAL EMOTION

The interpretive problem of underpinning a discussion such as this with
the distinction between normal and pathological is that they are typically
understood as mutually exclusive categories rather than as defining the

poles of a continuum (cf. Jenkins 2015a). Even if it is granted that there is a continuum between everyday anger and anger that requires treatment, is there a threshold that ultimately keeps them apart? The answer could be yes, but with the caveat that the need for treatment in no way delegitimizes the extreme or disturbed form of anger as human experience, or as an instance of emotion as a fundamental human process. This leads us back to our juxtaposition in chapter 3 of psychiatric diagnostic categories and categories of problematic life experience, which are not mutually exclusive. Anger is illustrative of how this is the case, as it belongs equally to both series of categories and, in fact, is a kind of phenomenological pivot between them. Anger is simultaneously a symptom in the domain of mental health and an emotion in the domain of life experience, and in the latter it is precisely a moral emotion (Rosaldo 1984; Lutz 1988). This dual interpretive framework allows us to avoid the convenient fiction of intelligibility that is interpolated into the lifeworld by diagnostic categories of "oppositional defiant disorder" and "intermittent explosive disorder." These categories provide labels for but not accounts of anger and by no means explain it—except in the spurious way that presumes that if something can be called a disorder it is understood as situated in conditions of mental illness that are divorced from spheres of the moral or the cultural. As outlined above, when it comes to mental illness, while we fully recognize the personal pain and anguish involved, such conditions cannot be conceptualized solely in terms of individual pathology. Given this line of thinking, the domains of both emotion and mental illness are properly understood as both cultural and moral. We are arguing not only that the anger of these youth is sometimes extreme and sometimes quotidian (and in practical terms this distinction may be culturally and clinically critical), but that aspects of symptom and emotion are mutually implicated and closely intertwined in constituting anger as a prominent aspect of their experience.

The notion of moral emotions has a history that includes debate about whether they really exist, which we will not address here. In contemporary cultural psychology and psychological anthropology, they are very much in evidence (Martin 2018). Haidt (2003) observes a general shift in morality research since the 1980s away from a nearly exclusive focus on moral reasoning and toward inclusion of moral emotions, along with a broadening of the domain of moral emotions itself. He identifies four families of moral emotions: the other-condemning, including anger, contempt, and disgust; the self-conscious, including shame, guilt, embarrassment, and pride; the other-suffering, including sympathy and compassion; and the other-praising, including gratitude, awe, and elevation. Haidt describes anger as an underappreciated moral emotion, sometimes treated more as a destructive and immoral emotion. He invokes Aristotle's understanding of anger as an honorable impulse to revenge for an unjustified insult to oneself or others, and cites studies that analyze descriptions of angry episodes to show that themes of frustration, blocked goals, and unpleasantness were thoroughly mixed with concerns about betrayal, insult, unfairness, and immorality. Depending on the circumstances and actors, the element of revenge in anger can be aimed at either violent or nonviolent redress of injustice.

Sorting out the symptomatic and moral threads in the immediate experience of anger can only be done against the background of several levels of cultural patterning. At the level of broad cultural values, for example, Menon and Shweder (1994) observe that when Anglo-American college students are asked which among the three emotions of shame, happiness, and anger is most different from the other two, they say either happiness, because it is pleasant while the other two emotions are unpleasant; or shame, because it is a diminishment of the self while the other two emotions, each in its own way, render the self expansive and full. Oriya people in India, comparing the linguistic equivalents of the same emotion words, say that anger is most different because it is destructive of social relationships and everything of value, while shame and happiness are the glue of social relationships. Our interpretation of anger among troubled adolescents must take into account the cultural presupposition that anger is about the self before it is about social relationships, but even more concretely it must attend to the situational relevance of specific values and expectations regarding affects such as pleasure, expansiveness, and relatedness.

At the level of interpersonal practice, White's (1990) work on Santa Isabel in the Solomon Islands demonstrates how emotion talk can be an idiom for asserting moral claims indirectly. Santa Isabel is a small, face-to-face community in which talk of anger in close or asymmetrical relations or in public is disapproved as potentially disruptive, while at the same time suppressed anger is regarded as socially dangerous. White describes the social practice of "disentangling" tense social situations by publicly "talking out" bad feelings in a way that reframes them and discursively transforms anger into either sadness or shame. Disentangling works insofar as these emotions can be applied to the same situation, but whereas anger implicitly leads to retribution, sadness implicitly appeals for repair of social relations. Working in such an ethnographic setting, one can construe

> emotions as sociocultural *institutions* that depend on both the cultural model and the interactive situation for their meaning and effect. . . . By recognizing that emotions are not simply expressed in social situations, but are in fact constituted by the types of activities and relations in which they are enacted, ethnographic attention may be given to the institutionalized discourse practices that shape emotional meaning and experience. (1990: 78)

While the language of institutions adds a social dimension to the more psychological understanding of emotions, and can perhaps be usefully generalized to comparative settings, one wonders: could White have arrived at this position if the interactive situation he studied was the emotionally insular North American household, defined by a relatively rigid boundary between public and private spheres, where young people were not initiated into a culturally instituted means of "disentangling" snarls in sociality but to an ad hoc, clinically inculcated, and after-the-fact repertoire of "coping skills"?

In Santa Isabel, revealing hidden feelings to defuse their destructive potential takes the form of narrative reporting and reconstruction of problematic incidents rather than cathartic release of feelings. This observation leads to yet another level of cultural patterning, that of the linguistic forms presupposed in the discussion and expression of anger. These have been exhaustively described for American English by Lakoff and Kovecses (1987). They argue that the combination of the metaphor "the body is a container for emotions" and the metaphor "anger is heat" results in a central metaphor that determines how anger is expressed and, by extension, experienced: "anger is the heat of a fluid in a container" (1987: 198). Thus, by extension and with relevance for our work in the American cultural setting, "In the central metaphor, the danger of loss of control is understood as the danger of explosion" (201). Lakoff and Kovecses elaborate a broad repertoire of additional anger metaphors, but of particular relevance is their observation that our cultural models of anger and insanity overlap in their mutual inclusion of agitation, leading to the metaphor "anger is insanity" and our use of the word "mad" as a synonym of "angry" (204). For these authors the fact that an insane person cannot function normally and is dangerous to others suggests the same of an angry person, but for our purposes we can observe that the metaphor also offers itself to literal interpretation, such that someone who is really mad really is mad. Finally, it is noteworthy that the "prototype scenario" of anger in American culture is essentially moral, constituted by an offending event that provokes anger followed by an attempt to control it and a failure of that attempt, and completed by an act of retribution upon the wrongdoer (211). In this cultural system, it would appear that anger, insanity, and morality are mutually implicated in a way that must be consequential for experience and its interpretation.

To understand anger as a moral emotion in a situation characterized by psychic distress requires a further step toward taking into account the needs and rights faced within an institutional structure, the evaluation of interpersonal relations, and the expressive repertoire of affect. Anger is moral insofar as it is a response to offense, harm, violence, injustice, insult, damage, cruelty, or abuse. As was the case with many of our interlocutors, the two young people we have discussed in detail in this chapter had specific issues or events about which to be angry. In such a situation, "extreme" anger might consist simply of an incapacity to handle the depth of an anger that is quite appropriate. Anger beyond propriety is not a homogeneous category, however, but can exhibit a range of phenomenological modulations. Thus, it can occur with unusual frequency or intensity, can be directed at inappropriate targets or situations, and can take the form of an almost permanent disposition. Even when disproportionate anger is provoked by the seemingly trivial, however, it does not entirely lose its moral character. Consider the list of reasons for being angry given by Hayley and her parents as presented in box 2. Hayley was a thirteen-year-old Euro-American girl who had experienced long-standing domestic insecurity and instability and whose KID-SCID diagnostic picture included ADHD, major and minor depressive abuse, fleeting and remitted cannabis abuse, adjustment disorder, depression, tension, anxiety, and ODD. Our documentation of reasons for anger would be of little interest if it were relevant only as the discourse of entitlement deployed by a "typical teenager," and of marginally more interest insofar as the degree of her rage transcended what could normally be expected in such a situation. What is more interesting, and central to our argument, is that even here the discourse takes the form of moral justification—that is, anger was a response to a perceived injustice or injury. By assertion and tone of voice, it was evident that the girl's statements made a moral claim, while her parents' utterances of the same form attempted to establish the unreasonableness of their daughter's actions. It is also the case that both this adolescent and her parents were perhaps atypically inclined to formulate and express

Box 2 Micro-moral Reasoning—Hayley, Female, Age Thirteen

Hayley

At home I became angry because

my friends were fighting

my parents were fighting

I was angry at everything (so I took pills on impulse)

my mom was not giving me a chance

my parents put me in residential treatment

they put me in without discussing it with me first

I had a boyfriend but my mom messed it up

In the hospital I became angry because

they only gave me four pieces of tape to hang my drawings

they made me participate in games with other kids (the games were fun but it pissed me off)

they don't give me enough drawing paper

they say there's a paper shortage but I saw paper there

they asked me if I wanted to talk about what I was mad about (I don't remember what it was)

they made me go to bed early since I didn't have enough good behavior points

Hayley's Parents

Our daughter became angry because

mom wouldn't take her to the mall

mom has been sick (and couldn't do things she usually would)

we tracked her down when she took off to a friend's house

mom was delivering her medication to the hospital (for no reason)

we refused to let her get eighteen ear-piercings

it's just a mother-daughter dynamic at this age

reasons for her behavior. Nevertheless, anger retained a moral underpinning within the tissue of interpersonal relations among family members.

On the other end of the spectrum from interpersonal to structural, we may consider, as the clinicians at CPC did, that there is much to be angry about in contemporary society. In the opening lines of their study of adolescent gangs in Montreal, Perreault and Bibeau (2003) invoke a smoldering and rumbling anger among youth who feel blocked from enjoying the good life. Basic needs for stability, security, and care are not easily met when not only children but parents and caregivers themselves are deprived of them. Schools subject to budget cuts, a mental health care system under the regime of managed care, and a legal system reeling under the burden of methamphetamine and heroin constitute the backdrop for the lives of many of our angry boys and angry girls. The 2010 murder in Albuquerque of a treatment foster care worker in her home by two adolescent girls in her charge, who drove away in the woman's car with her wallet and money, cannot be thought of only as a crime against that woman. It is also an event made possible by the structure of the mental health system and the cultural presuppositions that led the girls to their course of action. Rising anger accompanies increasing disparity, and as inarticulate as it often remains, some proportion of the anger we observe coincides with moral protest on this structural level. To be precise, our assertion is that one can be angry quite explicitly *about* a violent event or relationship, but one can also be angry implicitly *because of* structural violence (Farmer 2004a). This is violence that can undermine the possibility for young people to enjoy their rights to stability, security, warmth, and care. In this sense, structural violence should not be conceived either as the principal cause of anger among these most disturbed of adolescents or as a factor exacerbating their pathological anger, but should be understood as essentially built into, intertwined with, and refractory of an ethos that spans family, school, treatment facility, legal institution, and civic life.

Against the background of global moral protest and micro-moral reasoning articulated in a specific vocabulary of anger, these considerations lead to the recognition that one of the problems with diagnostic categories like oppositional defiant disorder and intermittent explosive disorder is that they define anger as a problem without necessarily taking the further step of examining in detail what the anger is about and how it is experienced. They are of value in requiring us to weigh the qualitative distinctions between justified and arbitrary anger, between measured anger and explosive rage, between extreme anger and anger as one among several symptoms of mental illness, or even between violent anger and impulsive violence that looks like but may not be experienced as anger. In the end, however, these categories direct our attention more to behavior than to experience, and more to illness as a phenomenon for the clinician or observer than as an experience for the person ensconced in a lifeworld. Success in addressing the question we have posed—the meaning of anger in the lived experience of troubled adolescents—has required us not just to ask what they are angry about, but to determine what there is to be angry about, what the anger feels like, what its modes of expression are, and what these modes of expression disclose about the structure and quality of lived experience. We have come a long way from the Inuit and Ilongot, though much more could be said about the angry adolescents in the Land of Enchantment.

CHAPTER 5

The Experience of Psychiatric Treatment

I was in [the hospital] for so long, it was like part of my daily
life. . . . After a while you just, like, the flame in you just dies
out after a while; they tame you.
—Kevin

I don't want to be like, "Oh, RTC [residential treatment
center] would be so good for me," 'cause, yeah, I've gotten
help there, but it didn't like fix me.
—Sherine

When we set out to describe the rubric "experience of psychiatric treatment," what do we mean by this phrase? It is the trajectory of each
person through the treatment system, the cumulative experience that
defines the subjectivity of each troubled youth as someone with a psychiatric disorder or disorders. Our scope is thus broader than a description
of *therapeutic process* in the sense of the interaction between therapist
and patient with its intimate dance of insight, symptom relief, setback,
and transference confined to the session of individual, group, or family
therapy. It is likewise broader than a *clinical ethnography* in which the
boundaries of the hospital circumscribe the interactions among patients
and between patients and staff or clinicians. The object of our interpretation is a narrative and existential trajectory superimposed on a developmental trajectory through adolescence in the context of family dynamics, educational advancement or failure, judicial involvement, and peer
relations. It includes multiple therapists, counselors, psychiatrists, and
foster parents engaged across multiple facilities whose environments the
young people are quite able and willing to compare. The phrase "psychi-

atric treatment" does not mean that all treatment is done by psychiatrists, but that the young people have been admitted to institutions whose purpose is to treat psychiatric disorder, mental illness, emotional disturbance, and behavioral problems. With their lived experience immersed in these extraordinary conditions (Jenkins 2015a), they are inculcated with the habitus (Bourdieu 1990) of psychiatric treatment in such a way that they often come to take the extraordinary as a normative feature of their everyday lives. Yet like the young people quoted in this chapter's epigraph, they are quite capable of judging their treatment as a way that "they tame you" or that "it didn't like fix me."

The treatment facilities in which the patients found themselves constitute an implicit hierarchy with the flagship CPC at the top. Twenty different sites were mentioned by patients and their parents over the course of the study, but there were eight in which the youth most often found themselves. Six of these were in the Albuquerque metropolitan region and two in the southern region of the state. These institutions varied not only along the continuum of care described in chapter 1 but also along the axis between what Hejtmanek (2014, 2016) has characterized as psychiatric custody and therapeutic process, terms that bear overtones of the carceral and the caring, respectively. Indeed, conditions in some of the facilities where we conducted interviews were sufficiently oppressive to be just as much forms of structural violence as are conditions of poverty, gender violence, gang activity, and the severe contraction of services under the regime of "managed care" (see chapter 1 and the book's closing remarks). Yet whether the experience leans toward the carceral or the caring depends not only on the character of the institution but on the different pathways into the hospital, including through the police, the courts, physicians, and families.

In this respect it is useful to contrast our study with the work by Hejtmanek (2014, 2016), which focused on therapeutic procedure, process, and outcome based on an immersive ethnography in a single "total institution" (Goffman 1961) where youth were interned by court mandate for periods of up to several years. Like the youth described by Hejtmanek, our interlocutors were subject to procedures of institutionalization, therapy, medication, and behavioral modification in the form of point and level systems, and like those youth they did not discuss their experiences or conceptualizations of their problems exclusively in terms of psychiatric frameworks. However, a different perspective is afforded when we shift focus from within a single institution to a trajectory among treatment settings, including movement among inpatient facilities, between inpatient and outpatient treatment, and between home and foster care. The very existence of these sometimes complex trajectories is an element of residential instability, and sometimes therapeutic inconsistency, that can potentially affect improvement in mental health as well as overall development. Available beds, determination of immediate need, and insurance coverage are factors that play into determining these trajectories, and indeed the interplay among these factors would be worthy of a separate study in itself. Moreover, being propelled through and navigating these complex trajectories has a formative influence on the subjectivities of these young people, and the evidence for this influence is their ability and willingness to generate comparisons across their experiences with different facilities.

TRAJECTORIES

The trajectory of each young person was distinct, with a beginning that in some cases significantly predated their participation in our study. CPC was the sole inpatient facility for 32 percent of the youth, though a number of them were admitted there more than once. Another 23 percent also had experience in one other inpatient facility either before or after being in CPC, and again sometimes on more than one occasion. However, fully 45 percent of these young people had at some point been in three or more inpatient facilities. In addition, 45 percent had experience of outpatient treatment at some point along their trajectory, 19 percent having begun their treatment trajectory as outpatients, and 17 percent being in outpatient treatment at the end of their participation in the study. A substantial proportion, accounting for 36 percent, had been in treatment foster care (TFC) in the course of their trajectory, 4 percent having had TFC as their first experience and 21 percent being in TFC at the end of their participation in the study. Juvenile detention was a part of the trajectory for 9 percent of the youth.

Given the complexity of their treatment trajectories, we begin with an attempt to catch a glimpse of the youth's experience through circumstances in which they and sometimes their parents drew comparisons among facilities (including juvenile detention) in which they had been inpatients/residents. At the least this indicates that the young people are not indifferent to their surroundings; at best it can convey a sense of what they find worthy of observing and what they find helpful or unhelpful. These comparisons cover a wide range of topics beyond where they felt they received the most effective help, such as which facilities had better food, more pleasant rooms, stricter rules, more structure, better school, more enjoyable activities, a safer environment, meaner staff, tougher peers, nicer friends, or fewer kids. Comparisons were often quite specific, including differences between cottages (e.g., acute and residential) at CPC or between different stays at the same hospital. The young people sometimes noted differences among inpatient and outpatient therapists and/or psychiatrists; among individual, group, and family therapy; between therapists and staff; and even between staff working on different shifts. In the case of two of our older interlocutors, we also heard comparisons of being in the children's facility and on an adult ward.

The same institution often provided a positive experience for some and a negative experience for others, and this sometimes varied for the same individual across different admissions to the same institution. Moreover, given that our protocol was to conduct three interviews at different points in time, a retrospective account could have a different valence than one rendered during or close in time to the hospitalization. For example, one young woman initially complained about CPC because the therapist listened to her parents more than her and the staff was mean, whereas during her second interview she declared it the most effective facility she had ever been in, remarking, "I know I said some pretty horrible things about it when you first interviewed me there." By the time of the third and final interview, she indicated that the group home she was currently in was wonderful and that "it made me one with myself," even though she had hated it when first admitted.

One of the comparisons that might (mistakenly) appear so obvious as to be trivial is the comparison of food. The institutional food was explicitly mentioned by 49 percent of the adolescents, with only two of them liking the food in any facility and one saying it was "not too bad but could have been better." There were several outliers, such as the boy who complained that there was simply not enough food at one hospital compared to another (but who received dietary accommodation for Ramadan as the only Muslim in the study) and the girl who feared her mother was intent on poisoning her and, being depressed about her weight, engaged in binge-purge behavior. Three reported refusing to eat at some point, and three explicitly used the term "gross" to describe hospital food. Three commented that one of the hospitals (the same one for all three) not only had better food but had a menu they could choose from rather than having to eat whatever was served.

Not all these comments can be attributed to the pickiness of teenage dietary habits. From the standpoint of lived experience, food and eating index a fundamental bodily process with an affective component related to emotional security and security of place—in that sense, all food is "comfort food." Hence, we heard that the food "tasted different from Grandma's or the hot dogs I make for myself," and "Hospital food was better than in juvenile detention but not as good as home." There were often combined complaints in which food was one factor among a variety of rules and conditions. For instance, the food was good but the beds uncomfortable; TFC was too strict because you had to ask for food, couldn't have a phone, and couldn't wear a tank top; the beds were uncomfortable and the food was bad except for the chicken nuggets; the rules had changed since a previous admission, to no longer allow bringing in food like cookies baked by the family; a certain level of privilege for good behavior included checking out a radio and ordering fast food once a week; you couldn't touch anyone and could barely talk to them, there was bad food, cold showers, and hard beds; there was a terrible wash [laundry], a terrible vacuum, and terrible food. The most comprehensive among such combined complaints was from one girl who said, "I didn't get the right kind of treatment that I needed, I was around girls twenty-four seven that all they wanted to do was fight and make drama, I had horrible food, the food fattened you so much, the beds were hard, you had to go to bed at eight thirty, um, there's a list."

From the standpoint of health, youth described food with words like "unhealthy," "fattening," "gave me cholesterol," "getting fat," and "everyone gains weight." We heard comments related to health from 19 percent, only one of these complaining that there was too much emphasis on healthy food and low-fat foods. One boy reported that "I was like, 'So you are punishing the healthy kids for the fat kids?' And they were like, 'It has to be healthy.' And I'm like, 'I don't think that I deserve to be punished just because other people don't really want to get off the couch.'" On the other hand, a girl who had an eating disorder, talking about the same facility, said that she liked the nutritional advice that her therapist was giving her, that they had a nutrition/cooking class every week, that she was being accommodated by being given a vegan tray for meals, and that she thought the food was healthier during her second than during her first stay in this hospital. For those youth who complained about weight gain, it is reasonable to presume that the quality of food intersects with the side effects of psychopharmacology, but for them weight gain is more associated with the hospital stay per se than with medication. Only one girl mentioned medication in this context, to reject it as a factor: "I gained so much weight in the hospital. They tried to blow it off, saying that meds make you gain weight. None of my meds ever made me gain weight before. It's the food. It's the food. But now I am back down to my usual. I gained, like, about ten pounds there. Maybe even fifteen. They are gone now."

If we can gain this much insight and identify this much complexity by considering the ostensibly simple issue of food, what do we discern by considering the issue of how these youth perceive treatment efficacy? Parallel to how we took a methodological step back from diagnosis to examine how they defined and understood their "problem" in chapter 3, our strategy here is to examine whether or not they experienced treatment as "helpful." Our guiding concept is *therapeutic process,* where process is distinguished from therapeutic procedure on the one hand and therapeutic outcome on the other (Csordas and Kleinman 1996). Therapeutic procedure is who does what to whom, the organized application of techniques with some goal in mind; therapeutic outcome is the disposition of these youth at a designated end point of treatment. Therapeutic process is our concern because it has to do with the experience of a person during (1) the course of a treatment event, (2) the course of an illness or illness episode under treatment, (3) a sequence of experiential or intrapsychic phenomena unfolding during treatment, (4) the exercise of social control on a patient, and (5) the exercise of ideological control on values in treatment by broader economic and social regulatory constraints on the therapeutic system. An open-ended investigation of how treatment has been helpful taps into the experiential nature of therapeutic process, allows the young people to use their own voices in expressing what counts as helpful, and recognizes that treatment can produce changes that are incremental in nature. With helpfulness as the minimal criterion of how young patients perceive treatment efficacy, we can span the broad range of treatment trajectories among this highly diverse cohort of troubled youth, a continuum ranging from multiple stays in multiple facilities to one stay in a single facility.

At one end of the continuum is Christopher, a fourteen-year-old Anglo-American boy with a history of sexually abusing other youth as well as having been abused himself. He was first hospitalized at age seven for several days that he described as not helpful because "they just found out what was wrong and took me home." At age eight he was hospitalized in another facility, which was helpful because they started him on medication and got his depression and hallucinations under control. The following year, at age nine, he was admitted two separate times to CPC, helpful because it "helped get me back on meds." He then spent a year and a half in a fourth facility, which he found humiliating but where there were some things he says helped him get his thinking straight. A third period at CPC helped him with suicidal thoughts, while experiencing physical restraint gave him the useful message that "I'm going to get put down every time I do that" there and at other treatment facilities, as well as at home. He was admitted to a fifth hospital, where he acknowledged benefiting from treatment by the outpatient psychiatrist who had been seeing him since he was small, who helped him by "talking and getting my meds straight," and whom he admired so much that he aspired to be a psychiatrist himself. Also, at this facility inpatient therapy was "going pretty good" and it was helpful to talk to the therapist, though sometimes he wanted to be alone, especially after incidents of head-banging. By the time he had been there a year and a half, he had come to describe treatment as helpful because

> they focus on your real issues. They don't focus on just one thing. They focus on everything. They look at it in a more broader thing, a broader perspective. They look at the big picture. They have us take a step back, a couple of steps back and take a look at our issues and what we've done and how we're gonna fix it.

Christopher indicated that this treatment had helped him decrease his level of self-harm and helped him realize the value of family. When his period of participation in the study concluded he was moving toward release to TFC, where he anticipated being able to see his family.

At the other end of the continuum is Kayley, a fifteen-year-old Anglo-American girl who had been in outpatient treatment since age four in the aftermath of her parents' divorce but whose admission to CPC was her first and only hospitalization. She said, "I think things I remember most about the hospital are probably the people I met there. And they were like one of the main elements that helped me get through it." She indicated that getting out of her home environment and confronting some issues really helped her get out of the state of mind she was in. While in the hospital she was able to begin the process of "pulling myself together" and take the first step in the "process of working on it." She explicitly stated that her peers in the hospital were not helpful to her treatment because they were either too serious or just seeking attention. Yet seeing some of them improve inspired her, even though seeing their ups and downs was difficult. Her overall claim was that "the person who went into the hospital was very different from who I am now." She remained in outpatient therapy and, on the suggestion of her therapist, had taken up the practice of karate as a kind of therapeutic technique.

What we see most clearly across the otherwise vastly different experiences of Christopher and Kayley is the ability and willingness to identify specific elements of treatment as helpful. Several additional instances will consolidate our sense of how these youth conceive and talk about what counts as help for them. By the end of his participation, fifteen-year-old Kevin said, "I think it helped me because it taught me how to cope with a bunch of things and it taught me how to be around people and how to act around them." It did so by forcing him to deal with being around peers he didn't like. He said his peers became his family, and once he got back home he felt a little strange, but

> I think that I am making such good progress even without therapy. It feels great because I am starting to feel normal . . . I think a lot of the therapy I had over the years is starting to kick in. And therapy has helped me realize that there is a lot more to life than just negatives and I finally appreciate the therapy and everyone that's backing me with everything that I do.

For Kevin, therapy including inpatient treatment had a cumulative and even delayed effect. His description is notable in that it simultaneously invokes making good progress, feeling normal, and realizing there is more to life than just negatives.

Samuel, a seventeen-year-old Hispanic youth who had trouble with alcohol abuse, was critical of the therapy at CPC because he did not feel like he was getting helpful advice to deal with his problems, comparing it unfavorably with a previous facility:

> I think the only problem that I had there was just that the therapy there isn't, like, intense enough, I guess. They don't make you look at your problems enough and the way I looked at it, it was just basically like going to summer camp or something, except without the wilderness. . . . But when I was in [a different facility], we had chemical dependency group for anybody who had any chemical dependency problems. They had groups to talk about stuff in the past, or just like all kinds of stuff for different things. And then I came here and we just have the two groups and they're not very helpful.

We observed above that hospitalized youth are often able and willing to compare different facilities, and in this instance, it appears that the comparison itself was useful for Samuel in formulating what was and was not helpful. As stressful and destabilizing as a trajectory among multiple facilities may be, it thus can have the advantage of affording the development of such a comparative perspective.

Nadine was a seventeen-year-old biracial African-American and Anglo-American among whose problems was a pattern of binge and purge eating. She compared the helpfulness of two admissions to the same hospital. She believed that the first time really helped her because

> giving me insight into my problems helped me realize what's going on with me . . . like they go into a lot of detail and so it just makes me realize a lot more of what I'm going through with my condition and how my behaviors affect me and stuff like that. . . . [The second time] some of the staff has been helpful but one of them hasn't 'cause they were like talking about how they would like binge and purge and just went into their money troubles and just like had really bad boundaries with me so I reported it and my therapist said she'd try and get something done . . . [but this time I've learned] a lot about nutrition and I've learned some more about like bipolar disorder and I've learned some more coping skills. I've learned a whole lot this time around [because] I'm a little more levelheaded and I'm a little more clear in my thought than I was last time and I mean just processing it a little bit better.

Nadine exhibits reflexivity in comparing her two admissions, including both helpful and unhelpful aspects of her hospitalizations. Contrary to the expectation that a second admission is invariably a setback, she suggests a cumulative helpfulness insofar as the first time she gained insight into her problems, while the second time she learned a lot that was helpful in managing those problems. She also clearly states that her clearer mental state allowed her to process treatment better during the second admission.

Neal, a fifteen-year-old part Hispanic boy, was largely dismissive of any hospital treatment:

> No, I think if the treatment helped there wouldn't be kids coming back here every three months going out and coming back in for three months going out and coming back in for two months, you see what I'm saying? . . . No, they're not doing anything, it's more me realizing I have it better at home than here. . . . Treatment doesn't do anything unless you want it to do something. . . . I've had to wake up on my own, I've had to wake up and see the light on my own.

Neal refers implicitly to the revolving-door phenomenon of repeated admissions that he knows is not unique to him. Whatever help he received was of a negative kind, in making him want to be at home rather than in the hospital. Recognizing that engagement in treatment is necessary for treatment to be effective, he rejects that engagement and insists that any improvement has to be achieved through his own autonomous effort to "wake up and see the light."

COPING SKILLS: CONTRASTING PERCEPTIONS

Our goal in the immediately preceding discussion was to show that troubled youth have the capacity to articulate what they find helpful in treatment and to compare that helpfulness across their treatment trajectories. This includes comparisons of different facilities and of different admissions to the same facility. It is also the case that the youth may adopt contrasting stances toward particular themes emergent in hospital experience. Thus, some say that treatment centers are too unlike the outside world and therefore are unable to help, while others experience them as a valuable time-out or vacation from the stresses of family and school. Some find it helpful to be in the company of other youth with similar problems, while others find their peers a bad influence or actually harmful. There are youth who think the hospital has too much structure, others who find the structure itself helpful, and yet others who do not like the structure (including point and level systems for rating behavior) while acknowledging the expectation that the structure will help them. Alongside those who objected that they were in the hospital too long (only a few thought they did not need to be there at all) were those who thought they would have been helped more by being there longer.

Prominent among the recurring themes that elicit contrasting perceptions, feelings, and attitudes is that of whether "coping skills" are helpful or unhelpful within the experience of psychiatric treatment. The term "coping skills" refers to practices and strategies of emotional and behavioral self-regulation that are taught in the therapeutic setting but that one can also independently learn to develop or improvise. These practices and strategies are expected to allow the youth to cope with stressors that antagonize them and exacerbate their problems by providing positive, healthier alternative behaviors. In conceptualizing these choices as skills, a patient is able to view their preferred strategies as subject to improvement with practice, allowing them to set active goals to improve their capability to successfully "cope." As a practice, coping skills are intended to give patients the power of choice, which subsequently should give them increased control over their mental health. A substantial proportion (26%) of our participants reported that they appreciate coping skills and actively employ them in their lives. They reported all-around positive perceptions of the skills, which they said allow them to better handle their stressors, and result in having easier, happier experiences. The most commonly reported coping skills were reading, puzzles, music (most often rap, when specified), walking, talking with friends/family, breathing, and journaling/poetry. Several young people described these skills as hobbies, a defense, a way to achieve a sense of normalcy, or a way to be happy. For some, they offered a method of reflection on one's behavior, enabling them to see when they have done something wrong. Some reported that these skills offer ways to maintain control and/or to calm down one's thoughts and emotions when they are angry or sad, due to internal strife or to exterior stressors such as being mistreated. Others reported thinking of the future and utilizing coping skills to avoid negative consequences such as blowing up at friends/family, returning to the hospital, or harming oneself. They thought of these skills as healthier coping mechanisms than other possible, less healthy responses such as lashing out, cutting, purging, punching walls, or taking drugs. One youth reported believing that these skills will be helpful for their entire life. To some, the power of these skills and their ability to help one cope is amazing, while others reported that these skills are useful but can only go so far to help.

Those who expressed negative perceptions (13%) described these skills as inapplicable, unnecessary, not useful, unhelpful, a hindrance, or said they just don't work. Many felt that doctors use the term "coping skills" excessively and were greatly irritated by this overuse, attaching a negative connotation to the term. One young person felt that these skills are solely for "crazies or whack jobs" and have nothing to do with them. Another had attempted to use coping skills to control anger but felt that these skills are stupid, lame, and embarrassing. While it is not clear that the youth lack coping skills entirely, it appears that they uniformly reject the institutional framework in which they are presented and the repertoire of acceptable coping skills presented to them. It is likely that some of them perceive coping skills as a form of discipline rather than a set of tools.

In three other instances, the young people expressed a mixed perspective. One person spoke about agreement with the usefulness of coping skills but wished to utilize coping mechanisms that are not safe or approved (playing with toy guns). Despite an overall acceptance of coping skills and willingness to adhere to the concept, the desire to cope with inappropriate methods is outside the conceptual framework of what a coping skill should be (i.e., a positive, healthier behavior). Two others connected "coping skills" with the use of medication and felt that while coping skills are useful, medication is also a necessary and useful component of coping. One boy felt that "coping skills can only go so far" and that medication is an important aid for what he is incapable of controlling. Another indicated that he would rather take medication than practice coping skills—if the medicine works, coping skills are not needed.

The varying experiences with and orientations toward coping skills suggest that they often play a significant role in the lives of these youth. Some reported successfully using the conceptual framework of coping to develop personal strategies that improved their ability to manage difficulties with mental health and consequently improve their quality of life. It is not valid with respect to this variable success to say that the illness of some youth allows them to embrace the practice of coping skills while the illness of others predisposes them to reject the entire conceptual framework as relevant to their lives. Temperamental differences quite apart from illness could play a part in why some embrace and others reject formalized techniques and practices. In general, however, talk about coping skills, learning and developing coping skills, awareness of negative coping skills, and rejecting coping skills comprise an integral part of the therapeutic milieu, an essential category in terms of which daily life is conducted in the hospital and which is then carried back home or to other institutions.

TAKING MEDICATIONS: EXPERIENCES AND MEANINGS

Another aspect of psychiatric treatment that elicits contrasting judgments and evaluations is psychopharmacology. The biomedical practice of prescribing psychotropic drugs for persons diagnosed with mental disorder has been commonplace for over half a century, and its ever-increasing frequency for adolescents is well documented and controversial (Thomas et al. 2006; Pescosolido et al. 2007; Behere et al. 2018; Schepis et al. 2019). According to household survey data collected in the United States between 2011 and 2014 by the US Centers for Disease Control and Prevention (Pratt, Brody, and Gu 2017), overall antidepressant use (within the previous month) in the general population increased to 12.7 percent among those aged twelve and over; among those twelve to nineteen years of age the rate was 5 percent. Females of all age groups were more than twice as likely as males to be prescribed antidepressants. Among those seeking health services, rates are far higher. Antipsychotic medications have increasingly been prescribed for adolescents and children; beginning in 2006, Olfson, King, and Schoenbaum (2015) conducted an analysis of patients ages one to twenty-four and found that antipsychotic use increased (from 2006 to 2010) among adolescents and young adults, especially among boys. Within the United

States, there is an acute problem of overuse and misuse of psychotropic medications prescribed to adolescents and children in primary care.

As ethnographically observed and interpreted for adult populations, "taking psychotropic drugs is not merely a routine and pragmatic process of the self" (Jenkins 2015a; see also Jenkins 2015b; Read 2012; Brown and Dennis 2017). "There is marked existential struggle and sociocultural contestation surrounding identity, power, and medication. The decidedly social-relational experience and meaning of medications requires elaboration" (Jenkins 2015a: 25–26). The complexity of issues surrounding the use of these medications is evident in our data for New Mexican adolescents, and here we address only the most basic aspects of that complexity. First is the basic question of how many were taking medications and the types prescribed. Second is their lived experience of taking medications with respect to whether they like the drugs, think that they work or are efficacious, and encounter social stigma for using the drugs.

To start, how many were taking medications and what types of drugs were prescribed? Methodologically, we must note that among persons with extensive histories of use of medical and psychiatric services, which include both inpatient and outpatient facilities, this basic information is challenging to ascertain. This is certainly true for persons whose average age is fourteen, and accordingly the medication histories of patients in our study were often provided by parents. None of these young people were without an extensive history of taking psychotropic medications; many began taking them in kindergarten (around age five). We asked about the full range of time during which the adolescent had been taking medication and also obtained data on medications being taken specifically during the course of our research. As table 6 starkly shows, the mean number of all classes of drugs *ever* taken in their lives to date was just shy of four per person, with atypical antipsychotics most common (80.9%), followed by antidepressants (68.1%). When we investigated which classes of drugs (antipsychotics, antidepressants, anxiolytics, mood stabilizers, and ADHD drugs) that the adolescents were taking *during* the time period of the study (table 7), the numbers changed only slightly, with 74.5 percent currently taking an atypical antipsychotic and 57.4 percent an antidepressant. Psychotropics for mood disorders were common (29.8%), as were those for ADHD (21.3%). There were sex differences (not shown in the table) in the classes of medications, with males more likely to be taking antipsychotics (44.7% vs. 34%) while females were more likely to be taking antidepressants (40.4% vs. 23.4%). As table 7 shows, at the time of our research contact, the mean number of 2.49 medications overall that patients were

TABLE 6 PSYCHOTROPIC MEDICATIONS TAKEN BY ADOLESCENT PARTICIPANTS OVER LIFETIME (N = 47)[a]

Medication by class	n	%
Antipsychotics		
Abilify (aripiprazole)	20	42.5
Clozaril (clozapine)	1	2.1
Geodon (ziprasidone)	5	10.6
Risperdal (risperidone)	14	29.8
Seroquel (quetiapine)	21	44.7
Thorazine (chlorpromazine)	1	2.1
Zyprexa (olanzapine)	8	17.0
Total participants taking one or more drugs in this class	39	83.0
Antidepressants		
Prozac (fluoxetine)	10	21.3
Celexa (citalopram)	1	2.1
Zoloft (sertraline)	14	29.8
Paxil (paroxetine)	3	6.4
Lexapro (escitalopram)	8	17.0
Effexor (venlafaxine)	3	6.4
Cymbalta (duloxetine)	4	8.5
Wellbutrin/Budeprion (bupropion)	10	21.3
Total participants taking one or more drugs in this class	32	68.1
ADHD drugs		
Concerta/Ritalin (methylphenidate)	12	25.5
Catapres/Kapvay (clonidine)	6	12.8
Adderall (amphetamine and dextroamphetamine)	11	23.4
Strattera (atomoxetine)	2	4.3
Dexedrine (D-amphetamine combo)	2	4.3
Total participants taking one or more drugs in this class	21	44.7
Mood stabilizers		
Eskalith/Lithobid (lithium carbonate)	11	23.4
Depakote (valproate)	3	6.4
Neurontin (gabapentin)	2	4.3
Lamictal (lamotrigine)	2	4.3
Trileptal (oxcarbazepine)	4	8.5
Total participants taking one or more drugs in this class	15	31.9
Anxiolytics		
Buspar (buspirone)	2	4.3
Klonopin (clonazepam)	5	10.6
Ativan (lorazepam)	1	2.1
Total participants taking one or more drugs in this class	7	14.9
Mean number of psychotropic drugs taken over lifetime	3.96	

[a]Data obtained from ethnographic and clinical research interviews.

TABLE 7 PSYCHOTROPIC MEDICATIONS TAKEN BY ADOLESCENT PARTICIPANTS
DURING STUDY (N = 47)[a]

Medication by class	n	%
Antipsychotics		
Abilify (aripiprazole)	15	31.9
Clozaril (clozapine)	2	4.3
Geodon (ziprasidone)	5	10.6
Risperdal (risperidone)	8	17.0
Seroquel (quetiapine)	15	31.9
Zyprexa (olanzapine)	5	10.6
Total participants taking one or more drugs in this class	35	74.5
Antidepressants		
Prozac (fluoxetine)	9	19.1
Celexa (citalopram)	1	2.1
Zoloft (sertraline)	11	23.4
Paxil (paroxetine)	1	2.1
Lexapro (escitalopram)	3	6.4
Effexor (venlafaxine)	2	4.3
Cymbalta (duloxetine)	1	2.1
Wellbutrin/Budeprion (bupropion)	5	10.6
Total participants taking one or more drugs in this class	27	57.4
ADHD drugs		
Concerta/Ritalin (methylphenidate)	3	6.4
Catapres/Kapvay (clonidine)	2	4.3
Adderall (amphetamine and dextroamphetamine)	6	12.8
Strattera (atomoxetine)	1	2.1
Total participants taking one or more drugs in this class	10	21.3
Mood stabilizers		
Eskalith/Lithobid (lithium carbonate)	8	17.0
Depakote (valproate)	1	2.1
Neurontin (gabapentin)	1	2.1
Lamictal (lamotrigine)	4	8.5
Trileptal (oxcarbazepine)	1	2.1
Total participants taking one or more drugs in this class	14	28.8
Anxiolytics		
Buspar (buspirone)	1	2.1
Klonopin (clonazepam)	5	10.6
Ativan (lorazepam)	1	2.1
Total participants taking one or more drugs in this class	6	12.8
Mean number of drugs taken during study	2.49	

[a]Data obtained from ethnographic and clinical research interviews.

currently taking was high; there were sex differences observed here also (not shown in the table), with boys prescribed more drugs (mean = 4.24) than girls (3.64).

Our second question concerns these adolescents' experience of taking medications, particularly with respect to whether or not they liked the medications. The answer to this question is far from straightforward, since typically there were mixed feelings and ambivalence. Overall, however, 62 percent reported that they liked their medications, 28 percent were fairly clear that they did not like their medications, and 10 percent were indifferent. These data are complicated by the observation that those who "liked" their medications did so for a diverse set of reasons. Much of this had to do with the relative emphasis they placed on main effects and side effects of medications (which they might regard as considerable or minor in significance). Some insisted that they liked their medications and that they perceived either no or insignificant side effects. Others reported liking the medications despite considerable negative side effects, as expressed by a fourteen-year-old Guatemalan-Chinese girl who said, "At first like I was kind of depressed and stuff but then I felt like a lot happier, like I just wake up happy and stuff . . . [but] the first day [I took it] it was like, um, I don't like it, cause the first day it made me like really hyper and I like really hated it." She also found that sometimes she would cry or feel sad for no reason and wondered if that was due to the medication; overall, however, she was insistent that she needed the medication and liked taking it as a means to "feel happy."

Concerning whether the medications were perceived as "working," the majority (72.3 percent) felt that they could perceive that the drugs worked based on effects they could discern, whereas 27.7 percent were convinced they did not "work" or have discernible helpful effects. Those who thought that the drugs "worked" (whether they "liked" them or not) described efficacy in terms of feeling better or of tamping down behaviors they construed as problematic, such as anger, violence, agitation, or depression. The following excerpt illustrating the perception that the medications "work" and are useful was provided by a sixteen-year-old Native American boy who struggled with extreme anger, generalized anxiety, social phobia, and occasional paranoia. During one interview, he jokingly referred to himself as a "psychiatric junkie," at which point his grandmother quickly chimed in to insist that he was a "*legal* psychiatric junkie." He said, "It's helping a lot. It's improving me . . . the meds are working, um, they help my depression and my, my hallucinations go away. It gives me a good feeling." He also thought the medication made him less likely to wake up or act out in a violently angry way, although he also thought that the medications worked to make him hungrier and drowsier than he liked.

The specifically cultural dimensions of taking psychotropic medications have been studied among adults (Jenkins and Carpenter-Song 2005, 2008, 2009; Ecks 2013; Martin 2009; Jordan et al. 2017). The influence of the medical and pharmaceutical imaginary has been formulated (Good 1995, 2007; Jenkins 2010a, b; Dumit 2012) in relation to forces of globalization on the one hand (M. Good 2010; Good et al. 2011; B. Good 2010), and to subjective experience of the self on the other (Good 1994, 2012). As with other aspects of medicine, taking medication is shaped by stark inequalities of care in relation to race, ethnicity, and income; these matters have only become more pronounced over time in the United States in the context of increasing income inequality and ethnic hyper-diversity (Good et al. 2005).

Compared with adult populations, far less ethnographically informed research has been carried out among children, although there have been pioneering efforts to pave the way for better understanding. Despite what many have presumed as the dominance of bionarratives, Elizabeth Carpenter-Song (2009, 2015) has demonstrated that such cultural formulations hardly eclipse families' nonpsychiatric cultural interpretations of mental illness in children (see also Floersch et al. 2009; Foltz and Huefner 2014; Kranke et al. 2015; Murphy et al. 2013, 2015; Narendorf et al. 2015; Chubinsky and Hojman 2013; Choudhury et al. 2015). What emerges prominently from this literature is the need to pay close attention to social stigma that attaches to mental illness and to taking medication among children and adolescents (Carpenter-Song 2009; Longhofer and Floersch 2010; Narendorf, Munson, and Floersch 2015; Pescosolido et al. 2007; Kranke et al. 2011). In addition to the social stigma meted out by others, the subjective experience of *self*-stigma (as noted for adults by Jenkins and Carpenter-Song 2005) is a phenomenon that has been identified ethnographically and through first-person accounts (Corrigan and Watson 2002). Kranke and colleagues (2015) completed a narrative analysis of twenty-seven adolescents with the aim of identifying modes of "empowerment" that teens can use to counteract social stigma they may self-apply. Globally, further research is needed with young people to determine the extent and types of social stigma that are present as well as ways to reduce discrimination perpetrated against those struggling with problems of mental health across the life span.

In our study, there is extensive ethnographic evidence of social stigma that adolescents perceived as directed at them by peers, family members, and others. The situation of teens taking medications, as with numerous other domains of lived experience that we examine in this book, is clearly a matter of struggle "not just *against* an illness and its symptoms but also *for* a normal life, *to* make sense of a confusing and disorienting circumstance, *with* intimate others, and *in* a world characterized by stigma" (Jenkins 2015a: 261). Analysis of our ethnographic interviews and observations revealed that a primary way in which the adolescents felt stigmatized was in feeling "less normal" even as they *tried* to become "more normal." Many struggled with perceptions by parents, family, and the broader community that their condition or illness is "not real." Some parents insisted that their child was just blaming "the illness" as a means to not take responsibility for their actions. Others called our interlocutors "crazy" just for taking medications, and extended family members would sometimes not allow them (or would convince them not) to take medication while they were staying with them. Extended or immediate family members often told them they did not need medications to get up every morning or to function every day.

However, as we have seen above in the adolescents' perceptions of their medication, they often countered with an agentive insistence that they knew they needed it, and the *primacy* of this experiential knowledge was often framed in contrast to knowing what it is like to be off medication. Often the latter meant trouble for them, trouble they were usually not willing to risk by refusing medication. For them, the utility of the medication was behaviorally oriented insofar as they wanted medications to make them less mad, or not so rude, or happy, for example. There is also the sense that medications can "give control" back over one's body. This is important, as one person put it, even though medications are limited in "not being able to heal [their] disorder parts." Still, given residential instability and frequent hospitalizations, many valued medications for allowing them to feel stable or to feel that they have the capability of controlling themselves. Some emphasized the need to keep quiet about their experience in the presence of those who would judge them or think they were "crazy," and some also feared that the side effects of medications might make them "look crazy." Yet more striking were adolescents' assessments of the trade-offs of medications, which usually came down on the side of describing the experience of taking them as worth it.

THEMATIC PORTRAITS OF TREATMENT TRAJECTORIES

We have gained significant insight into how troubled young people experience psychiatric inpatient treatment by attending to how they compare the various facilities in which they have found themselves and talk about how treatment has or has not helped them. However, we have yet to examine how some of the themes we have touched on are woven together for individual persons. We need to develop a richer sense of treatment trajectory as a kind of existential movement. In order to do this, it is necessary to take a closer look at several selected patients as they are thrown, to borrow Heidegger's term, into a world where stability, care, well-being, and healing are highly precarious. Accordingly, in what follows we present neither brief vignettes nor full case studies, but unique portraits of the treatment trajectory of four among these youth. We have designed these portraits to be sensitive both to lived experience over the course of multiple hospitalizations and to narrative intersubjectivity between afflicted youth and engaged parent/guardian.

"I'm a Psychiatric Junkie"

One of our older participants was Robbie, a young Pueblo Indian male who was seventeen years old when he first began with the study and nineteen when he completed participation (we briefly met him in chapter 3 p. 104 as someone who readily endorsed psychiatric diagnosis). He lived with his grandmother, brother, and sister in a remote rural area; the children's mother was absorbed in drugs and alcohol and their father had not been present since Robbie was three years old. The grandmother attended meetings of the National Alliance on Mental Illness and did her own internet research on Robbie's diagnoses. She was strongly supportive when Robbie's siblings were hostile to him at times; he regarded them as "completely clueless about my disease and all that, so I have to look elsewhere [for support] if a situation happens." Prior to his first hospitalization he had been seeing a psychiatrist for several years because "I was not, like, socializing very well and I was getting harassed by the people at school." He had been admitted five times to CPC since age fifteen, punctuated by admission to another facility at age seventeen. In talking about his earliest hospitalization, he referred to "incidents at home that led up to that one intervention where I was taken to a hospital and learned the tricks of the trade of having a psychiatric disorder."

This was by no means a cynical comment, but rather a sign of engagement in the therapeutic process. What Robbie meant when referring to the "tricks of the trade of having a psychiatric disorder" in fact had three elements. The first had to do with what he called his disease:

> Because of the way the disease has shaped me over growing-up years, I live by a different set of codes and principles growing up that normally, that normal people don't normally believe in. And which contradicts what my great grandma believes and all this and that. Sometimes I have to suck it in, and bite the dust or bite the bullet because I'm the kind of person that rather likes to talk to people ever since the hospital's taught me this value, ever since I've been talking with people from all around the state, you could say.

This passage indicates the challenge posed to Robbie by his own sense of exceptionalism and the struggle to explain his experience to others, here in the context of a value placed on communication with others that he attributes to learning in the hospital.

The second aspect of these tricks of the trade involves his embrace of psychiatric medication. Robbie's grandmother worried a good deal about her grandson's potential exposure to the street drugs and gang violence that had consumed his mother, noting she was relieved that he had not become involved in that world. In this context, the following humorous exchange describes the way in which grandmother and grandson characterized the situation:

GRANDMOTHER: He's done really good, he's legally on drugs.
ROBBIE: That's right. *I'm a psychiatric junkie!* [*laughs*]
INTERVIEWER: [*laughs*] *Psychiatric junkie?!*
G: Legally.
I: *But legally.*
R: You hear that!? Psychiatric junkie! [*laughs*]

An added element of humor comes from the fact that Robbie had a truly diverse set of medication experiences. He had at various times been on different medications (e.g., Abilify, Seroquel, Geodon), had at times been off his medication regimen, claimed to have developed "immunity" to several medications, and on one occasion reported having an allergic reaction that required hospitalization in order to readjust his medications. Overall he said that medication "gives back the control over my body" although, poignantly, it "can't heal my disorder."

Finally, there are tricks of the trade that have to do with therapeutic language in the sense of a lexicon of terms encountered in treatment settings:

> When I first got here to CPC for the very first time I was like bombarded with all these therapeutic terms and like overfilled my head overloaded and it kind of made me upset because of the way they like, the way their attitude and all is with therapy and all. It must be like these kinds of hospitals that use complicated words. I didn't get them at first but eventually I came along. It's like, it's like a different lifestyle and persona you live here while you're in these hospitals because you have to act appropriate, you have to like therapeutic terms and all that. I mean it's so different from when you live in the outside world. . . . I'm so mature and I'm so responsible for myself I already know what to do and everything and like when they try to [give] advice for how to deal with the outside world, like how to deal with arguments with other people, not all of it (I should say not most of it) applies in the outside world, so you still have to just think for yourself and actually make your own judgment.

The therapeutic terms he gave as examples included that his problems were "psychiatric," being given a "time out," being subjected to a "team call" for disruptive behavior, progressing through behavioral "levels" in the residential cottage, and being "redirected" for doing something wrong. From this young man's subjective stance, his own increasing maturity was a value underlying insight about his distinctive codes or principles and about the importance of therapeutic terminology. As examples of his maturity he cited his own voluntary admissions, his description of acting as a role model for peers, and developing enduring attachments to staff. Perhaps most telling about what he called the exhausting struggle with episodes combining a "migraine-type headache" and a repetitive "thought process disorder" that made him feel as if he was "going crazy and insane" to the point that he could "end up in the loony bin" is precisely that he apparently *did not* equate his multiple hospitalizations with being in the loony bin.

The issue of therapeutic language is less one of discursive operators, as we found with terms specifying psychiatric diagnoses, than one of a technical vocabulary or institutional jargon. As reflected in what young people say, the terminology can be analyzed into two categories. First are terms referring explicitly to therapeutic process, such as "coping skills," "triggers," "anger management," "treatment goals," "responsibility," and "processing." These bridge the space between inpatient and outpatient treatment as well as the space between functioning in the institutional setting and in everyday life after discharge. Second are terms referring to behavioral regulation in the inpatient setting, such as "line of sight" (observation of a patient who is or might be suicidal), "key 15's" (observation of a patient at fifteen-minute intervals), "HRP" (high-risk precautions), "PI" (peer isolation), "crisis teams" or "c-teams" (which intervene in violence or confrontation), "restraint," "silent program" (no talking with peers), "points and levels" (for good behavior and rewarded with privileges), "matrix" (a small rule break), "corrective" (a major behavioral problem), "to take a tag" (to remove points), and "transition" (between staff work shifts on the unit). Patients incorporate these vocabularies, and the terms quickly become a part of everyday life in inpatient treatment, varying somewhat from facility to facility.

Robbie insisted that he typically volunteered to be admitted, including for a recent episode in which he had checked himself into an adult unit shortly after turning eighteen "just for another medical tune-up."

Well first off let's say this, I personally was the one who admitted myself, with my grandma taking me on again as a treatment guardian. I grew resistant and scared because it was the first time being in an adult unit. It was more like coldhearted and basically I panicked because it seemed like real mean and the role of the staff of any psychiatric ward is to maintain a safe environment but the methods I had were questionable and then they eventually led to me being scared because at the time I was still at the point where I was easily intimidated by those who had a psychiatric background such as doctors, mental health technicians, because of the methods I have been subjected to as in a children's ward before. I thought I knew the system but it was a whole different thing and I was entirely scared. For one they don't give you the same kind of attention the children's do like they won't sit down and help you and all that. In fact, at times to subdue the intimidation and fear I want to sit down and talk to the staff, kind of like just let it out and they did at first but they wouldn't stay for more than three or four minutes and all they just said was that "you're not the only one we have to care for." In fact, I wasn't even granted or no one was granted at all individual therapy, the only kind of individual achievement I got was the psychiatrist and even then the psychiatrist only wanted to check about medical progress, like how is the medicine reacting, et cetera, then I would leave. It was more of group therapy but unfortunately the treatment I needed at the time was individual which made me grow really scared and I just wanted to get out. I thought at first about it was a mistake but in my room I was conflicting in my mind that I have to stay here because if I just leave now without getting the medicine at least on a normal basis where I can last. Even now, even today I feel a little edgy about adult wards because it's not proper treatment they're giving.

While being in an adult ward put Robbie's tricks of the trade to a serious test, his reflectiveness is evident in acknowledging the conflict between being scared and feeling the need to stay long enough for his medication to be rebalanced.

During the follow-up interview, Robbie explained that over the years he had learned to be more attentive to and understanding about his "disease," which had allowed him to improve. CPC, he claimed, had been helpful in this regard:

> When I first got the disease, I'm being honest, honest, I quite frankly didn't give a damn about it. But because of the therapy and the people I've met at UNM it pretty much made me realize that my life is destined for more. But unfortunately I didn't take it too seriously at the time which led to my second hospitalization. I had to get intense psychological rehabilitation to master and eventually understand and control the disease.

He described life with his "disease" as one of "trial and error" where "new challenges in life pop up" and have to be faced. He tried to use "preventive measures" such as "taking deep breaths" or "chronicling," along with his medication. Robbie felt that his condition had improved over the past year or so and attributed this to what he termed "chronicling." This was similar to journaling, although he said that he often did the chronicling in his head. It entailed a kind of self-talk and self-analysis, especially with regard to his behavior and mood. It was not entirely clear whether this was something he had learned at CPC or had come up with himself, but he said he learned these "preventive measures" both in his experiences at CPC and through his everyday personal life experiences. Given what we noted above about Robbie's analysis of therapeutic terminology, he was quite clear about his preference for the term "preventive measures," insofar as "I'm one to admit I really hate the term 'coping skills.' I understand the purpose of coping skills. In fact, I rather say my coping skills are hobbies. But the reason why I hate that term, not the actual method—I do the method of coping skills. I hate that term 'coping skills' because it's really used by the doctors way, way too much. . . . The hell you guys talking about?"

Robbie continued to see both a psychiatrist and a therapist following his last hospitalization, though according to his grandmother he had trouble developing and sustaining relationships with therapists and psychiatrists. Robbie agreed and attributed this partly to the fact that they are from the "city," rather than the reservation:

> But yeah it's just that my previous psychiatrist, we couldn't get along and that's what ultimately ended the relationships. I mean, we were honest about the disease and all that but it was just a matter of getting along. Even now

my therapist and my psychiatrist are not from this reservation, they're from the city . . . because they were from the city they didn't know our way of socializing out here and ultimately led to arguments so I decided I'm just going to get a new one.

Robbie's problem with particular mental health professionals neither diminished his commitment to a psychiatric model nor precluded the possibility of seeking traditional Pueblo healing. Although he had not done so during the time of his participation in the study, both he and his grandmother said they had considered it. However, he recognized a potential conflict between the alternative medical systems insofar as "medicine men are some of the most skeptical people of all Native Americans. Since they believe in their own spiritualism ways of healing rather than outside-ways, as slang term would put it, 'white man ways.' No disrespect."

"When I Get Mad I Start Banging My Head on the Wall"

We now return to Taciana, the fourteen-year-old Native American girl we introduced at the beginning of chapter 1. Her trajectory began with TFC at age five when she was removed from her house by social workers "because my mom wasn't taking care of me like a parent should." For two years "they gave me all the help I needed and I went to school, and learned a lot from that school." Following this she was placed with another foster mother, who regularly slapped her and whose grandson attempted to rape her, till she was removed from the home. Returning to live with relatives, she was in outpatient treatment at the reservation Indian Health Service hospital before being admitted to CPC for a suicide attempt. She reported having volunteered to come to the hospital anticipating that it would help, and two weeks after her admission reported that "I've been here at the hospital and it's really helping me, I am not sad anymore. I am feeling happy, just it's really helping me and I'm really glad I came." By the time of her second interview she had been transferred from CPC to another residential facility, and we quote her at length below for the sake of her vivid comparison of life at the two places:

It's more structured and more organized [here]. And you have to really follow the rules because if you don't they'll get onto you about it. And then, [they] give you a goal that you have to follow. And you have your own room that you have to share with a peer, and you can cook on the unit. It's just huge here, and you get to go to school—right now I'm going to summer school. And we get to play, like, recreation ropes course, and volleyball, soccer . . .

we just have games. And we don't go out as much [as] at CPC. At CPC it was like a lot of people are nice there. They gave you respect and they took care of you twenty-four seven, and you got to go out daily. You could eat meals three times a day, there's always snacks. And there was movie time. You wanted to stay in your room you could, and [if you wanted] to go outside, you could. But here it's more structured. And, like, for me it's a bit difficult. Because when certain peers get to me, I don't ignore it, I just let them get to me and, and that's when I lose control. Then I start getting mad. And that's why I wish I was still at CPC but then all they could've done is send me back here. When I get mad I start banging my head on the wall, or I'll start cutting on myself, or I'll try to choke myself with my jacket or with my shoestring. That's why they took our shoestrings away. [But I like] the staff, they're nice, and the food [*laughs very slightly*], and the rec time we have. I usually like to go to ropes course, and if I don't wanna do that I'll go play basketball or soccer or volleyball, or just take walks, or read my Bible. [The structure is] the hardest thing, but right now I worked my way up to level two, so you get privileges.

At CPC I was always happy. And I was cooler over there. Well, over there at CPC they were nicer and you got, you got to have a lot of privileges, you got on level right away. They would give you your space and the kids were nice. They were polite and they treat you with respect and the staff were nice. They weren't strict. You could have your shoelaces and your makeup and everything. And here it's more strict because the program director is hard on us. And she's always getting mad at us and she's usually telling us that we do wrong things and that we should focus on ourselves and that's what I'm trying to do but other kids here, they're like always putting you down for who you are. And they're always cussing at you and telling you that they don't like you and that you're doing a bad job. And the staff make lies, and, I don't know, it is just different here than it is at CPC. Like they'll, they'll lie [about] what you're doing. If you don't do your chores, they'll give you a zero for it [*sighs*] and if you're being rude to peers they'll give you a zero for it, and they won't give the other person a zero. They'll just put it on you and they say that you did something when you didn't. [That's] just the staff and the kids. The therapists help you.

Mention of therapists is almost an afterthought in this description, but Taciana saw her social worker and also met with a therapist once a week. In addition, she had family sessions with her mother and father during which "we share our feelings and what we like and what we don't like, and what we want to change and what we accept from my dad and what he accepts from us." She indicated that she would have preferred to see her therapist every day rather than once a week.

In this facility, Taciana's typical day started at 6:30 with a shower and breakfast, then chores followed by a "goals group":

Like, we have to pick a number [from] zero to ten [and rate how we're feeling], zero is the worst and ten is the greatest, they just ask you what your day is, [about] your anxiety, your depression, your self-harm, your frustration, aggression. We do it three times a day. We do our chores and we just wait for the therapist to come around. And we usually watch movies about drugs, how it could affect you and what can happen to you while you're pregnant and stuff. It really helps me. We're doing a lot of outings and things. Going to feed the homeless and going to watch new movies. And sometimes we'll go fishing or we'll go watch racing cars or basketball games. We just go all over the place. [*Note that this apparently contradicts her earlier statement that there were few outings compared with CPC.*] And we have speakers come in on Mondays, Tuesdays, Wednesdays, and Thursdays. . . . And the males they come over to our side and talk about their experiment with alcohol and drugs. So, we're telling our stories. And the [guest] speakers talk about their life story and their childhood. [*Note that this facility is particularly attuned to youth who have experience with drugs and alcohol.*]

In daily life, peer relations are as immediately relevant as those with staff, and Taciana commented about the other girls on her eight-person residential unit housing two girls to a room, indicating that they were split into two hostile camps of four against four:

They [four of them] respect me. They're nice to me. They share things with me. [Except] D, I don't really get along with her, we just don't talk to each other at all. And when she talks to me, I just ignore her. Because I gotta remember that I'm mad at her for things that she's been saying about me. And I'll turn my back on her, and start talking about her. . . . [The other hostile] girls [are] telling me what to do all the time and telling me that I'm not pretty enough to have the boys see me and everything. And I tell them I'm not here for the boys. I'm here for my treatment. And they're always making up letters and sending them to the boys and saying that they're my letters and I tell them that it's not my handwriting. They always try to lie their way out. I get into arguments with them. Like when I tell them what they're doing wrong they get mad at me. And then when they tell me what I do wrong I get mad at them. So, it's like we tell each other things that we're not supposed to be doing and we get mad at each other for it. And we get put on silent program where you can't talk to anybody, you just have to focus on yourselves. And you have to copy pages out of this [Narcotics Anonymous] book, from page one, word to word . . . it's really stressful and I get tired of it. It's frustrating and I also cry a lot and I usually think about dying because the way they [peers] treat me and it's like I don't like it. And some of them make me like cut myself. And tell me to like die, just do it. [At CPC] they were nice. They would give me feedback on how I'm doing and they would ask me questions, if I'm OK and if I got anything that I can harm myself with. They helped me. They'd tell me, give it to me, you're not gonna do anything with that. And I just give 'em my things that I was gonna hurt myself with. And when I would cry they would hug me and ask me what's wrong and I would usually tell 'em. They were just helpful.

Again, in this passage, Taciana returns to comparison of her current life with life at CPC. Her description of losing control of herself in the hospital evidently has to do as much with the stress of peer relations as with any illness process or pathological symptoms per se:

The last few days I've been having c-teams [crisis intervention] where, when I go crazy they call the c-teams. They just say c-team whenever someone's going off. Like, I bang my head now on the wall. When I do that they call a c-team. And they like restrain you. [It's been happening] for the last couple of months. When I first came here I was doing OK. I was on level and everything. And then I moved to unit 2. First, I was on CT4, then I moved to unit 2. I was there for about two months and I started messing up. A lot of girls started hating me and they started lying about things and I started getting mad. And I started cutting and I started banging my head, and I started trying to hang myself again. [I started banging my head] because I saw my friend do that at CPC. I saw her do that and I thought it was OK to do that so I started banging my head and [peers] would ask: "Why do you do that?" and I would tell 'em it's a coping skill, but they tell me that it's not good for me because I'm gonna mess up my vision and mess up my head and mess up my brain. And I started banging my head when I get mad and I told them it's to release stress but they said I could handle it another way.

This is a vivid example of how coping skills can appear in descriptions of the lived experience of hospitalization, though not in the way that a clinical perspective would understand as positive coping. A more successful coping skill for Taciana was the one she devised on her own, combining indigenous Native American tradition with a technique more common in Euro-American culture:

[I keep some blessed Native American corn] that's really special that we have to take care of. That's why I tell them [staff and peers] not to touch my corn. And so they can get scared of it. When I get mad, I usually hold it by me and they usually won't come toward me. So, it's like protection that I use. You just hold it up and toward them and they just run away. It has power but I just don't know how to use it. I just talk to the [Native American] godfathers while I'm in treatment, don't let them [*breathes in*] do any danger to me and I also ask them to help me be nice. I asked my staff to help me out when I get mad and I have time-outs when I'm about to go hit somebody. I just go talk to my cornmeal and my corn, I talk to them. They help me. This is what you have to do, if you wanna get mad or when you wanna do this, you have to do this. You wanna do that, you have to do this first, before you go ahead first and get in trouble. . . . [*Holding up a ball*] This is like a stress ball I use. [I squeeze it] when I, when I get mad. [Sometimes I've had] corn in the one hand, and the stress ball in the other hand. It was weird. I don't know, I had this feeling. Like, I'd gotten lifted up or something. And like I got this feeling, went down my body . . . like something good touched me. I was just playing with the ball. And then I got my corn and I saw me holding two. And I just squeezed them, [and felt] something touches me. So that's why I do it every morning before I wake up. It just gives me a better day every day.

Partly by chance, Taciana has created a syncretic personal practice of empowerment and protection that draws on simultaneous invocation of indigenous spiritual beings and the commonplace North American concept of stress reduction. This practice is emblematic of her ongoing struggle and resilience. It is profoundly embodied not only in its use of particular symbolic objects, but also in the feeling of being touched and lifted up. It is deeply imaginative not only in the juxtaposition of cultural and therapeutic traditions, but also in the moment of seeing herself as she held the corn and the ball.

Given the struggle of her everyday existence, it appeared that for Taciana treatment per se made up a relatively small part of her routine. Her attitude toward treatment was generally positive:

> [It's helpful] just talking with somebody about my problems. I mean, I have a lot of problems. And it's really hard to deal with them so I just talk to someone that I'm comfortable with. . . . [Hospital treatment has] helped my hallucinations. I take medicine for it. And it's helped me. I haven't been hearing things or seeing things for the last couple of months. . . . [Treatment is] getting me to eat. Like I get hungry and I'll start to eat. At CPC I would usually refuse to eat. I would throw my plate away. But their food is good over there, [*laughs very slightly*] and it isn't over here. [The most important thing about my treatment is] my schoolwork. I got A's and B's. [What I didn't expect was] trying to hang myself with some shoestrings I found in my room. I tried hanging myself to a doorknob. And to the shower thing, shower pole. And I was put on line of sight, so whenever I'd go into the bathroom I would have to count and leave the door cracked open. And I got scared. I thought I was just gonna die, but the girls came and they untied the string and they were crying because they're like why are we treating her bad. We shouldn't be doing this 'cause now she's just wanting to kill herself. [I'm surprised] getting c-teams every day and cutting myself. I told CPC people that I was never gonna to do that again. And I happened to do it again, just to feel pain when I needed it. Yeah, when I got mad I wanted to feel pain so I usually cut on myself.

As we have seen before with other youth, Taciana offers a matter-of-fact description of how she surprises herself with her own behavior, poignantly reflective about a regression from a previous level of improvement. By the time of her final interview, however, Taciana had a post-discharge plan to return to TFC, where she would rejoin her biological brother. She had met her foster parents, with whom she had already been shopping, to the movies, and ice-skating. She said that they "have a lot of rules," and that the mother is "calm, really true about things, really helpful, believes in God, really focused on us kids." Taciana reported that she liked calling them Mom and Dad, and noted with anticipation that they regularly took the children to Disneyland.

"Most of Them Really Did Care. I Could Tell"

Maria was a young woman of Hispanic background who had been hospitalized a number of times since she was fifteen. She entered the project at age seventeen and concluded her participation when she was nineteen. Her mother narrated the early history of her hospitalizations, beginning with an admission to CPC when "she was cutting, starving herself, throwing up, smoking weed, not going to school, driving me nuts [*laughs a little*]." Maria had already talked to her school counselor without her mother's awareness, and by the time the mother herself called the school the counselor recommended admission to CPC. From there she went to another inpatient facility and then to a brief TFC placement that ended when she fell in the shower and injured her head. The fall sent her back to the second inpatient facility and then to a third inpatient facility for several months, this time away from Albuquerque, in the southern part of the state. Her mother reported that although she could not visit often, they did therapeutic work on their relationship, and after a trial visit Maria was allowed to return home, though to her sister's rather than her mother's house. Another two-week inpatient stay at a fourth facility took place shortly after Maria's baby was born and she had a serious episode of postpartum depression with psychotic features.

Her cumulative experience with multiple facilities doubtless allowed Maria's mother to critically identify what she did and did not like about treatment. She "didn't like the way they had her drugged up all the time" but was pleased with being able to speak "with her counselor just about every day and they gave me a little tour of it, it looked OK. You know, I got a good feeling about that." Nevertheless, Maria's mother had some blunt complaints about therapists:

> To tell you the truth, this last therapist that she had, I wanted to choke her. I mean, her job is to sit there and listen, not blab. And she was literally cutting me off, cutting me off, cutting me off. I wanted her to know how I felt, what [my daughter] had done, and where I couldn't save her, where I couldn't stop it. And, um, she just "blah, blah, blah." She didn't listen. And her psychia-

trist called me and I told him. I says, "You know, that woman is no—I don't know where she got her degree." And there was another one, too, at [another facility]. Oh my God, I wanted to choke that one, too. You know, she was looking at me like this was all my fault. I probably have my role in it, just like any other parent, but I'm willing to take responsibility but not sit there and watch you point your finger at me. That's not what you're here for. . . . And then the one she had [in the other place], I like her. I could tell her anything. She would be on the other end [of the spectrum].

Maria had her own reflective narration of her treatment trajectory, comparing different facilities and making it clear that she did not always concur with her mother's assessment of therapists:

You know what, CPC is probably the best treatment place I've been in because the staff was just awesome. They're just on top of it, like, and most staff people you can tell if they're just there because it's a job or they're there because they care. And most of them really did care, I could tell. So that made it really good. And my therapist wasn't too bad. I heard my mom saying stuff about my therapist, but sometimes that's just how people are. People are different. I didn't think she was that bad. There was times when she maybe said things that were pretty off, but overall she was a good therapist.

Maria said that her first hospitalization came when she began self-cutting and developed an eating disorder, and "did a lot of that stuff basically without thinking, like I was more into the boys than the treatment and I was trying to go out with boys that were at the treatment center and getting in trouble at school." This resulted in her being sent to TFC, which she did not like, and she asked to be taken back to the hospital. She was instead sent to a residential treatment center in the southern part of the state, where she stayed for two months. She said,

It was awful. I was there with sixteen other girls, you know how that can get. I don't really get along with girls, so a lot happened. I was getting into fights. I didn't like the fact that girls were going out with girls. I don't want to say that I'm homophobic or nothing, but I just felt uncomfortable. I was still a virgin and they're like all talking about sex, and I was—like, I'm not saying it's their fault, I'm just saying that they just put it in front of my face, in front of me.

Although she "loved" her therapist, she acknowledged that she was only playing the part in order to earn her release, rather than truly seeking help. While Maria judged that two of the facilities helped her, two others "just opened the door into all this stuff, like when I was around all those other girls, I started learning different things."

By the time of her second ethnographic interview, she had yet another hospital experience to report:

> I was eighteen, I went to an adult unit. It was maybe early September when I went back, and that was because my mom was really worried about me. I had started with my eating disorders again, I started starving myself and then I was starting the bulimia again. My mom was just really scared. She didn't know what to do. I was eighteen, I felt like I could do whatever I wanted and I didn't have to be put back in the hospital, but my mom did whatever she could to get me back in there. And I ended up going and I think that's when I really snapped, also. Because that was, like, what? The eighth time I had been in the hospital and I just didn't want it anymore. I didn't want all that weight, to be in there.

Maria thought that her mother had wanted her out of the house because "of course, eating disorders are dangerous and stuff like that," but that her mother had claimed Maria was cutting herself when she was not, in order to get the hospital to keep her longer. In fact, this admission lasted one week. On this adult ward she felt awkward and out of place, again doing what she was told and telling therapists what they wanted to hear in order to get discharged. She determined to stay out of hospitals and residential treatment, no matter "how big I get." This hospitalization was also unsatisfactory because "I wasn't hearing much about any of my problems, it was just kind of everybody just talking about theirs. It was more independent than it would be at CPC, or [another facility], or any place like that. And I just, basically, wanted to get out of there. I wanted my son back. And I got him, I got out of there."

In retrospect, at this second interview, she was willing to evaluate her own engagement in treatment during most of her hospitalizations as "just doing whatever I had to do to get out. I wasn't really working on myself." She reflectively said that this attitude was

> why I keep getting off my meds, because I feel like I am OK, so I don't need them, I don't feel like taking them every day. But in reality, I need them 'cause when I had postpartum depression, I did not miss a day, I was on top of it. I was so scared of being that way again. I was scared of getting those thoughts, I was just terrified. I know how important they are now, but [back then] I wish I would have really stayed on them.

Over a long trajectory, through multiple treatment settings, Maria had incorporated an appreciation for the necessity of medication. She also continued to comparatively evaluate her experiences at different treatment facilities, with respect to both their environments and her own engagement:

It feels like those places kinda made me worse. I learned a lot more from there. This girl told me when I was in one hospital, "You are cutting yourself the wrong way, you are supposed to cut down." Like, wow, I learned that there. I learned a lot of things when I was in those hospitals. And then again, I know that there are people there helping, but I just felt like it didn't really help me. Because when you don't want to be somewhere, you are not going to do what you have to do, you are not gonna try and get better, you are gonna try and get out of there, no matter what.

In this second interview, she also thought back to her very first hospitalization, reiterating that

I was just doing all kinds of bad stuff, I was going out with boys and just, doing everything that I wasn't supposed to do. [Another facility], I would say that was the worst. I was just so dumb when I was there. I was experimenting and just . . . doing weird things [*embarrassed laughter*], and then I started dating girls, and started getting in trouble, started fighting. It wasn't even about me anymore, I wasn't cutting myself or anything, I was like, taking my anger out on other people. I feel like putting somebody like me in that setting, just wasn't the right thing. I would say CPC was the best. I really put myself into that one, and [another hospital] was good too. I really liked all the staff, and my therapist was really helpful, and I think it was better that we were separated from, how should I say it? I know that not every girl is boy crazy, but I know that when you are boy crazy, that you are going to focus on boys, not going to focus on anything else. And that's when I had the postpartum depression, I was totally out of it. So they were there for me when I was there.

Maria's reflections on her past treatment are self-reflective and nuanced. She does not complain about ineffective treatment, but acknowledges her own lack of engagement in settings that could have been helpful, and holds that it was not the right thing to put someone like her in other settings that may have made her condition worse. Likewise, she does not blame the bad influences of peers in some of these settings, but acknowledges her willingness to be influenced by and experiment with "doing weird things," being "boy crazy," dating girls, and getting in fights. Her comment that in one facility another resident instructed her about the proper way to cut herself is an important glimpse into the kind of knowledge circulated in the institutional peer culture of adolescent inpatient mental health treatment.

It was not until her most recent hospitalization, about which we spoke at her third and final interview, that Maria acknowledged a truly satisfactory experience, having been admitted through an emergency room to another facility in the southern city of Las Cruces.

I finally got a straight answer 'cause I never really knew what my diagnosis was. I knew that I was depressed, but I didn't know that I have psychosis. [I had been waiting to get an appointment] 'cause I didn't want to be an inpatient. I've been an inpatient so many times and I just didn't want to go through it again. But going through it actually showed me a lot, because I'm in denial about a lot of the stuff I've been through. I kind of say that it could've been worse, or my life could've been worse, it shouldn't be as sad or I kind of try to downsize it but really, I went through a lot. I didn't think I was going to have to go all the way to Las Cruces 'cause I had been there before a long time ago. So I was like, Oh God, I don't want to go that far, 'cause I want to be able to see my son. And being there showed me that I need to be on my medication, 'cause that's usually how it happens. I go off of them because they have a lot of side effects like weight gain and stuff like that. I don't want that, but without them I'm not gonna be functional. It was because my therapist talked to me more [than before]. Because at first, I was so delusional [*laughs*]. I kept asking everybody, "Do you think I'm crazy?" I just . . . seeing myself like that, so delusional, and then going from delusional to where I'm myself again it just opened my eyes. Because the medication was, it was, a lot of it was 'cause of the medication. And because I told them. 'Cause a lot of the stuff I was thinking, like I was keeping it to myself 'cause I thought I was crazy.

During this hospitalization her therapist at first thought Maria had bipolar disorder, but a psychiatrist listened to her describe some of the thoughts she was having as feeling like someone else was putting them there. Toward the end of this weeklong stay she asked what her diagnosis was, and the psychiatrist told her she had post-traumatic stress disorder and psychosis. PTSD made sense to Maria in the context that she had been sexually molested when she was eleven years old by one of her mother's boyfriends while her mother was unconscious in an alcoholic blackout, but psychosis was still more disturbing:

And the post-traumatic stress disorder, I was like, "OK, you know that I have that," but then psychosis, I started thinking about Andrea Yates, 'cause she had psychosis and all kinds of stuff and she killed her kids. And them telling me I had PTSD—'cause I was telling him, when I see stuff on TV like about molestation I start feeling weird, I start feeling very uncomfortable and like grossed out. My body actually feels grossed out too. They're telling me that that's the PTSD, I never realized that that's why I felt like that ever since it happened to me. So, that's another thing that I realized at [the hospital this time]. When I first was there I just didn't really care, I just kind of said whatever I had to say to get out of there, but this time I was like really in it. Participating in all the groups and you know, talking with the therapists and stuff like that, it really helped me.

This account of the most recent hospitalization includes a series of developments that appear to give Maria satisfaction and describe her engagement in the therapeutic process: thinking through the implications of depression and psychosis, coming to understand the diagnosis of PTSD in a way that corresponds with how she feels on a bodily level about having been sexually molested, consolidating her appreciation of psychiatric medication despite its side effects, being in denial of troubles she has been through, and, for once, fully engaging group and individual therapy.

Again, in the case of Maria, we see a young woman whose trajectory through multiple hospitalizations cannot be understood merely as a continued series of setbacks—she learned progressively and incrementally how to take advantage of the help offered there. This included learning to use and value "coping skills":

> [What I learned most from those places is] probably coping skills. I still use those. I always try to find new ones. When I am really depressed, they told me, crying can be one of your coping skills. If you need to cry, you cry. But then again, I find myself crying too much and then it just . . . gets worse. Also going for a walk. Just playing with my son. Playing with my son helps a lot 'cause he just makes me happy no matter what. I still love to write. Writing has always been one of my coping skills. I have always been into poetry. I used to share a lot of my poetry there with everybody. And, as I got older, my poetry started being, it's less dark and . . . like, suicidal and stuff like that. Because I was in that phase, where I was writing suicidal poetry and drawing scary pictures of people hanging and bleeding and stuff like that. It's really kinda scary stuff.

Although exposure to so many different institutions created stressful instability, Maria had the internal resources to learn by making comparisons and evaluations across her experiences at these diverse treatment centers. Motivated in part by fear of being separated from her son, her trajectory traced an arc from reckless behavior in the hospital, with only the gesture of going along with a treatment plan in order to get discharged, to what appeared to be a reflective engagement with therapeutic process that included an understanding of the implications of her diagnoses, the value of psychiatric medication, and the usefulness of coping skills.

"Wow, Maybe I Do Have Issues"

Amy, a shy fifteen-year-old Anglo-American girl diagnosed with bipolar disorder, had a treatment trajectory complicated by a tendency to run away from wherever she was. She underwent nine inpatient admissions at five separate facilities punctuated by a period in TFC, and finally was accepted into a group home. Her mother described this trajectory:

> Um, the first one was [a residential facility], which was crap. The staff didn't care, most of the people who worked there seemed to be gang-affiliated themselves. It was very, very poorly run, and her therapist and me didn't get along because you couldn't find two people more from different worlds. And at that time, she wanted me to put her in treatment foster care and I was like, "No way, I'd never do that." [That place] wasn't real effective. She ran away from there, they got her back, she was in the partial, and they were getting high outside and smoking cigarettes and having sex outside, you know, at the treatment center. Not good. And so, the next one was [a residential facility]. It was very, very structured, very clinical, very hospital-like—the only problem was it's in Las Cruces, so it was really hard being that far away. We went down there, of course, a few times to visit and have a few sessions. Weekly, we had conference-call therapy sessions and, um, she did well there. [Insurance stopped covering that.] Of course, she deteriorated a month after she got out. Then [another residential facility] was OK except it was too easy to run away from. She went to party. She ran away from there with another girl and they went somewhere in the South Valley and stayed with some guy and didn't do much of anything. Oh, she decided—that's what she did—pierced her tongue. Herself! [*laughs*] I couldn't get her to go back at the time, and being wimpy as I was, I just let her come home and just said, "OK, let's try it again." And that was a year ago and it's been downhill ever since. [She's been here at CPC for acute visits] I think about four times. It is well run, people care, and, you know, since we've done this so many times, I told them when she came in, "I want to be part of this, because she's my daughter and I've been caring for her for years and I'm her main caregiver." And they call me and make me aware and discuss it. I think they're doing a really good job all things considered. And it's safe. It's very safe. I mean, you don't see kids running around getting high or carrying on. I wish their food selection was a little better. It's not very healthy. And she's got a massive weight problem and the food is not healthy. I think they need to work on the nutrition part of it, but that's minor, I guess, in the scheme of things.

Initially Amy did not like CPC. She described her experience as follows, while acknowledging that it was better than her first inpatient experience:

> I think people try to help and they don't really know how to help here. And they just think they know it all and they really don't. [They could be] listening to my part in it, you know, instead of my parents' part in it and listening to me 'cause I'm the one who has the issues. And they don't really do that. I think the best one that I was in was [another treatment facility]. They actually listened and they helped and they . . . not everything is my fault that I've been through, and, some of the things that my parents say are not always correct. I don't think [my therapist here] is the best therapist in the world, she doesn't listen to me. She kinda listens more to my parents and like, I'm the one with

the issues. . . . I can follow the rules, but sometimes, you know, the staff here are kinda mean and they just, they're mean. [But] I've been to, like, a really crappy treatment center before and that was [yet another residential facility] and they don't do nothing there. Here's a little better, but, I don't know, I don't really like it. There [it] was kind of ghetto and this is more, like high class-ish. I haven't been here for a real long time, so I don't know if it's going to help me or not. I've gotten in more trouble since I've been off of it here. I guess I'm rude and just mean and stuff, but I don't really see it. I got a 91 last night. I don't know how, 91 out of 100. So, if you get below 90 you're no privs, that means that you have to stay in your room for free time and stuff. So, I got a 91, close to no privs, and I just don't get why.

At this point in her interview, Amy began to complain about being disciplined for rudeness to her peers and for not being social. She said that was stupid and that she would prefer being told what she was doing wrong rather than having points taken away, because "like, how am I ever supposed to learn like that? [Peers] bug sometimes 'cause being with other people who have issues and living with them, it just bugs sometimes." Rudeness on the part of staff was a parallel theme as Amy narrated the loudness of a staff member while she was talking on the phone to her mother. When she asked the person to please be quiet, the staff member "just blew up on me and got kind of mad and said that she has other people to deal with and she can't help it if she's loud or not and it just made me mad. It was stupid." Amy felt like she had to "bite my tongue" and suppress a response even though in a therapeutic environment one should not have to do so. "You're supposed to, like, tell them what's going on, but I'm afraid to 'cause they're just rude. I swear, they're so rude. I don't even know why."

By the time of her second interview, Amy had changed her mind about CPC in a way directly relevant to her understanding of and engagement in therapeutic process. She thought it had provided her most effective treatment to date, and was explicit about this in remarking that "I know I said some pretty horrible things about it when you first interviewed me there. [But I] got a lot more support. People actually cared. There were a lot of people to talk to. It wasn't just one person. A lot of support and understanding." Her mother concurred, saying, "I think because of everything that has happened, we've been there so much and we had begged and begged for help for so long, um, there were a few doctors who actually, personally really do care. And they made a definite personal effort, you know. I think that made a real difference."

In the course of Amy's treatment trajectory, she spent a period in TFC. Her mother reported that several potential families had rejected her after reviewing her dossier, to which the girl's response was "That sucked. It was like, 'Wow, maybe I do have issues.' You know. It was a pain. And then finally I got the right family." Her mother was frank in the assessment that she and her husband needed the respite of TFC. Speaking shortly before the placement began, she said:

> After her last admission, the reality was "Either you make the effort and do what you have to do or your parents won't be able to maintain you at home." The community family team, C-F-T, came to the house and we were getting nowhere and we discussed that treatment foster care is probably the next step. Amy understood that but she deteriorated and wouldn't make an effort. Also, I'm at the end of my rope. I can't do it. I cannot maintain her at home. I cannot do whatever she needs to get her to function. I'm not equipped for it. And it's not fair to the rest of my family, especially my son. . . . [I feel] like crap. I feel horrible. I don't want it to be this way. I wish I didn't have to. See, since the beginning, I've always asked every doctor, every therapist, just tell me what I do to deal with her and her behavior. And I've done everything they've told me. 'Cause they don't know. You know, every little project they've given us to do, we've done. She didn't but we did. If she would decide—I mean, I know she's sick, but she's not incapable. If she owned her own illness and owned her own emotions, realized she had some power in this, I think that would make a big difference. I don't think anyone else at this point can do anything but her. And she knows the system *really* well. So she knows how to play that as well. But right now, she's a little unstable to play anything, 'cause she's been off the lithium and they just started her on lithium and Adderall today . . . at this point, she's not functioning. She's not OK. And whether she can make it in a family or in a regular home-based program, I don't know. Your guess is as good as mine. But what I saw today, she's not OK. . . . [My husband feels] horrible. But we have no choice. We just wish this wasn't our reality, but at home it's too difficult. I mean, we've taken two vacations since she's been gone and we never could have taken vacations because we just couldn't take her anywhere. Her behavior is too embarrassing and it's too high maintenance and she can't relax and just have fun. I don't think she even knows how. Unless we lavish her with gifts—then she's good. That makes her happy.

The final arrangements were made during a meeting at CPC in which all parties discussed whether the placement would work. Amy's mother was impressed at how "they really tried to match her, they just didn't pick anybody from the clear blue sky. So they really try to make it work." Amy herself expressed both awareness and apprehension of what lay ahead:

> It's just like the last resort. The last option. We've never tried it before, so yeah. I don't want to. But since I'm going, I might as well make the best of it anyway. I don't want to live with some other family that's not my own but

before I came in here [to CPC], we talked about it and I guess I was supposed to come in here and then go to a TFC. [It makes me] nervous. . . . [I met the family yesterday.] They kinda bothered me. Well, I liked Martha, who's the mom. She's pretty cool. They're old. Old people and don't do a whole lot. They sit around and kinda do stuff in the house. But the dad kept on telling me about this ex-patient from just before me, everything he would tell me he would relate to her. Yeah, like he doesn't care about anybody's sexual orientation, 'cause she was a lesbian and even though she wasn't his real daughter he would say she was his real daughter. I don't know, that's some stuff I didn't really need to know, but. . . . Yeah, actually they live [practically] right across the road from my house so if I ever got mad I could run away to my house, but I wouldn't do that. For thirty days I am not allowed to talk to my parents, which is going to be really hard. But if I do good in the first two weeks that I'm there, I can talk to them in those two weeks. I don't know if I'll make it, honestly . . . I hope [I do] so I don't have to come back to these places [inpatient facilities]. Teaching me rules, like in the house, so when I go home it'll be just doing my chores and stuff.

Particularly striking in this situation is the expression of frustration combined with care on the part of Amy's parents. Equally striking is Amy's self-reflectiveness combined with evident attachment to her family and uncertainty about whether she can "make it" in the next stage of her treatment trajectory.

We were able to interview Amy eight months later, after her term in TFC—which, although expected to last six to nine months, ended up totaling only three months. She reported that her attitude became more positive after the first month and that

it was pretty interesting because they had two kids, one was four, one was five. The five-year-old was an autistic boy. So, it was really kind of interesting. You know, I got to see an outlook on somebody else's life. 'Cause being autistic is not easy. You know, I mean, we'd go places and [the boy] would freak out because he felt so nervous and stuff. And then the girl was growing up with an autistic brother, so she was a handful, too. But it was pretty interesting. I got to see how other people lived, who I didn't even know and I got to come live in their house. It was like, uh, a life-changing experience. . . . I went on passes a lot. My mom came to visit me a lot . . . it started out on the weekend. Sunday for a few hours, and then it would be all day Sunday and then we gradually transitioned into spending the night at the house. And then we'd follow up in the family group how that went. . . . [Beforehand] I didn't want to go. Oh, God, I hated the idea. I hated everybody. Whoever wanted me to go, I just hated them. But it turned out really good. I got to see what it's like to live with a new family. You know, people I didn't know. And I got to see what it's like for someone who has way more issues than I do deal with their issues. And how everybody has struggles, 'cause, um, it was pretty hard in that family, 'cause they had an autistic son and their daughter was just a raging ball of fire. I saw a whole bunch of things. I met new people in school. I've just got so much support. And the family was so different from us because they're real quiet—not real interactive. And we're pretty lively.

Amy's ability to reflectively compare family environments appears to have made a real difference, especially with respect to "someone who has way more issues than I do." For her family, the test came with how they together handled the stress of moving to a new house shortly after she came home from TFC. Amy saw it this way:

> It was interesting because I just found out we were moving and, uh, I was so excited because I wanted a new start. That's why we cut my hair and, like, did all that stuff. Just for a new beginning. And it worked out great . . . [but it was] stressful! Oh, my gosh. Everybody getting mad at each other. It was hard to come home to that, well, it wasn't really horrible, but everybody was kinda mad and so stressed out. And it was a test, I think. Like, God put me through that test just to see if I could handle it and I did. We made it. We're all still alive. We didn't kill each other, so . . .

While not killing each other may seem like a low standard, there is no denying that relocating a household can be maximally stressful even for a smoothly functioning family.

By the time of her final interview, Amy had progressed to treatment in a group home, which in her view surpassed the effectiveness of CPC. She specifically distinguished between the hospital's contribution with respect to medication and what she understood as her treatment per se:

> [The group home] is very trustful, it's very down-to-earth. A lot of treatment centers these days, they tend to sugarcoat it and make it not really what you did a big issue, but here they help you more and that's a treatment center that's helped me. They don't sugarcoat it. If you do something wrong, they'll let you know you get in trouble for it. Like, you get grounded or something like that. . . . A lot of people run and go somewhere else. They don't usually come back. I was lucky they accepted me back [after I left], but a lot of people are there a couple of months and then leave. Three months' average and then leave or go home. [The length of time] is different on everyone's basis. It just depends on the person and how their treatment is. . . . The group home, you're in the world. They take you out. You do things like a job and stuff. You know, that's why when you get in trouble and they take things away it sucks. At CPC, you're just stuck in a little, little bubble. I mean nothing's really big. And yeah . . . CPC was one step in my journey. One stepping-stone that made me come to this point. CPC also helped me with the medication thing, it didn't really help me with the treatment, but they got me on the right medication, the right path. They took me off my lithium to see where I was, all my meds, to see if I was, if everything was working and oh! It was working! Oh

my gosh, I don't know it's kinda like how I was in jail [juvenile detention] without the lithium. I was just like, "Ahh!" I was very emotional and stuff. And that's how I get when I'm off my lithium, but when I was in jail, it was ten times worse but at CPC I was just like, "Ahh!" so aggravated and so irked. They helped me with the med part and when I was manic and stuff, that is what it was there for, and it helped me with that, getting stable again, but the [group home] was the real treatment center to help me with everything. I wasn't really ready [to develop coping skills at CPC]. [The group home] made me come to terms with a lot of things, not just the med thing. I had the med thing down, I just needed that other part. I think I came to terms, they just pushed. I don't really honestly know how to explain it. It is just something that kind of happened and, you know, I was ready for myself to change.

Amy acknowledged that adjusting to the new environment was really hard. Noting that she was currently on a pass to see her family, with plans to return that night, she said that things were in fact wonderful, that she saw everything in a different light, and that things were going to change for the better. "It made me one with myself. It made me realize who I am and that I can't change who I am, but I can be a good part of who I am, you know what I mean? I don't have to be bad, I don't have to do bad things. I can be me in a good way." This had come about because they had taught her and talked to her, but she also had to learn it herself. Although she hated the place at first, she had to

come to terms with myself and teach myself that I can't be bad, it hurts my family. And I guess you can say I opened my eyes a lot more than I had been. . . . I think now that I am on the right kind of meds, I think meds have a lot to do with it . . . [but] it's not all the medication, it's yourself has to do with it too. I think it's more yourself than the medication.

In this respect she said she had learned to take the initiative to talk to someone, to relax, and to calm herself, as well as to initiate contact with her psychiatrist about her medication.

I take on—what is that word? *Assertiveness* for myself and make sure either if it's my meds or if it's me, I talk to someone. I use my own coping skills: I take a break, I relax, I lay down, I think about something else. I walk out, go outside, something to take my mind off of—or talk to someone if I need to talk to someone. I just realized that it helps so why not use it when you feel like you're going crazy? My treatment is so different from a lot of the others and I taught myself that. They teach the kids to realize what they are doing and to, you know, their behaviors are not OK. For me, I know my behaviors already and it's like what I need to do to prevent myself from slipping. That's what my treatment is, to learn how I can prevent myself from falling.

Amy's mother concurred with her positive assessment of the group home, saying that

> they have really been wonderful and they take a personal interest in Amy and that really means a lot to me. And they don't let her get away with crap. I mean, there's no excuses [like] a lot of other treatment centers. It's not the idea that "well, you're crazy. You're bipolar, you know, poor baby, it will be OK, you know. Here, take a med." It's like, "Take your meds, you have a problem, but if you don't take control of your problem, your problem takes control of you." Bipolar is no longer an excuse. Because if she did something wrong, she wouldn't take responsibility, saying, "Oh, my bipolar is kicking in." You know, it's like, come *on* . . . she cycled constantly [*imitates sound of bouncing*]. She'd make my head spin. And the dangerous behavior."

Amy was articulate regarding the influence of peers in the therapeutic milieu of the group home, reminiscent of her earlier comment about the challenge of living with other youth who also have "issues":

> Oh my gosh! It's drama, you know? Because it's so, because the way the facility is so down-to-earth that people take advantage of things and it's just a lot of drama. I'm not in that drama [but] a lot of times my name comes up in the drama and I think that's because I am there and I'm a leader. I mean, I have done bad things too, but the people there are drama. A bunch of girls, I live with twelve girls and plus there are eighteen boys on the other side, plus staff. . . . When I don't work, on weekends, it's pretty laid back, you know? We go places. People just hang around and sleep. We do chores in the morning and we do it at night. We sweep or clean on Saturdays. The weekdays, people, they go to school. People there, you know, who are still in school. I took my GED, so I don't go to school. The people wake up, do chores, get ready, go to school, that's pretty much it. Come back, do chores, we go to NA [Narcotics Anonymous] on Wednesdays . . . usually the people that come in there are all, "Oh my god, I hate this!" They'll go to their rooms, slam doors. After they calm down, I think that's a day later, that's when Mr. Jake comes in and he will talk to you, "What do you think you did wrong? Why'd you do that?" They let them blow it all out before they talk to them and I think that helps too instead of trying to calm down. If it gets to a point where they are punching holes in the wall and stuff, they'll calm them down and stop them, but the whole thing is they have to come to terms with themselves, why they are acting like that and then after they will ask you, but I think that helps people too, you know. Not just "Oh, are you OK?" You know? [My new roommate is] also from Albuquerque and she, she doesn't have her shit together; she wants to run, she wants to go away and I'm like, "That's up to you. You can do what you want to do." She's been in jail since she was thirteen, she's now fifteen and she been in jail, in and out. I try to be the voice of reason, I can't always, it's them who have to help themselves.

After a month in the group home Amy had cycled into a manic episode and went, as she said, "on the run." Her mother explained that she had been doing well enough to move to an independent-living building next door, which is the next step to freedom, but which was too much for her daughter—she expressed this by imitating the sound of a rocket taking off. Amy described a house of four residents, each with her own room, commenting that

> a lot of people don't make it through independent. We just had a girl not that long ago come back from independent because she left the house and smoked weed and stuff, so it's not for everyone. I mean, you make your own food and you do your own thing but a lot of people aren't ready for it. I was in independent. They said that if I didn't get a job and do my things right, because I was starting to slip again, that they would put me back in the group home and I was like, I can't go back, so that's when I ran. Now I'm not in independent, I am back in the group home, but it's the best thing.

Despite her reflexivity and insight, and despite ongoing support from her family, Amy's struggle to have a life endured. Perhaps more clearly than with any of our other interlocutors, her treatment trajectory was characterized by alternation between advances that she felt were genuine and setbacks that were beyond her control.

A WORLD OF TROUBLE

While they are inpatients, the youth with whom we have become acquainted are confined within an institutional milieu that has a distinct architectural space and temporal regime. They are within an interpersonal milieu populated by staff, peers, and occasional visitors. They are also within a rhetorical milieu characterized by a discourse of diagnosis, medication regimes, psychotherapy, behavioral management techniques, and coping skills. We have seen how adolescents moving through the inpatient psychiatric treatment system are often able to compare and evaluate the facilities in which they are placed and to make observations about how helpful or unhelpful they may have been. At times these comparisons are somewhat predictable, such as which places had better food or more pleasant rooms. Our interlocutors were also willing to observe which places had stricter rules or meaner staff—consequential insofar as there is more contact with staff than with clinicians and insofar as everyday routines can create positive structure and stability or be experienced as oppressive. Occasionally comparison included which places were easier to run away from, regardless of whether a youth was able to articulate why she or he might choose to run, or whether the youth was running away to get back home or to get away from the institution. Interaction with peers is another critical feature of the treatment milieu. The density of the inpatient population and how many children shared a room are not insignificant, but it was also evident that some facilities were perceived to have tougher, more "hardcore" youth or "gangsters," and occasionally a participant indicated that other kids seemed to have "more issues" than him or herself. The influence of peers ranged from their being sources for learning self-destructive behaviors, to people with whom one could talk about shared problems, to people with whom they had made friends regardless of whether they ever saw one another after they left the hospital.

The treatment trajectories of these youth often pass through a number of different settings. Each treatment form along the continuum of care structures lived experience by creating a distinct kind of subjective polarity, with the home environment as a point of reference, and each has a distinct temporality defined by duration of separation from the home environment. Hospitalization creates a polarity between mutually exclusive locations, where admission and discharge mark a boundary of accessibility between home and hospital. The duration of separation is defined by acute versus residential admissions, and the trajectory can span a range of facilities public and private, sometimes far from home. Treatment foster care creates a polarity between family milieus, one ostensibly healthy and the other either unhealthy or at least temporarily incapable of sustaining the troubled youth. The standard duration of TFC is six to nine months, but it may be only another stop along the treatment trajectory rather than a step toward return to the family of origin. Living in a group home creates a polarity between peers and parents as primary reference group and, to a certain extent, between autonomy and authority. The duration is indeterminate and the next step on the trajectory is undetermined, be it home, independent living, or rehospitalization. Outpatient treatment creates a polarity of departure and return: going out to a therapy appointment and then returning home. The duration of separation is only for the length of the therapy session, and there may be no separation at all in the case of family therapy. All of these settings are explicitly *therapeutic* and stand in polar contrast not only to the youth's home but also to both the *carceral* alternative of juvenile detention, which many of the young people face because of having been arrested by the police, and to the *peda-*

gogical alternative of school where many of them are engaged only irregularly, often not at grade level, and sometimes without the continuity of being in the same school from one year to the next.

The ethnographic importance of mobility among treatment forms as a trajectory and not just a shuffling of persons from one place to another is highlighted by recalling that home is not merely one of the stops on this trajectory. Tapping into narrative intersubjectivity by juxtaposing accounts from adolescents and their parents/guardians helps remind us of the primacy of home as the existential point of reference for hospitalized youth. Critical here are convergence or divergence of parent/guardian accounts with patient accounts, as well as issues of family dynamics and sibling relations. In this respect, an additional note about treatment foster care is in order. TFC is not just an alternative to an orphanage or a partial remedy for abandonment. The other family in TFC is not a surrogate or replacement but a mirror, a touchstone, and a point of comparison. It is not only implicitly an example of how family life should be lived but also a way of introducing perspective into the therapeutic process, creating a kind of stereoscopic vision of what a family is by concretely introducing the awareness that not all families are the same. It invites comparison and hence engenders reflection as the troubled adolescent becomes not just the object of treatment but the subject in observation of his or her new surroundings. It is both a time out, in the sense of a respite from conflict and stress in the family of origin, and an initiation into possibility as new patterns of relationship, rule, affection, and activity are superimposed on the pattern that had become taken for granted by the child.

In introducing this cohort of youthful psychiatric inpatients in chapter 1, we saw a wide range of household composition and socioeconomic conditions. The final additional factor we will observe here is that the emotional and interpersonal milieu of these households not infrequently includes the *presence of siblings and parents/guardians who experience emotional distress, psychiatric disorder, or physical illness.* Among the adolescents who participated in our study, twenty-four (51%) had parents/guardians who reported that they had some kind of illness. Twenty-three of these parents/guardians reported mental illness in particular, and among those, sixteen endorsed depression, including four who reported suicidal ideation. In three families both parents reported mental illness of some form. Furthermore, nineteen (40%) of the adolescents had one or more siblings who either were diagnosed with mental illness or had been in therapy. Given constraints of space and the limitations of our data, we can only point to the complex significance in lived experience of such overlapping and crisscrossing treatment trajectories. Likewise, we can only point to the degree to which parents/guardians can become overwhelmed and fatigued by the demands of care (Danely 2017; Kleinman 2019). This is a circumstance we have noted several times in passing, and it is especially salient in households burdened with multiple members who are troubled. It deserves respect, empathy, and recognition as an intimate part of a family's experience of psychiatric treatment.

Hospital treatment can be disorienting for patients and parents alike, insofar as institutional environments differ, the length of stay may be unclear or indeterminate, and a diversity of staff, therapists, and other clinicians come into play. Such disorienting influences are likely to be exacerbated given preexisting instability in life circumstances and severity of illness. The accounts of treatment trajectory we have provided in this chapter deal with issues of lived experience not often enough brought into focus in trying to understand the lives of troubled adolescents. Examining treatment trajectories also serves to expand the scope of therapeutic process well beyond what happens in therapy sessions and to understand it as a profound modulation of everyday life. Family separation, residential instability, interpersonal flux, diagnostic uncertainty, gaps in the continuity of care, becoming accustomed to new therapists, and changing medication regimens are all critical to whether afflicted youth have a chance at getting better as they move toward adulthood. In chapter 6 we will look explicitly at the future as a temporal horizon and the prospects of having a life for these troubled young people.

Having a Life

I am just the kind of person who always has hope. I mean, when he first gets in trouble, or starts getting bad, I lose that, but it always comes back.

—mother of Ted

As we all are saying, they hoped she wasn't too old to change . . . I was more hopeful and less not hopeful, but now I'm like fifty-fifty, because, excuse me, I'm afraid. I don't want her to be like her father [deceased] . . . I didn't want her to wind up dead at the beach because she just can't stand her life anymore . . . it's gonna be hard, you know, cause she's still fighting things too much so—cross my fingers and hope.

—mother of Nadine

I'm hoping that this, with these people, they're helping him out.

—grandmother of John

Throughout this book, we have attempted to portray the lived experience of troubled youth and their families against the background question of the kind of life they have, what it means to have a life that is severely disrupted, and what it takes to have a life. We have examined the social context of treatment, the family milieu of youth and their families, the episodes that bring them to inpatient treatment, the way they define their problems, the powerful force of anger in the lives of many of them, and their treatment trajectories through the mental health care system. What remains is to ask what we can discern from their own subjectivity—the structure of their experience as expressed in how they talk about that experience (Jenkins 2015a; Csordas and Jenkins 2018)—about the prospects for their developmental trajectory toward adulthood. In this respect, a critical element of having a life is having a sense of the future—or more precisely a sense that there is a future. Our analysis suggests that the most relevant issues are (1) how hope and worry are articulated in the immediate present and (2) how their temporal orientation defines a foreclosed or open developmental horizon. The manner in which these issues point to the possibility of "having a life" is our topic in this final chapter.

We have seen that even some of the most distressed and developmentally challenged youth can exhibit reflectiveness about their problems and the extraordinary conditions in which they live. One strategy for identifying how they orient to their futures is to determine what they worry about. In table 8, we present results from the Adolescent Health Survey (see appendix) showing the most common worries reported by adolescents in the study. Most striking is that the two leading worries (in terms of the proportion who worry quite a bit or very much about these issues) are loss of a best friend (51.1%) or a parent dying (50.0%), while the two worries endorsed least often have to do with personal tragedy (dying soon, 23.3%; getting HIV/AIDS, 23.3%). Worries about personal appearance ("my looks," 48.9%; being overweight, 34.9%) and peer perceptions (how well other kids like me, 37.2%) are also prominent. Economic concerns are among the prominent worries (my family not having enough money, 44.2%; getting a good job when I'm older, 37.2%). Worries about the broader society are also represented (all the people who are poor and hungry, 34.9%; violence in our community, 27.9%). There are two critical points in evaluating these results. On the one hand, we can infer that issues of loss, violence, and death are closely connected with the emotional distress that is so prominent in their lives as psychiatric inpatients, even if not in an overtly causal way. On the other hand, identifying these worries reminds us that for them there are issues of concern that go beyond their illness experience per se—or, to put it another way, that the scope of their concerns and apprehensions are not limited to their symptoms and treatment.

THE CHALLENGE OF HOPE

Preoccupation with worries may dampen possibilities for hope among these adolescents. Their narratives rarely speak directly about hope; however, this is a complex and subtle matter for interpretation insofar as, for

TABLE 8   WORRIES EXPRESSED BY ADOLESCENT PARTICIPANTS $(N = 47)^a$

	n	%
I worry about losing my best friend		
Not at all	11	25.6
Very little/somewhat	10	23.3
Quite a bit/very much	22	51.1
I worry about one of my parents dying		
Not at all	9	21.4
Very little/somewhat	12	28.6
Quite a bit/very much	21	50.0
I worry about my looks		
Not at all	13	30.2
Very little/somewhat	9	20.9
Quite a bit/very much	21	48.9
I worry about my family not having enough money		
Not at all	7	16.3
Very little/somewhat	17	39.5
Quite a bit/very much	19	44.2
I worry about how well other kids like me		
Not at all	9	20.9
Very little/somewhat	18	41.9
Quite a bit/very much	16	37.2
I worry about not getting a good job when I'm older		
Not at all	12	27.9
Very little/somewhat	15	34.9
Quite a bit/very much	16	37.2
I worry about all the people who are hungry and poor		
Not at all	13	30.2
Very little/somewhat	15	34.9
Quite a bit/very much	15	34.9
I worry about being overweight		
Not at all	19	44.2
Very little/somewhat	9	20.9
Quite a bit/very much	15	34.9
I worry about the violence that happens in our community		
Not at all	14	32.6
Very little/somewhat	17	39.5
Quite a bit/very much	12	27.9
I worry about dying soon		
Not at all	13	30.2
Very little/somewhat	20	46.5
Quite a bit/very much	10	23.3

TABLE 8   *(continued)*

	n	%
I worry about getting HIV/AIDS		
Not at all	22	51.1
Very little/somewhat	11	25.5
Quite a bit/very much	10	23.3

ᵃNot all participants completed all items on the Adolescent Health Survey (Resnick, Blum, and Harris 1989). N may be less than 47 for some items; percentages are based on number reporting for each item.

a variety of reasons we discuss further below, these youth may not easily or consciously be able to articulate it. Overtly, it is primarily the parents and guardians who engage in discourse about hope. While the theme of hope is in no way exhausted by overt and literal use of the words "hope" or "hopeful," it is useful to focus on circumstances in which parents speak about it explicitly. We must be cautious in assessing the significance of word use, however, both insofar as absence of the word does not mean absence of hope (see below) and in distinguishing between when the word is used spontaneously and when it is uttered in response to its use by an interviewer. In this respect, responses are not necessarily entrained by the interviewer's word choice, as in this exchange between Amy and her interviewer about the upbeat prospects of returning home to live:

OK. So you sound really hopeful.
AMY: I am very hope—I am very excited.

Even the most direct and "leading" query can lead in a variety of directions and pertain to the immediate or more distant future, to hopes circumscribed by the illness or hopes that point farther ahead beyond it. For example:

So what are your hopes for Alex?
ALEX'S MOTHER: Hoping that they could find a medicine that is going to keep him somewhat stable—at least that he's not that aggressive. But him getting better? I don't see it happening. They would have to come out with like a miracle drug and up to right now, there is no such thing. All the medications they have put him on, from what they've told me, um, most adults don't take those dosages.

In this instance, "hoping" appears faint at best and the response is an occasion for the boy's mother to comment sharply on the prospects of her son's improvement and the efficacy of psychopharmaceutical treatment. Specific inquiry about hope leads in an unexpected direction in a response by the grandmother of another youth:

What do you hope for your family now?
SELENA'S GRANDMOTHER: That they live a long life instead of running away. I wish I could run away. I said to myself, I said, one of these days, I'm gonna run away. But, you know you will run away when you die. Then you run away. But I'm not gonna do it any time soon. Because they still need me.

Given these caveats about the possibility of gaining insights on the theme of hope from the interview format, it was more typically the case that reference to hope emerged integrally in our conversations. Let us examine further how these interlocutors spoke of hope.

Diego's mother speculated about prospects for her son's recovery (from severe psychosis) in terms of hope: "I have a feeling it may be ongoing. And might be lifetime. But I have real hope that it's temporary. I am hoping it's not permanent, but I guess, you know . . . I think about it a lot. And I guess my biggest worry is working." "Permanent" and "temporary" here define two potential states of a temporal and developmental horizon that determine whether illness is ultimately experienced as an interruption or as an integral element of life, and whether productivity in the form of the basic ability to hold a job is in question. This mother elaborates as follows, later in the same interview:

I shouldn't live with "what if, what if, what if?" Right now, we are just taking each day as it is. I can't plan anything, because I never know when . . . has he gotten better since the last time? Oh, definitely. I hope he never goes back to the way he was before. I don't know. I try not to feel guilty, because I know I couldn't deal by myself. And I keep telling myself that. But honestly, I feel like it's never gonna go away and in the same token he doesn't have to get an education.

In this passage hope constitutes not a horizon but a plateau; it is a hope not of going forward but of not going back, and she embraces the sense of permanence not as a worry about her son's future ability to work but as an acceptance that he may not complete his education.

A mother spoke following her daughter Anne's hospitalization for a suicide threat, using "hope" in three ways at different places in the same interview:

I don't know if you just got to wait and hope for the best, and I don't have a lot of faith in it really, to tell you the truth, in her having a normal life. . . . We're just going to have to wait and see with Anne. Like, I don't know. Have to just, go with the flow, I guess. Hope for the best . . . I'm not sure. It doesn't seem—I don't know, I'm just here waiting. I'm hoping one of these days the light bulb is going to come on and she'll be OK. But as of right now, it's not on [*laughs*]. It's still dim! [*laughs*].

Lack of faith, going with the flow, and the lightbulb coming on are intriguing modulations of hope in the mode of ambivalence, where hope for the best is tempered by the possibility of the worst. Integral to this situation was not only a troubled child but also a severely vexed relationship between mother and daughter.

In the final interview, when the situation had improved, hope figured much more prominently and in a different register, and Anne's mother talked about how illness affected her daughter's educational progress as follows:

She lost a lot of hope and she dropped out, you know. She just started crying and telling me the truth about how she felt about school. She didn't want to let me down and stuff. And so we talked about it a lot and like now, it's like, you know, you're gonna get your GED. You have to be in classes for your GED. You have to have a job. You can't just be here, hanging out, you have to be doing something with your life. She came a long way; she's been doing really good.

Here hope plays a critical role as a mediator of the mother-daughter relationship and as a determinant of whether the future can be open or closed. Specifically, Anne dropping out of school is described neither as an effect of psychiatric symptoms nor as a function of laziness and lack of will, but as a result of losing hope. The implication is that hope can be domestically and intersubjectively managed, whereas dealing with symptoms and character traits may be beyond the capacity of the mother-daughter relationship. Hope played an additional role in the family dynamic, however, because the patient's father had also been diagnosed and struggled with mental illness, and he could not relate to his daughter with emotional intimacy. Anne's mother said, "I tell her, you know, 'Don't get your hopes up too high because your dad is as old as me, forty-one years old and still don't know love.' So we're hoping that by us helping him a little bit it will give him some kind of hope." Here again, hope appears as the crucial missing element that could be transformative. In a final variant, her daughter spoke in the same idiom of hope when referring to prospects for a younger cousin who had been sexually molested and was herself significantly troubled: "Mom told my auntie, 'I have hope because of Anne. Because Anne changed, I have hope that Linda can change.' And that just, that touched me a lot because even, all those bad things I went through, I can help somebody, you know? I can give hope to people who were like me." Seeing herself as a symbol of hope for others was based on her perception that she had succeeded over the course of two years and several hospitalizations in becoming a "different person."

Ambivalence is also thematic in the following words from the mother of another young girl, Jess:

> I am hoping that she does come out, you know, the way we think she should, but you know, I don't really have a really high expectation of that. I don't think she's, you know, she'll come out great the first few months or whatever, and she ends up going back to the same thing. So, maybe this long term will help her, you know, but I don't know, I really think that we're gonna end up being together the rest of our life, her and I, just trying to take care of each other. This is the thing. So. We'll see what happens.

In this instance ambivalence about the future is thematized as hope in explicit contrast with expectation, and the possibility of short-term improvement is framed by the likelihood of a long-term need by the troubled girl for continued care.

The parents of Kevin were evidently hoping not so much for their son's improvement as for some kind of help:

MOTHER: Well, that's where we're at, trying not to lose hope, trying to stay positive. We still haven't gotten any information on support groups for Asperger's from anybody that we've asked to meet with, there's . . .

INTERVIEWER: *Is that just because they're just not out there, or people just aren't giving you the information?*

MOTHER: People just aren't giving us the information yet.

FATHER: There's people out there.

For Kevin's parents there is a concrete horizon of hope, defined by the sense that there is information available somewhere, but a passive waiting for someone to provide that information.

The grandmother of Michael expressed hope for his improvement virtually in passing, focusing instead on the pragmatics and necessary tools for survival outside the hospital: "He's just not proactive in his recovery. And my figuring is Michael is gonna be eighteen in September. If I don't do anything now or at least give him the tools to get well, even if he doesn't get well when he comes out, which I hope he does, at least he will have these tools." Likewise, Samuel's mother had her hopes fixed on obtaining a specific kind of treatment, while expressing concern that her son must understand he needs to "do something": "One of the things that I want to see is that if we're going to be able to get that family therapy going maybe it'll help. In a way to get Samuel to understand that he needs to do something. So I'm, I'm hoping that that's gonna happen because I'm just scared that he's gonna go back to what— I mean, he was, he was terrible. I hope he sticks with this program." Both these examples direct hope to the availability of and access to treatment, while adopting the stance that recovery, or at least avoiding relapse, is contingent on a "proactive" use of "tools" and the intitative to "do something" and "stick with" a treatment plan.

For the mother of Ruben, the expression of hope was centered on access to the ideal and idyllic treatment center:

> It was a wonderful treatment center . . . and the only problem that we had was that he could only stay nine months. They only took kids up until a certain age, up until adolescence and it was borderline for him to even be admitted, but they went ahead and took him. It's a wonderful beautiful setting, not anything like [the hospital] where he started out, it was completely different and I felt such, such hope for him when I went there and met with them. And I just prayed and I hoped, kept my fingers crossed that they were going to accept him, they had to accept him. They had a waiting list. They used animals as part of the therapy for kids, actually adopting baby goats, at a certain time of the year. And so each child had their own baby goat to feed, to nurse and that helps with the trust issues and also being responsible for something, for the animal's well-being, and I can totally understand all that.

Aside from hopes about a promising therapeutic milieu, Ruben's mother also identified inner transformation as a target of hope. She recalled a violent episode in which her son punched a hole in a wall:

> He went outside and he was crying. And I remember sitting there and just thinking, I was just feeling so horrible and so bad and he came up to me and he said, "I am so sorry." And you know, there have been those moments when I truly believe. That's what gives me hope, for him, that he truly feels in his heart that "I'm sorry." He has never had empathy, never been able to put himself in someone else's shoes, or be sympathetic and caring. There has always been a little hidden agenda of his and what he wants. And that has been his driving force—"How will I benefit from that?"

This is one of the few instances in which hope is articulated explicitly in relation not only to overt behavioral change but to emotional connection, and here specifically with remorse and empathy. Recognizing her son as highly intelligent and manipulative, Ruben's mother finds hope in a moment she perceives as one of authentic emotional insight and responsibility on the part of her son.

Whether or not help is available and forthcoming, the possibility for change is another area of indeterminacy that can be outlined by the figure of hope. The mother of Nadine told us that

> if she's going to start all this [treatment] she needed to start when she was much younger and get more help when she was much younger, so I don't know particularly what's going to help her now and I don't want her to come to something where the state actually says she has to take medication or something but I hope not because I told mother I just want to make sure she stays out of jail and I don't know what's going to happen but I always like to say more of an almost scared straight type of thing [*laughs*]. She says she realizes one day she could accidentally really hurt someone. I'm still hopeful that she will go ahead and keep going and take, but on the other hand that she may slip sometimes and there may be years where she has to be on Social Security disability. I thought with mental illness it was like any other illness, like you had heart surgery then you rehabilitate, it may take a few months but then you're fine [*laughs*] but I said, it doesn't seem that with mental illness, it seems like she's always going to be rehabilitating type of thing and it takes a long time. I didn't think it took so long. I thought, OK, now she's cured [*laughs*] . . . I guess I'm 50 percent hopeful, 50 percent not hopeful because when I first found out I just thought OK there's a miracle cure, I'll give her some medication, she'll take it and then she'll be fine and she can go to cyber academy, she can catch up and still be graduating when she's supposed to and all that type of thing. . . . It's gonna be hard, you know, cause she's still fighting things too much so—cross my fingers and hope.

For Nadine's mother, hope is almost quantifiable, and one can envision a virtual hope meter with an indicator needle swinging between scalar ends of hopeful and hopeless. Immediately relevant to this configuration of hope are age limits beyond which the chances for improvement decline. Over the horizon of these age limits loom the possibilities of state-mandated medication and incarceration, the chances of finishing school or lapsing onto disability relief, the apparent impossibility of a miracle cure and the potentially disruptive effects of foster care, the mortal fate of her daughter's father (afflicted with bipolar disorder and passing on a genetic susceptibility), the need for the young woman to stay off drugs and on medication. It is hardly surprising that her discourse ends by suggesting, with the mention of crossed fingers, that her daughter's future is perhaps as much a matter of luck as of hope.

As in the preceding case, drugs also played a dominant role in the purview of John's grandmother:

> I'm just hoping he stays off of drugs. It's just a worry, a problem, just thinking that they're out there doing drugs. That's what scares me, that he'll come back and—the same guys that were giving it to him will start up again. I hope he thinks harder on his own and doesn't take anything that they give him because we're not always out there with him to know what's going on. . . . I'm hoping now that this, with these people, they're helping him out. He'll know what it is to have to do chores and do what he's supposed to do. And he'll come back doing that. Hopefully he still stays that way because they said he was really helpful over there, that he cleans his room, he's real good cleaning.

Compared to the mother of Nadine, who had been unaware that her daughter was smoking so much marijuana, this grandmother is aware of her grandson's life on the street and his exposure to people who provide drugs. What she has to say is balanced between hope for what he won't do (drugs) and what he will do (chores). For her the two are implicitly linked as the inverse sides of irresponsibility and responsibility.

The parents of Neal had a penchant for impassioned expression, and they had several children in the mental health system with rather dramatic problems. Hence the apparent incongruity when one of the boy's two mothers said, "It's been like a death of our dreams and our hopes, for the outcome of our children and our efforts have . . . really, probably, not changed much." In other words, they carried on caring for their children the same way, regardless of the death of their hopes. These parents were also uniquely attuned to the institutional convolutions of the mental health system and to the possibility that those might be addressed by the results of our study, such that we were drawn into the idiom of hope with the comment that "I just hope that something comes from this and somebody pays attention . . . and that eventually things change, because, you know, it means . . . lost families and . . . young people . . . not being able to realize their potential in the system as it is." In fact, despite the statement about the death of hope, this parent elsewhere was articulate about her hopes:

> I mean, my hope for my boys is that they'll get housing, they'll live independently to a certain extent, pursue some education interest or part-time jobs,

they'll get food stamps—and that's kinda sad when you are like, I really hope that happens [*laughing*] you know? But it's OK. I mean, I just want them to have some fulfillment. I want them to function to the best of their ability, and if that means that's what it is and they are happy, and they are safe and not hurting other people, then that's OK.

As for Neal, his only explicit articulation of hope was in response to the interviewer's query about whether, when he was discharged from the hospital, he expected to "get along better" with his parents: "I hope so. I can only hope so."

Ted's mother, when asked whether she had hope that things would get better, responded as follows:

> I am just the kind of person who always has hope. I mean, when he first gets in trouble, or starts getting bad, I lose that, but it always comes back. Sometimes that's a good thing, sometimes that's not such a good thing because I really get disappointed and hurt. It's a cycle and it's very hard for me. I have finally come to the realization that he's probably going to be ill for the rest of his life, to some degree. I really thought that he would grow out of a lot of the stuff, but I think I finally decided that it's not going to happen [*laughs slightly in a crying way*]. At this point, I just want him to go to college. . . . A lot of times, mental illness gets worse around your twenties. I hope it won't happen. I mean, if I thought that he was going to get worse or be unable to function, I don't know how I would do it. If that was the case, if I truly believed that, I would probably be wishing for his death. For his sake, not for mine. You know what I mean? Please just, rid him of all of the suffering.

This passage is striking in the stark contrast between the avowal of being a person who always has hope and the radical consequences envisioned if she ever lost that hope. It is equally striking to see the temporal scope of perpetual and terminal hope compressed into the more quotidian time frame of a cycle of losing and regaining hope based on whether her son gets in trouble or "starts getting bad." We also see here, for the first time, a relatively common variant of speculation about whether the illness is temporary or permanent, framed in terms of the possibilities that the child could "grow out of it" and that it can "get worse around your twenties." This particular iteration of hope is crowned by the poignant expression of desire, realistic or not, for the son to go to college. By the time of the final follow-up interview, his mother said, "I've just kind of lost hope on Ted being able to change very much," though this did not include giving up on the possibility that he might complete a GED, get a job, and eventually marry.

A final variant of hope was expressed by the adoptive father of Christopher: "I always have hopes for him. I mean, he could have a much worse diagnosis than what he has. What he does have is treatable. I mean, he could be schizophrenic bipolar." Treated clinically for depression, from our research diagnostic determination Christopher met threshold criteria not only for depression but also for PTSD, anxiety disorder, substance abuse, and psychotic disorder. In such an instance it could be argued that parental awareness of a comprehensive diagnosis might do less good by its presentation of knowledge than harm by its message of foreboding and overwhelming obstacles to well-being.

Risky and Roalistic Hope: Incongruous, Eclipsed, Panged, or Latent?

These accounts show that hope is more explicitly articulated by parents and guardians than by young people. How might we understand this? We might suggest either that the youth are not necessarily aware that hope is a relevant possibility or that the struggle between hope and hopelessness is not salient in a way that they can *consciously* articulate. After all, given the fragility of their conditions and circumstances, perhaps from their subjective social positions this is a realm of experience that they *dare not* articulate verbally. Perhaps the risks for future disappointments loom too prominently. Perhaps the risks of open defiance of parents, guardians, and other adults are too great should the youth simply state they cannot bear any more time in parental custody and are privately counting the days until they can legally flee and get out of town. Perhaps the psychological chasm of separating themselves from already fraught relations with their only known kin is so threatening that hopes and farewells are guarded tightly from all. Given our predominant reliance on narrative and observational ethnographic data, we can make no claim of knowing for certain. Another consideration is that these youth are not fully aware how precarious and serious their situations are in the absence of a stable or secure point of reference or comparison. Knowing how badly off you are, having a realistic sense of the problem or even that there is a problem, is a condition of possibility for hope coming into play in the first place. It would be myopic not to reiterate that thirty-two (68.1%) young persons had made a suicide attempt or had a preoccupation with suicide (see chapter 3: table 5). Relatedly, recall that the KID-SCID data showed the prominence of depression among this group (57.4% overall, 81.8% for girls, and 36.0% for boys), and that feelings of hopelessness often figure prominently in such formulations.

Other researchers have shown that children ages eight to thirteen who were psychiatric inpatients demonstrated that contrary to the "view that children may be unable to conceptualize the future well" (Kazdin et al. 1983: 505), "children's negative expectations of the future can be reliably assessed and are related to current psychopathology" (1983: 509). Based on standardized instruments, they determined that "suicidal children showed significantly greater hopelessness than nonsuicidal children" (1983: 508), while at the same time there were no significant differences between them and nonsuicidal children in depression and self-esteem. Yet another study showed that among a group of 180 formerly hospitalized adolescents, "both severity of hopelessness at hospitalization and greater expectations of later suicide attempts were associated with increased risk for posthospitalization suicide attempts" (Goldston et al. 2001: 94). Depression was a somewhat stronger predictor of later suicidal behavior than was hopelessness, but hopelessness was strongly predictive of posthospitalization suicide attempts among those who had attempted suicide previously (2001: 97). In contrast, "'reasons for living' serve as a protective factor against later suicide attempts" (2001: 98). To round out this picture, a third study showed that inpatient youth who rated high on hopelessness "tended to perceive their families and peers as providing little support, to express their anger overtly and aggressively, and to demonstrate more negative emotions than youngsters with low hopelessness scores" (Kashani et al. 1997). These quantitative studies indicate that there is indeed something at stake with respect to hope and hopelessness among youth who have been hospitalized. Yet for both the suicidal and the nonsuicidal study participants, the relation between hope and the possibility of a future cannot be exhaustively captured by such measurements.

Beyond whether adolesents and parents articulate or opt out of explicit talk about hope, there are a variety of ways in which hope is conceptually salient to the problem of having a life. A cognitive psychological approach to "hope theory" conceives of hope as the perceived capability to achieve goals, including a sense of successful agency in the form of goal-directed energy and the availability of pathways to those goals based on planning. Hope can be distinguished from optimism, self-efficacy, self-esteem, and problem-solving and can be measured as either a state or trait among both adults and children. In this conceptualization, hope is a way of thinking, with feelings and emotions being derivative and playing an important but contributory role (Snyder 2002; Snyder et al. 1997; Valle, Huebner, and Suldo 2006; McMillan et al. 2007; Venning et al. 2009). From the standpoint of educational sociology, implementing a "philosophy of hope" for marginalized youth includes cultivating a positive culture, a focus on possibility, a community of hope, and critical reflection (Te Riele 2010). Contemporary philosophers and social theorists have examined hope from a variety of positions (Marcel 1951; Bloch 1986 [1959]; Godfrey 1987; Rorty 1999; Harvey 2000; Zournazi 2002; Hage 2003; Badiou 2003; Waterworth 2004; Lear 2006; Eagleton 2015), ranging from reflections on the nature of hope as a human phenomenon or capacity, to hope in specific domains of human activity and endeavor, to hope on the macrosocial and political level for issues such as indigenous cultural survival and viable alternatives to capitalism.

The quotidian and limited versions of hope expressed by our interlocutors underscore our decision to cast this work at the scale of lived experience. The immediate context of hope and its frustrations is defined by everyday affliction and vexed interpersonal relations, as well as by the institutional constraints of managed care and the continuum of care within the mental health care system. Parents/guardians who participated in the study have also expressed critiques of the health care system in various ways, though we do not have space here to take these into consideration. In this respect, our concern with the immediacy of lived experience and the possibility of having a life under extraordinary conditions leads us to the small but significant anthropological literature on hope (Good et al. 1990; Crapanzano 2003; Miyazaki 2004, 2006; Zigon 2009; Mattingly 2010). This literature sometimes deals explicitly with suffering and illness experience, and even when engaged with broad sociopolitical issues it leans toward the immediate experience of concrete persons. We agree with Crapanzano's suggestion that hope is best understood not as an emotion, but instead as "an emotionally and morally toned descriptor of an existential stance or attitude" (2003: 26). If hope can be thought of in this way, what if we thought of anger—specifically of the all-consuming type we encountered among angry boys and girls in chapter 4—in the same way, as not only a moral emotion but as an emotionally and morally toned existential stance?

This would create an interpretive/existential axis between the burdened hope (with anger seldom expressed) of parents/guardians and the endemic anger (with a muted articulation of hope) of the adolescents.

In contrast to anger, one could argue that the reason hope remains inchoate among these youth is that one of hope's essential conditions of possibility is already having a life. In this view hope is "the temporal structure of the background attitude that sustains an already accomplished social life . . . [and] the fidelity to the social life trajectory on which one finds oneself" (Zigon 2009: 254, 262). Likewise, the manner in which people realize their own possible selves "depends very much on where and how they live, and who they already are" (Parish 2008: ix). From our standpoint, it is entirely problematic to say who the young people already are, or that they have anything like an already accomplished social life. Their troubled early life, their conditions of social precarity, and their illness itself can militate against both hope and selfhood.

If continued aspiration in the face of structural violence and foreclosed opportunity is a form of cruel optimism (Berlant 2011), one must also entertain the possibility that hope may not always be a positive thing. Working with African refugees in the United States, Haas (2017) goes beyond the evaluation of active versus passive hope to pose the question of whether there can also be a destructive hope. While struggling to sustain life in an immigration limbo, hope becomes "risky—and is potentially destructive—in that it disallows consideration of an alternative ending . . . the risk of hoping is not just psychic but existential. The disconnect between the object of hope—the granting of asylum, and the reality of the situation—a high probability of denial, renders hope itself precarious" (Haas 2019b). While the circumstances of mentally ill adolescents are different in many ways, they have to deal sometimes with otherwise reasonable hopes that for them may be unrealistic, and sometimes with delusional hopes that have little chance of coming to pass. None of this is to say that hope is futile for the cohort of adolescents we have introduced in this work. It is to suggest that research that may pick up where we leave off should be sensitive to the conditions of possibility for hope, and cognizant that although hope may be a positive existential stance, it is no solution in itself.

Particularly relevant to our concerns is anthropologists' identification of cultural dimensions of hope in cases of chronic illness. Although they deal specifically with adult oncology rather than adolescent mental health, Good and colleagues (1990) identify critical cultural features of the

American "discourse on hope." This includes a strong emphasis on will, such that "if one has enough hope, one may *will* a change in the course of disease in the body" (1990: 61). The theme of will is evident among our interlocutors, who not infrequently invoked their own need to take responsibility for their circumstances and adopt an active role in getting better. In chapter 2 we observed a variation of will in this sense among the Native American youth who, in a notably higher proportion than Anglo or Hispanic/Latinx young people, reported entering the hospital of their own volition. In Good and colleagues' discussion of cancer treatment, the clinical maintenance of hope also relies on the importance of *disclosing* the diagnosis (in contrast to masking it as in some other cultures, such as Japanese and Italian) in the context of a *partnership* between physician and patient. In this sense, a discourse on hope is linked to the prominence of what we have called the discourse of diagnosis among the study participants. From the standpoint of oncologists, instilling hope was important; yet for them hope was not necessarily a force that affects the course of illness but something to be "staged, given in calibrated, achievable, and realistic bits" relevant to quality of life, pain control, managing side effects, and consolidating the physician-patient relationship (Good et al. 1990: 72). This corresponds to another cultural feature of hope that we have analyzed in our data, namely that it is not understood as an abstract capacity or trait of hopefulness but in terms of specific and pluralizable hopes and dreams, hopes and fears, hopes and desires, hopes and prayers. One hopes that something good and nothing bad will happen.

In another anthropological account, Mattingly (2010) deals with the manner in which African American families with children who have serious chronic physical illness cultivate a "blues hope" characterized by a realism that transcends the polarity of pessimism and optimism. This form of hope is located not in biotechnical practices or discourses, but instead "in highly situated practices of people struggling to live with chronic medical conditions. Hope most centrally involves the practice of creating, or attempting to create, lives worth living even in the midst of suffering, even with no happy ending in sight" (2010: 6). This practice of attempting to create lives is an essential part of the struggle we have identified in the lived experience of our interlocutors, and is quite distinct from suggesting that they are in situations that can be summarily characterized as "tragic" or "sad" and about which we must "do something" to save them. Prior to lamentation or intervention, the spotlight we have focused on how the term "hope" appears in the ethnographic interviews allows us to understand it as contributing to the constitution of lived experience, a background condition of everyday ethos that may or may not be elaborated in practice or utterance.

What remains is to address the prospects for these young people of having a life by recognizing the narrative role of the future in the present. In this sense, narrative is not just the telling of a story or a recounting of the past, but part of constructing the present and conditioning a future. That which is spoken is, in itself, part of a narrative thread that weaves together, more loosely or more tightly, the fabric of a life. Mattingly's use of the phrase "narrative phenomenology" (2010: 41–45) includes a sense of "narrative" that refers to the narrativity that pervades the unfolding and understanding of events and action as well as the interplay of motives and motifs that promote or conspire against having a life, while her use of "phenomenology" corresponds to our specific concern for immediacy in the lived encounter with affliction and precarity. In the case of our interlocutors, listening for hints of a developmental and biographical trajectory beyond their trajectory through psychiatric treatment cannot simply be about their career plans (or absence thereof) and "what they want to be when they grow up." It must also be about how their words (and those of their parents/guardians) outline a temporal horizon of challenge and struggle. Such a stance allows us to observe, for example, how rare it is to hear reference to our young interlocutors as "disabled," a term that minimizes temporality, but how it is not uncommon to hear that they are "immature," a term with an inherent dimension of temporal unfolding. Outlining the struggle to have a life and articulate a future is the task we take up in the next section.

TEMPORAL HORIZONS: FROM ONE DAY AT A TIME TO STANDING BEHIND ONE'S GOALS

Although hope defines an existential stance, and hence an examination of hope allows us insight into who these young people are, our approach so far has been overtly literal in the sense of focusing on the words "hope" and "hopeful." We have noted that these are words used more often by parents than by their afflicted children, and that they are also sometimes used in stereotypical or rote expressions. We can broaden the scope to obtain a sense not only of hope but also of what might be in store for them, and when we take this step our ethnographic data allow an analysis that more strongly brings in the young people's sense of the physiognomy of the future, indeed of its possibility. This includes an understanding of how their future and its temporal horizon changed from one time to another over the course of our interviews. Such an analysis is of particular salience in a society such as that of contemporary North America, where orientation toward the future is a cultural value, where people don't stop thinking about tomorrow, and where a premium is placed on "looking ahead" and "moving forward."

Critical to evaluating the material that follows is the idea of a temporal horizon. Horizon is a perceptual metaphor common in phenomenological description and based on the literal horizon, which constantly recedes as we advance toward it. In the metaphorical sense, we can interpolate a horizon that is closer and more constricted or farther away and more expansive, and can apply it to a sense of temporal trajectory and biographical coherence. For members of the study cohort, the temporal horizon may be suffocatingly close or comfortably in the distance; it may be fully foreclosed, such that seeing beyond it is virtually inconceivable, or susceptible of being surpassed such that anticipation, expectation, and planning are possible. Whether temporality in the registers of hope and inclination toward the future is bound within the horizon of affliction or extends beyond it is consequential for the young person's trajectory both developmentally and within the treatment process, for who they are and are becoming, and for having a life. From this standpoint, we have grouped the adolescents' characterizations of the future into five categories, ranging across a continuum from a relatively foreclosed to a relatively open temporal horizon. These categories are (1) constricted horizon with unelaborated future, (2) constricted horizon with elaborated future, (3) ambiguous horizon with inarticulate future, (4) open horizon with continuity and progression toward the future, and (5) open horizon with resumption of interrupted progression toward the future. Although in previous chapters we have selected among the adolescents to elaborate various topics and themes, in this final analysis we offer a brief account from each of them out of respect for the unique situations of these troubled youth as they struggle to have a life.

Constricted Horizon with Unelaborated Future

Although it cannot be said that for this group the temporal horizon was entirely foreclosed, there is little sense among them or their parents of seeing beyond the immediate present.

- **Taciana's** orientation toward the future was temporally constricted to the immediacy of where she would live after discharge from the hospital, with her brother or in foster care.

- **Ian** expressed the goal of finishing high school "so people can't say I didn't finish and call me stupid." He wanted to become a gangster rap music producer and drive a Ferrari. He said he was taking life one day at a time but anticipated that he would get into more trouble.

- **Diego** said that things are going to be all right and avowed that he had no plans or concerns yet. His mother said they take each day as it is and can't plan, but she thought he might be able to achieve working in a music store.

- **Katie** said she wanted to finish school and work, remarking "that's as far as I've gotten." Her mother attested to hope but remarked that "this is not gonna end nice."

- **Jacob** did not speak about the future; his mother had "no idea" what would happen but wanted him home and wanted happy kids.

- **Ruben** said he wanted to go to college so that he could make money because he is "materialistic." His mother thought he would not "turn it around" and that he is manipulative.

- **Allison** was both "yes and no" about high school, saying that she was fed up but needed education. She wanted to become a forensic anthropologist like on the TV show *CSI*.

- **Andrew** looked forward to being back with his dad and and said he will continue therapy "just to make sure I am being safe."

A temporal orientation toward "one day at a time" dominates this existential stance, with little sense that the horizon will recede at any time, or that it will only be necessary to take life on a day-to-day basis *until* conditions change. Possibilities remain unelaborated. Aside from the comment by Andrew about needing therapy "just to make sure I am being safe," there is little sense even of dealing with an illness. We suspect that this is not because the illness is irrelevant or unacknowledged but because it so fills the field of everyday life and coincides with everyday hardship that it is virtually an invisible medium through which these adolescents move.

Constricted Horizon with Elaborated Future

For this group of young people, the temporal horizon has expanded so that a future is visible, but frustratingly so because at the same time the constraints of illness become more palpable.

- **Alan** did not have a response at the first interview, but said at the follow-up he might want to be a mechanic because his uncle said he would be good at it. In the final interview he expressed interest in working in the zoo with animals. His mother said that as long as she's alive and maintaining the house and his medications, he'll be OK, but if not, he'll be crazy on the street.

- **Kevin** did not respond, but his mother (a professional herself, in an allied health care field) said that almost all his problems were short-term management issues. He was involved in an activity (running cross-country) and needed to learn social skills for success.

- **Quincy,** in his second interview, said he wanted to go to college so that he wouldn't have to work in a minimum-wage job. He was worried about medication stigma at a job interview. At his final interview he was oriented toward a job in fast food or at a mall, maybe college, but nothing further into the future. His mother at first was worried about his impulsiveness and the possibility of jail. At final follow-up she thought he would need treatment "forever" but can learn to manage his hallucinations and other problems. Then she said that she expects treatment and medication to continue but not necessarily forever.

- **Mickey** wanted to move into a new apartment with his mom but worried about leaving his grandmother behind if they did so. His mother at first stated that he needs to be regulated on medicine and raised the possibility of him becoming self-sufficient, but was concerned about the consequences of his illness. At final follow-up she mentioned the goal of a GED.

- **Dave,** a temporarily homeless boy who could not keep his dog, at his first interview was looking forward to having a place to live, his mom having a job, and her boyfriend having a job. He wanted to go to design technology school, to become an auto mechanic, to hang out with the right people, and to "be myself." CPC was a respite for him and at follow-up his goal was to stay in for nine months in order to get the most out of the program, then to go into the Job Corps.

- **Natalie** was, at her first interview, both excited and nervous about going home from the hospital because of the responsibility for maintaining good behavior. Her mother expected her behavior to continue as it had been and said she would likely kick her daughter out in two years. Natalie and her mother were interviewed together at the first follow-up, and together they anticipated her high school graduation and possible enrollment in community college for auto mechanics, at the same time mentioning financial support from disability insurance. At final follow-up, Natalie's mother wanted to move out to their ranch and emphasized that she was taking things one day at a time.

- Selena wanted to be an actress and did not know whether she would graduate from high school. At follow-up she predicted she would be arrested more than once during the next year and that this was not preventable. At final follow-up her mother said she would attend college at the University of New Mexico (UNM).

- Ted initially expressed a desire to become a designer of video games but said he would end up being a lawyer or a doctor. He said he does not want to graduate high school but "has to," and that he is oriented toward easy money and going to heaven. By the time of final follow-up he said that in order to be well, "something has to click" for him, and that treatment is no help. He wanted to graduate but had no plans except getting out of treatment. Computer graphics or video game design were his aspirations. In her initial interview his mother described herself as "a person who always has hope"—if he doesn't get worse. In her final follow-up she said that indeed she had lost hope. He would be better on his own but was still sixteen. Yet she articulated goals for him of completing a GED, getting a job, and getting married.

- Nielsen, both of whose parents were diagnosed with bipolar disorder, said at his first interview that he was already better and was planning to move with his sister to Japan to attend college there, but had no thoughts about what he would do subsequently. At follow-up he reiterated this, saying that they had been planning for Japan for the past six years, and that his brother was part of the plan as well. At the time of her first ethnographic interview, Nielsen's mother acknowledged improvement in the sense that he now thinks before he acts, noting that he had hurt his mother. She wanted him to go to college, get a job, and be productive but thought he would be this way for the rest of his life and needs to be able to recognize his signs (cues of his own maladaptive behavior) like his father. She has told him that "you're going to work at McDonald's the rest of your days." At follow-up she commented that he was provocative in the sense of "pushing people to their limit."

- **Debra** initially wanted to become a criminologist because she was fascinated with serial killers. At follow-up she articulated the goal of obtaining a GED. In the final interview she said that she could always work somewhere and that she likes kids. She did not want to work in fast food all her life, but maybe in a call center.

- **John** thought he would have to remain on medication for "a little while." He was oriented toward college but didn't know what he wanted. At follow-up he said he wants to break the cycle of paternal abuse for his kids. He had started driving and wanted to get a job to help his family, eventually to become an airline pilot. At final follow-up he said he had started to make better choices than last time, about 90 percent favorable choices, although he acknowledged that it could get worse, and he had about 85 percent control over that. The issue was choosing his own consequences: "I'm not going to die in treatment." He said he wants to have a car, leave his small town, and move to Denver so he doesn't go back to his bad habits. He wants to be a carpenter because he likes building, but maybe not, because he has trouble with math. He doesn't think about the next day, because "you never know what will happen tomorrow." There's "nothing important as long as I'm getting by," and he was "just coasting." John's mother at first acknowledged telling him "I can't help, you need a counselor." She said she hopes he does something himself, and mentioned Denver as well as "passive detention." At follow-up she was concerned that he doesn't "mess up" with friends or at the hospital before his discharge. At final follow-up she said she wants him "to be a good kid" when he comes home after probation and treatment, to get a job at Baskin Robbins, earn his own money, stay off drugs, go to college, and move to Denver with his sister. She said it's hard when he's away at Christmas, because you "never know if you'll be here next year."

- **Travis** initially wanted to earn a GED and attend college to become a graphic designer, specifically video game design, and move to California because the opportunities were there. He thought taking medication was temporary, maybe till age twenty-one. His mother spoke later during final follow-up, reporting he was back from Chicago, which was too tough an environment for him, and would maybe attend a school for mechanics. He had been "gypped" of change by his circumstances and would likely end up doing kitchen work. He'll finally start to grow up because he's "hugely immature."

In these instances, having a life is not out of reach, and possibilities are somewhat more elaborated, but there is little sense of ambition or striving, and goals are either limited or unrealistic. There is a lingering sense that no progress will be made or that whatever progress has been made will be lost.

Ambiguous Horizon with Inarticulate Future

This group of interlocutors ambiguously articulated a temporal horizon that appeared to shift nearer or farther away over time from one interview to the next.

- **Michael** was preoccupied at first with the trial of his abusive stepfather, but at times he expressed interest in being an archaeologist or a NASA scientist, finding a way to slow down aging or a cure for cancer, and earning a PhD. In the first interview his mother said she didn't want his quirks gone but just wanted him to be stable. In the third interview she said that if he can get his crap together he can have a normal life, but on the other hand, "We don't do normal around here." A long-term perspective is evident in her statement that his dreams will save him, but at the same time the immediate goal was to get him out of special education.

- **Hayley** at first did not want to think about or "dwell on" the future, notably using a phrase that is typically applied to the past. However, in follow-up she was oriented toward the prospect of moving out of treatment foster care and in with her grandparents. She expressed the desire for a normal life and the opinion that therapy was annoying. At the final interview she definitely wanted to go to college, to become either a trauma nurse or a nurse at CPC. Her parents expressed rather stereotypical hopes for her future at first, but on follow-up they were notably vague about the future.

- **Neal's** initial goal was to get a girlfriend. At follow-up he wanted to get a job and continue school. He observed that he looks older than he is and can't live up to people's expectations. His mother said at the first interview that the doctor was extending Neal's stay at CPC while they struggled for approval of a group home for him. At follow-up his mother's goal was a supportive living situation or treatment foster care and, eventually, independent living. At final follow-up she referred to the "death of dreams and hopes" but reiterated the goal of supportive living outside their home, saying that some kind of isolative work (that did not require much social interaction) was possible for him, referring specifically to underwater welding.

- **Anna** expressed a future orientation only in the initial interview, when she specified her desires for a successful discharge from the hospital, to finish high school, and to become a veterinarian. Her mother was tentative, saying, "How hopeful can you be?" She mentioned the merger of science and religion in their Mormon religious faith, and also that her daughter needed to "find a talent."

- **Valerie's** profile is very close to that of Anna. She made future-oriented comments only in her initial interview. She was "trying to get my life straight" so that she could attend UNM, become a veterinarian, and have a family. Her mother worried that she would get raped or beaten, given her current behavior patterns, and wanted her to finish school and stay out of the kind of trouble she was in.

- **Scott** wanted to finish high school and move to Japan to become a rich and famous anime artist, and to have a family with his girlfriend. He wanted to be successful like his father, who makes t-shirts; he said he doesn't how his father is successful, but he must be because he is happy. At follow-up Scott wanted to visit his girlfriend, get his license and a car, and graduate early. In the first interview his mother acknowledged his dream of being an anime artist. She mentioned his plan to kill his parents and the idea of him moving to Iowa. She expected that "he won't outgrow this" and worried about his independence and the expense of medication. At follow-up she said that his "I hate you" response any time she disagreed and his blaming his

parents for trying to ruin his dream of being an anime artist
bothered her, as it would "any parent that cares about their kids
or the future." She said she believes in her heart he doesn't mean
it, but at the same time there is resentment and "I don't know if
we will ever overcome all of that and actually have a relationship." At final follow-up she wanted him to be emotionally
healthy and not think that his mom hates him. She had promised
to take him to Japan if he graduates, because of his love of
anime.

- **Jess** said that the cycle had been getting worse rather than better
repeatedly over a year, and she couldn't talk to her mother. She
wanted to go to college, become a medical assistant, and have a
family. At follow-up she said, "If I'm more social at the end of
summer maybe I can stop [treatment]." She was still oriented
toward college and becoming a registered nurse in an ER,
meanwhile working in the zoo or an animal shelter. In her final
interview she expressed the desire to become a nurse because she
likes helping. She acknowledged the need to continue therapy
and epilepsy medication in the future, though insisting she would
be "done with" inpatient treatment once she was discharged.
Her mother spoke of the future at follow-up, saying that Jess
would be in the Team Builders program for the rest of the
summer and then would be homeschooled and would start with
a new therapist. At final follow-up she said she has no high
expectations for her daughter and that they will be together for
life. She predicted Jess could go to college but would not be able
to work successfully, though she would encourage her to try.

- **Ben** expressed a desire to finish high school, get a good job, and
become a custom skateboard designer. His mother acknowledged
that they talked about potential careers for him, including
skateboarding, counseling, truck driving, operating heavy
equipment, or becoming a mechanic. Counseling stands out in
this list as a residual influence of psychiatric treatment; it may
not be a concrete goal, but rather an indication of Ben's positive
orientation toward the therapeutic process. In the only follow-up
interview completed in this case, his mother made it a point to
say that Ben was going to take motorcycle classes with his sister,
indicating both a degree of positive social functioning and a
collaborative and supportive sibling relationship.

- **Sherine** expressed a desire to become a social worker. At the second interview she had expectations of being assigned a behavior management specialist and attending a different school, but felt she might be "on the verge of going back" to CPC. At this time her goals were either to attend beauty school, become a social worker, or pursue music because "I sing." At final follow-up she said, "I know I need treatment but don't know if I'm ready for it." She said she has many things to live for but can't handle school, is interested in cosmetology, and will go "wherever life takes me." Her mother initially said that only God can help, that high hopes are unrealistic, and that Sherine will never get better. At the first follow-up she was afraid of her daughter going to jail, and particularly that having her picked up without warning would violate the trust in their relationship. At the final interview she was oriented toward a residential treatment center for her daughter but didn't want to have to drive far to visit.

These young people and their parents were ambivalent because they were challenged with reconciling ambitions and hopes with perceived possibilities and limits that were also in flux. The gap between possibilities and limits seemed to be somewhat intimidating or anxiety-producing, to the degree that this gap was immediately perceived. There was a sense that the bottom could drop out of whatever aspirations they allowed themselves to entertain, with overtones of impending failure if not tragedy.

Open Horizon with Continuity and Progression toward the Future

The youth in this group have a temporal horizon defined by a sense of developmental continuity and progression.

- **Robbie** had a constrained ability to interact with others but was sufficiently aware of this as a problem that he articulated increased sociability as an explicit goal. He wanted to earn a GED, become capable of living independently of his grandmother, and enter the Job Corps. He noted having come to realize that his life was destined for more than the disease with which he was afflicted, a statement that both defined his situation in terms of "disease" and resisted the definition of disease as a foreclosed horizon for his future trajectory.

- **Stacey** wanted to go to college, to be happy, and to move from the Native American reservation where she lived to a place where there are "less witching people around." When JHJ asked her how much of a problem that was, she got up from the kitchen table and pointed out the kitchen window, saying, "Right there [*pointing to a house across the yard*], and over there [*pointing to a different house*], they're everywhere, and getting younger all the time. These days, could be three or four years old."

- **Dustin,** paraplegic due to a severe injury, wanted to work with computers or in a pharmacy, and he recognized the need to graduate high school. By the time of follow-up these goals had shifted toward working in animal science or becoming a veterinary assistant. His mother did not anticipate that he would be capable of independent living.

- **Amy** was quite aware that a number of her family members had been in jail as adolescents. She wanted "to do good for myself and my family and not hurt anyone anymore." She wanted to get a GED, attend UNM, become a social worker, and have a family and kids. She expected to have to stay on medications for the rest of her life but wanted eventually to get off them. A long-term goal was to write an autobiography and to make money. She said, "My whole goal in life is just to have peace."

- **Anne** said in her first interview that she wanted to be a pediatrician, or a lawyer to help the innocent, or a social worker to help kids, and a poet. At follow-up she wanted to finish high school and go on to college and become a pediatrician. At the final interview she said she hoped to get her GED soon and was taking medical classes with the continued goal of becoming a pediatrician. She worried about her mom and other family members using drugs.

- **Mariana** initially wanted to erase her gang-oriented family past because, she said, she was looking toward the future, not the past. At follow-up she expressed a plan to finish high school, to work as a masseuse while in college, and to become an architect. There was no parental input about the future.

- **Sarah** initially said she was afraid to drive but wanted to start at age twenty. Her goals were to complete a GED and become an art teacher. She made it a point to mention that her boyfriend had been calling her. At follow-up she was still oriented toward completing a GED and also enrolling in the American Indian Arts Institute at a community college to become an art teacher. Her mother expected that she would always need medication and therapy.

- **Alicia** said at her initial interview that she planned on not finishing high school, to live with her aunts on the reservation, to have twenty kids of her own, and to be a midwife. At first follow-up she was oriented toward enlisting in the Marines as both her parents had before her. She wanted to be in aviation, first attending a military academy and then UNM. She wanted to move to Albuquerque with some friends, then later to Los Angeles to live with her father's side of the family, where she would attend the University of California (UCLA) to get a doctorate in aviation. Her mother was initially somewhat negative about the future, expecting that Alicia would be involved with law enforcement and that she would eventually have to raise Alicia's kids. She was more positive at follow-up, saying that Alicia planned to marry and was "trying to prove she can do it" in school and in the military. At final follow-up with both together, Alicia was oriented toward going to tribal college to study nursing and was planning to marry a serviceman stationed in Germany. She was concerned about having kids, and she and her mother both felt that the bipolar disorder was "not going to go away."

- **Christopher** was learning German and wanted to go to Germany. He was oriented to becoming a psychiatrist because it is "cool to help" people. At first follow-up he was taking it "day by day" but wanted to become a psychologist because he was interested in how the mind works. He attributed his problems to brain chemistry and wanted to study neurology. He also acknowledged having had a role model since he was little, referring to a psychiatrist whom he liked. At final follow-up he was "starting to like life" and was oriented to "not hurt anyone or myself." He wanted to help other teens with their problems and become a psychiatrist. In the final follow-up his adoptive father said Chris can "fight through it." Having read articles on "functional schizophrenics," he felt that his son could eventually live on his own with psychosis and delusions, though he will need continued counseling.

- **Tom** wanted to become a firefighter, to finish high school and attend college to become a fire medic. At follow-up he was oriented toward a summer job at Burger King and wanted to move to South Dakota to finish his probation while living with his grandparents. At the final follow-up he said he would put himself in counseling if he needs it. He wanted to finish probation and pass the test to become a firefighter, which he had already failed once. His mother, at the final follow-up, said his goals were a diploma, then to become a firefighter, and that this was particularly good insofar as putting a troubled child in uniform reverses stigma.

- **Matt** and his mother both initially mentioned UCLA as his targeted college. At follow-up he wanted to study microbiology because microbiologists make money and find new things. He had a host family in Los Angeles and was part of their Christian group. He was interested in helping others. He was planning to quit school to help his mother, but she told him to stay in school. In her follow-up interview his mother again referred to UCLA but also mentioned mysteriously that she had "a different dream for him" that was to be a surprise.

These youth are well able to articulate their goals—which, compared to those we have considered so far, are relatively more specific and notably more professional. They refuse to be defined by their illness and accompanying disability, while not denying either. Their realistic stance toward their prospects is noteworthy, and we can surmise that realism in itself opens possibilities by sidestepping the bottomless vortex of fantasy.

Open Horizon with Resumption of Interrupted Progression toward the Future

For this final group of young people, the horizon of expectation and possibility appeared open in a way that was relatively independent of their illness or that had some potential to transcend the constraints of illness.

- **Maria,** in her second interview, expressed a desire to be a counselor "for kids like her" or a nurse. At her final interview she expressed the goal of earning a BA in counseling or psychology. Her mother envisioned her "tripping and falling but getting back up."

- **Nadine,** at her first interview, was aspiring to attend an Ivy League university to become a surgeon or a research scientist. Her mother emphasized her high school awards, letters, and activities, including sculpture and orchestra. At the first follow-up she acknowledged that the future would be stressful but that she wanted to become "some kind of doctor." Her mother said that maybe she could grow out of her bipolar disorder but noted that her dad hadn't. In the final interview Nadine expressed concern about the logistics of her medication, the Social Security disability program, being at college without the support of a therapeutic team, and finances. She was oriented toward medical school but also liked the fine arts. She noted that she has been stable and expressed confidence that she would be able to handle college, though she expected continuing with psychiatric care, medication, and psychotherapy. Her mother noted that she would be attending New Mexico State University and was hoping it would be OK, praying that Nadine could stay on her meds and away from drugs. Having been hospitalized and having spent time in treatment foster care, she had lost a full year to bipolar.

- **Dana,** during our first interview in the hospital, indicated that she wanted to go home but did not want further counseling or therapy after discharge. At her first follow-up, she was oriented toward going to college, earning good grades, and getting a car. During her final interview, her goals had become more specific, including becoming a lawyer and learning languages. Her mother's initial observation was that she was not homicidal and not an addict, so she could probably make it to college. At follow-up, she observed that her daughter was "standing behind her goals" to become a lawyer and have a big house. In the final interview she reaffirmed expectations for college but indicated that Dana "will never be 100 percent."

- **Linda** lived in a relatively comfortable middle-class household, although in a highly conflictual relationship under her aunt's guardianship because her mother was incapable of providing responsible care. She had participated in a transitional living program for youth as a step toward getting away from her aunt. She considered attending UNM, but by all means she wanted to leave the small town in which she found herself. At her first follow-up interview she was planning a move to live with her grandparents in California, where she would also be able to be in contact with her mother. She felt she had her priorities more in order, while acknowledging a risk of relapse because of the difficulty of breaking old habits. She looked forward to outpatient therapy and high school in California, as well as to becoming an art teacher and a specialist in tattoo arts, while acknowledging worry because while she was regarded as intelligent in New Mexico, she might not be recognized as such in California. At her final interview she appeared well adjusted in her new home, expressing a coherent interest in working backstage on costumes and sets for movie productions and editing videos, with a sense of possibility enhanced by the knowledge that her grandparents had a college fund ready to support her. The effect of this change of scene was evident in guardian interviews, during the first of which her aunt expressed an end to her tolerance for being beaten by Linda and was exploring expensive residential treatment programs for her. At the first follow-up the aunt told us of the plan for Linda to go to California to live with her grandparents and, if that was not successful, to one of a number of costly facilities in Utah that specialize in the uncontrollable offspring of well-to-do families. By the time of the final guardian interview, Linda was studying theater set design in a California community college and preparing to transfer to a four-year college to pursue her passion for art. Whereas her aunt thought a more restrictive environment would be better for her, Linda thought more freedom was the solution, and when her research participation ended, the more laissez-faire living environment with her grandparents appeared to confirm the young woman's intuition about her own potential trajectory.

- **Kayley,** in her initial interview, acknowledged having wanted to become a veterinarian but, in part because of her own experience of emotional distress, had decided she was now interested in psychology. Her mother expressed confidence that she would completely recover and go to college in psychology. At the first follow-up, Kayley and her mother together expressed her immediate desire to transfer back to a regular high school from the "short-cut school" where she was making up missed credits. Her mother expressed the view that psychotherapy is good not only for depression and panic, as her daughter had experienced, but in general for relaxing, and Kayley acknowledged that she had always been encouraged to engage in therapy by her mother. By the time of the final interview, the young woman had identified the local college in which she wanted to enroll to study social developmental or counseling psychology, saying that although she used to worry, there were a lot of ways to go toward the future. Her mother said she thought her daughter would do well, though "probably not as well as I think she can."

In contrast to the preceding group, affliction and hospitalization for these young people constituted an *interruption* in their developmental trajectory and biographical coherence. Their subsequent temporal orientation was characterized by *resumption* of their former stance toward the future. Even if their expectations were somewhat diminished, they appeared to avoid the foreclosure of their horizons. Notably, they appeared to have more resources and more confidence, and they had started from a somewhat higher socioeconomic and educational baseline than many others.

Several general observations about this analysis are in order. First, it is evident that convergence between parent and child in orientation toward the future is by no means absolute, so that phenomenologically they are at times working within different temporal horizons. Second, there is evidently change over time across the relatively short one to two years captured in our data, and this is not only change in career plans but can indicate contraction or expansion of the temporal horizon itself. Third, there is an apparent association between how articulate, aspirational, and optimistic these interlocutors are and the socioeconomic plateau from which they begin. Complex as it would be, one can envision teasing out the relative effects of class habitus and illness severity in defining temporal horizons among the youth and their families. In terms of actual jobs foreseen, within this cohort commonly cited types that define the opposite poles of aspiration are fast-food worker (not just as a teenage summer job but as an occupational ceiling) and health care professional (23% of these young people mentioned either mental health professional, doctor, nurse, or veterinarian). The latter category is particularly salient because these young people had been so intensively exposed to the mental health care system.

Also relevant is the degree of realism, such that depending on the individual and family circumstances, the most outlandish and most conventional aspirations could be equally unlikely. The one young man who indicated he might want to become a psychiatrist was evidently influenced by the admiration and respect he expressed for the psychiatrist who had treated him from an early age, but his illness was sufficiently chronic that it was highly unlikely he would have the opportunity to pursue this goal. Unrealistic for different reasons was the aspiration of another youth to become a famous rap music producer and drive a Ferrari. His was among the most socially and emotionally precarious of circumstances, living in a poor neighborhood with two brothers who were violently mentally ill and a grandmother who was the sole thread holding the household together. Of all the youth, given the nature of his illness and the precarity of his life, his aspirations were the most grandiose and delusional. Finally, not to be discounted alongside realism is truthfulness. A number of these youth were described by parents (and occasionally acknowledged themselves) as being a liar, manipulative, or willing to say whatever they think clinicians expect to hear. It must suffice to say that to a certain extent our analyses have had to be premised on taking the words of our interlocutors at face value.

TOWARD THE FUTURE

We must take a step back from these observations in order to elaborate some theoretical and existential implications of our analysis of temporal horizons. A useful starting point is Minkowski's (1970 [1933]) analysis of lived time in relation to what he viewed as psychopathology. Minkowski distinguished among the *immediate future* defined by perception and apperception, the *mediate future* where hope and desire reside, and the *remote future* extending to the generational and even the cosmological. Within this framework, the temporal horizon of these youth may most likely become foreclosed at the boundary between immediate and mediate future, and this boundary is precisely the experiential locus of the five forms of horizonal structure we have identified. The temporal horizon may, in principle, also become foreclosed at the boundary between mediate and remote future, but in Minkowski's terms engagement with the latter is an aspect of "ethical life" that may or may not be reasonably expected of, or fully elaborated in, youth at the developmental stage of these adolescents, whether they are afflicted by mental illness or not.

From this standpoint, we suggest that these five forms of relation to the temporal horizon together constitute a structure of *temporal subjectivity,* a system or matrix of possible horizons situated at the boundary between immediate and mediate future. This temporal subjectivity partly defines the existential circumstances of the young people we have worked with. With respect to the analysis of future orientations we have just presented, each capsule vignette is an incipient narrative of future experience for one of the adolescents, a possible story of a "possible self" (Parish 2008) that invites the phenomenological technique of imaginative variation (Husserl 2013 [1931]) with respect to what is in store for each young person and anticipates a "narrative emplotment" (Mattingly 2010). Within this structure of temporal subjectivity each person's temporal horizon can become more constricted or open, more unelaborated or elaborated, over time. The idea of a horizon that can be constricted or open also evokes movement that is more or less constrained, and indeed these vignettes often include reference to going places as well as becoming something. Here a relevant image is that of Gabriel Marcel's (1951) *Homo Viator,* asserting that it is in our nature as humans to be wayfarers or travelers in both literal and metaphorical senses, en route in the direction of hope and away from captivity.

The capsule vignettes of temporal horizon and future orientation we have presented allow us—perhaps require us—to define the existential condition of hope in terms of possibility. As Stengers suggests,

> we have all the reasons we wish to despair—to think is to succeed in not following those reasons, one way or another. Thus I would say that hope is the difference between *probability* and *possibility*. If we follow probability there is no hope, just a calculated anticipation authorized by the world as it is. But to "think" is to create possibility against probability. It doesn't mean hope for one or another thing or as a calculated attitude, but to try and feel and put into words a possibility for becoming. (Zournazi and Stengers 2002: 245)

The possibility for becoming is, in the terms we have been using, the possibility for having a life. The variety and manner in which youth have articulated their lived experience throughout our ethnographic work and in the pages of this book indicate that they are by no means slaves of probability, and that despite their troubled lives they are capable of thinking and thus creating possibility. It is the dynamic between probability and possibility that also underlies the importance we have given to balancing our use of psychiatric diagnostic categories as an etic framework for understanding forms of affliction across individuals, and the existential ethnographic imperative to allow each struggling person to be defined by their own life experience. This balance constitutes a fundamental principle of psychiatric anthropology, recognizing that the imposition of diagnostic categories as a stamp of identity defers to probability at the expense of potentially masking possibilities of becoming and having a life.

These possibilities are never fully foreclosed, because becoming is a fundamental human process. As Parish says,

> human beings pursue their own possible selves. It is how they enter life. I contend, simply enough, that human beings try to grasp what and who they are, could be, and must be, as they make their way into and through life . . . [It is a question of] the possible selves that people assemble, their efforts to venture into life on the terms these provide, and what, in the end, they are able to do with these possibilities. (2008: ix)

It remains to be seen what each of the members of our cohort is able to do with those possibilities. Possibility is not presented to them in the form of making the most of opportunity, but in the form of an engaged struggle to have a life. This includes those who describe anger that is deeply existential and those who recount repeated suicide attempts, for they do not always and necessarily use an expressive idiom of hopelessness or despair. Indeed, from an existential standpoint, perhaps the very struggle of facing anger or surviving a suicide attempt carries an incremental coefficient of hope. In terms of possibility and probability, some of these troubled youth may have already beaten the odds.

Closing Remarks

In this research, we have been struck by the centrality of struggle in the lived experience of the youth, families, and mental health professionals involved in inpatient psychiatric treatment. Although it is certainly valid to describe much of what we have seen as suffering (Kleinman, Das, and Lock 1997), the activity of struggle (Jenkins 2015a) is both empirically urgent and theoretically compelling. Both suffering and struggle are fundamental human processes in the face of adversity. While we have consistently sought to avoid sentimentality and refrain from dramatizing their experiences, any empathic engagement with the youth must recognize the palpable anguish among adolescents and families living with psychic turmoil and social adversity. No less must we recognize the deep sense of care and frustration on the part of CPC therapists given bureaucratic constraints on therapeutic practice (cf. Benoit 2016).

The looming features of structural violence evoke a sense of disquiet as we return to the relation between psychiatric research diagnostic categories and narrative ethnographic data. While we have both used the SCID in a number of projects, more than ever in the SWYEPT study we feel the tension between the methodological usefulness of these categories as minimal descriptions and their unsatisfactoriness as a systematic series of pigeonholes. Their adequacy in providing accounts of or accounting for illness and distress is partial at best, as is their identification of treatable syndromes. We stand by our endorsement of the methodological value of rigorously collected SCID data—including reflection on the narrative data in the interviews themselves rather than only their coded categorical results (Csordas et al. 2010)—to construct a rudimentary etic analytic sorting by gender, types of condition, and comorbidity. Yet diagnostic description is patently inadequate to apprehend the complexity, messiness, and difficulty of the lives of these youth.

In order to best capture the immediacy of lived experience, we have stayed close to the words uttered by our interlocutors. We have constantly faced the methodological paradox that while at times we felt we were presenting too much of what they said, simultaneously we realized that what they said only scratches the surface of our full set of ethnographic materials and of their lived experience. Our method throughout this book has been to alternate between elements of individual case studies and themes common across the cohort of adolescent patients: individual admission narratives and types of narratives, individual definitions of the problem and engagement with a common discourse of diagnosis, individual experiences of profound anger and anger as a recurrent theme, individual treatment narratives and typical treatment trajectories, individual orientations toward the future and a common matrix of temporal subjectivity. In sum, case studies are to thematic analyses as the subjectivity distilled from individual experience is to a collective form of subjectivity based on a commonality of experience—a commonality in these cases defined by having spent time as a psychiatric inpatient.

There is a dynamic between subjectivity and institutional structure that plays out under the impress of extremity and precarity. The institutional structure of managed care and behavioral health corporations wields significant control over criteria for admission and clinical practices in a manner that dictates the kind of therapeutic care that can be offered and engaged by patients and healers. While the clinical team at CPC—New Mexico's largest public, not-for-profit mental health care center—may be fully aware that a particular therapeutic modality is needed to initiate the process of healing for these youth, such treatment may be precluded by limits imposed on lengths of stay (e.g., two or three days). This begets a triaging and enforced rationing of forms of care, though all the while clinicians know well that these are highly likely to be insufficient in light of obstacles that patients and caregivers are facing.

Recall that in our study the average age of the participants in this study is fourteen. By that age, 70 percent had already been hospitalized (most multiple times), and some were rehospitalized during the course of the study. The infelicitous and clichéd reference to such youth as "revolving door" cases makes this practice appear commonplace and expectable. In fact, it is unacceptable. The revolving door is a violation of the dignity of these youth (Dedios and Anderson 2014),[1] whose actual conditions of life are nothing less than extraordinary. Owing to economic restrictions and the constricted availability of adequate behavioral-health residential facilities, things often get worse as a result of placement in facilities where training and quality of care are typically not experienced as therapeutic by the youth. This is the institutional backdrop for our concern about the trajectory of the lives of troubled youth living on the edge of experience under conditions of extremity and precarity. As medical anthropologists, it is clear to us that from the standpoint of critique it is best to take aim at the political structures of profiteering, fraud, and abuse by behavioral health corporations and state-sponsored collaborators that conspire against patients, families, and health care providers.

Under developmental conditions of hardship for these youth, "ethnography has the power to show suffering" and "to invite us to examine it" (Parish 2008: 126). Moreover, since "suffering is a cause of *self*-awareness," it "requires us to understand selves as active agents in their own lives" and constitutes a "fundamental problem for cultural theory and for self-psychologies" (2008: 126). This line of thinking is coterminous with the "possibility of having a better life" (Myers 2015: 4), whereby the driver of recovery is "moral agency, the ability to be recognized as a 'good' person in a way that makes possible intimate connections to others" (2015: 13). Recalling our discussion of anger as a moral emotion, and with a concern for the conditions of possibility of having a life via the development of moral agency, it would not do justice to the lives of the youth to express pity for "these poor kids" and then move on.

Indeed, examining extraordinary conditions of struggle in the face of precarity (Jenkins 2015a) is critical if we profess to care about people who exist in those conditions. Such work invites us to extend and continue our examination of fundamental human processes in comparison with how those processes are expressed under other conditions and circumstances, including our own. The move to elevate struggle to a theoretical status alongside suffering as a fundamental human process emerges from the nature of our ethnographic encounters. Those encounters reveal the value of supporting struggle by means of engaged empathic listening and narrative interpretation of lifeworlds that can lurch from quotidian at one moment to harrowing at the next. If there is an aphorism to be derived from this stance, it is "Recognize suffering, support struggle."

For these troubled youth and their families, our hope is that this monograph may lead to a degree of understanding of the possibilities and constraints of human conditions. We also wish the work to serve as an ethnographic foundation that can inform engaged interventions. As a matter of subjectivity, we have emphasized that it is really about the possibility of having a life. Also evident is that the pendulum of suffering and struggle swings widely and frequently between moments of hopeful engagement and moments of being desperately overwhelmed or out of control. Likewise, it is clear that subjective possibilities of hope and transformation—when marked deeply by the impress of social extremity—are largely contingent on the availability of institutional-structural pathways and environments to take care of lives, establish well-being, achieve equity, and ensure equanimity.

The scarcity of such pathways or environments for education and health care in the United States, a nation marked by stark economic inequality, is as deplorable as it is unacceptable. Given the immediacy of the need, it is problematic that the lived experience of these suffering and struggling youth is largely unknown to the broader public. There would be no reason for this were we not in a society that hides its afflicted, particularly its afflicted youth. Moreover, this lived experience is mostly unavailable for social, psychological, or cultural theorizing. We feel fortunate to have obtained funding for a study of living humans in communities with real-world circumstances. However, support for ethnographic research of the kind we have presented has all but vanished. Finally, lived experience is virtually unattended to by policymakers. We are not policymakers, but we offer our work to those in a position to make use of it or collaborate in making use of it. Our claim is that the details of real lives as we have described them are worthy of far more attention and care.

At the beginning of the project we asked clinicians how the knowledge we intended to produce might be of help or interest to them, and they said they wished they could find out what eventually happens to the young people they cared for and cared about in the hospital after they are discharged. The director of CPC narrated a story of encountering a former patient in a restaurant where the young person was working, and how gratifying it was to learn that he had achieved a degree of stability in his life. In this work, we have responded to CPC clinicians' queries about what happens to young people once they are discharged by examining their trajectories through psychiatric treatment and beyond. Throughout our ethnography the real question, the hopeful question, is not the passive one of what will become of them but the active one of what they will become.

Indeed, the notion of trajectory with its connotation of having been launched on this trajectory without foreknowledge or consent recognizes and amplifies what Heidegger (1962 [1927]) identified as the condition of thrownness (*Geworfenheit*), the existential condition that we all share as we find ourselves already being in the world. This is vivid for most of the youth and their families who struggle to determine whether or not, and to what extent, their lives are like those of other teenagers, and, even more starkly, whether to continue or attempt to end their lives. Yet, in a way, we have not fully responded to the clinicians' desire to know what happens because those young lives are still young. To whatever extent we have been able to describe their lived experience and subjectivity, we must explicitly say that the end of our book can only be understood as the potential beginning of another, and the sequel is one they are already writing themselves.

Methods and Procedures

The core of our methodological approach was ethnographic interviewing and naturalistic observation following protocols developed in our previous work on psychiatric disorder and therapeutic process in other completed studies (with Mexican-descent populations, Salvadoran refugees, Puerto Rican migrants, Euro-Americans and African Americans, and residents of the Navajo Nation).

I. ETHNOGRAPHIC INTERVIEWS, OBSERVATIONS, AND LONGITUDINAL DESIGN

Open-ended interviews were carried out by psychological/medical anthropologists from the research team in treatment facilities or family homes except when interlocutors requested to meet in places such as a park or coffee shop. The interviews concentrated on everyday routines and life events, family background, origin and understanding of the problem/illness, pathway followed into the treatment situation, expectations of treatment, experience of treatment, interaction with staff and other patients, medication use, school and peer relations, religious involvement, and expectations for the future. Because the interviews were open-ended, many additional topics emerged that were unanticipated but important to the interviewee. Ethnographic interviews varied in length (from two to three hours). We carried out parallel interviews, most often in the family home, with the adolescent and parent, guardian, or primary caretaker (i.e., the person with whom the young person had the most face-to-face interaction). These interviews provided data on household composition and demographics, kin and social networks and resources, religious and ceremonial activities and affiliations, and understandings of the patient's problems and/or illness.

During home visits we complemented interviews with naturalistic observation, the methodological mainstay of social scientific approaches to describe and analyze social settings (Bogdan and Taylor 1998; Denzin and Lincoln 1998; Lofland and Lofland 1995; Luborsky and Rubinstein 1995). A key element of naturalistic observation is the relatively unobtrusive recording of ongoing events that would be occurring independently of the observer's presence. While the presence of an observer invariably alters the behavior of those observed to some extent, observer effects tend to attenuate over time.

In order to understand participants' developmental and therapeutic trajectory, we incorporated a longitudinal component by repeating these interviews and observations after six months and again after a year. Some of these interviews took place in homes, while we followed others into a variety of clinical settings in which they were placed following discharge from CPC. Because of logistical complications, for some interlocutors the time between interviews was lengthened such that some did not complete the full series for nearly two years. We were particularly concerned with (1) changes that the youth perceived in their problems since our last visit; (2) the extent to which they perceived these changes as attributable to treatment; (3) accounts of any other ritual, medical, or psychiatric intervention they had sought for their problem since then, and what they found significant about it; (4) accounts of any other problems that had arisen since then for the patient or for a family member, and of what had been done to alleviate them; and (5) changes in family circumstances and interpersonal environment, work situation, attitudes toward illness and health, religious commitments, and current health status.

In addition to these ethnographic methods, once, as near in time as possible to the beginning of each patient's participation, we administered three standardized instruments designed to assess psychiatric disorder, distress, and behavior as described below.

2. THE STRUCTURED CLINICAL INTERVIEW FOR *dsm-iv* CHILD VERSION (KID-SCID)

The SCID is administered by a mental health professional (psychiatrist or clinical psychologist) trained specifically to conduct the assessment according to established protocols and to achieve research reliability for the ratings in accord with criteria of the American Psychiatric Association's *Diagnostic and Statistical Manual of Mental Disorders* (DSM-IV). The rigor and time involved in conducting a SCID interview (one and a half to two hours) and subsequent rating and writeup far exceeds that generally in clinical diagnostic practice. SCID training is undertaken at specific centers (Ventura et al. 1998). Our SCID-trained research clinicians included a child psychiatrist and a child psychologist.

The interview consists of an open-ended information-gathering component used to elicit a lifeline narrative and separate algorithmically structured modules exploring mood, thought, anxiety, and substance-use disorder symptoms across the patient's life span. The SCID assesses clinical status across four of the five dimensions (axes) of psychiatric clinical status (developmental and personality disorders are excluded): (1) primary psychiatric disorders; (2) relevant medical disorders; (3) severity of psychosocial stressors; and (4) level of adaptive functioning (Spitzer et al. 1992). We used the version of this instrument adapted to assess additional psychiatric disorders that occur primarily in childhood. This KID-SCID integrates all available diagnostic information including a careful clinical diagnostic evaluation, and includes the same psychotic disorders module that is found in the adult SCID (Hein et al. 1998).

To augment the SCID results specifically for this research project, we developed a brief clinical protocol to elicit our research psychiatrist's or clinical psychologist's narrative assessment of the adolescents. Because the SCID interviews were typically carried out in homes of the youth following their discharge from the hospital, our research clinicians were able to observe adolescents and their families in their domestic context and to make narrative observations of all that they saw and with whom they interacted, and to provide their descriptions of the home and neighborhood along with their SCID diagnostic summaries. This also allowed interviewers to refine any reservations or caveats in reference to the SCID criteria or thresholds for achieving symptomatic, temporal, and functional criteria for any given disorder. A great many subthreshold observations were made; given the rigorous criteria for any given diagnosis in terms of the number, duration, and severity of symptoms, the SCID can be understood as remarkably conservative in its determination of clinical psychopathology. In addition, research clinicians were able to provide cultural commentary on the applicability of SCID criteria in light of the research team's ethnographic knowledge (e.g., Native Americans' sensorial experience of relatives and ancestors, Mexican/Latinx/Hispano bodily experience, or Anglo/Euro-American cultural tendencies toward individual attribution).

3. THE ADOLESCENT HEALTH SURVEY (AHS)

Developed by Resnick, Blum, and Harris (1989), this instrument contains 162 items related to issues such as physical and emotional health; peer, family, and school relationships; substance use; diet and eating disorders; sexual behavior and orientation; antisocial and high-risk behaviors; worries and concerns; health history and health care utilization. The measure has been widely used in research involving adolescents and has been administered to over forty thousand youth in Minnesota and Alaska. The questionnaire is self-administered, requires a fifth-grade reading level, and takes approximately one hour to complete.

4. THE CHILD BEHAVIOR CHECKLIST (CBCL) AND YOUTH SELF REPORT (YSR)

These were developed by Thomas Achenbach and are well-established measures of child behavior, the construct validity of which has been supported in numerous studies (Achenbach 1991). These 112-item checklists are used as dimensional measures of emotional/behavioral problems and social competence. Items are scored on a three-point Likert-type scale representing the informant's perception of the frequency of behaviors. The measures contain identical scales, including a total problem behavior score, two "global" problem behavior scales of Internalizing and Externalizing, and eight "narrow-band" clinical subscales including Withdrawal, Somatic Complaints, Anxiety/Depression, Social Problems, Thought

Problems, Attention Problems, Delinquency, and Aggression. Raw scores can be converted to *t*-scores for each of the scales based on population norms. The Achenbach measures have been utilized extensively in research on children and families to assess a range of psychopathological behaviors in youth and adolescence. Their psychometric properties have been analyzed intensively; Achenbach (1991) states that this work suggests that development of separate norms for subgroups within the US population may not be necessary because of a lack of statistical differences.

Notes

CHAPTER I

1. "Subjectivity is the relatively durable structure of experience that is yet subject to transformation based on changing circumstances and modes of engaging the world" (Jenkins 2015a: 9–10). This approach to subjectivity allows for identification of the conditions (social, symbolic, material, subjective) under which subjective and objective phenomena are conceptualized as equally "real." In the case of contemporary medicine, often symptoms are considered meaningful only if they can be identified as "real" pathology by means of biotechnological evidence. Such an approach denies the equivalently "real" experience of hearing voices or seeing visions as a matter of first-person subjectivity even, and especially, if this reality is not shared with others.

2. This literature explores a wide range of topics, including gender and sexuality (Burbank 1988, 1995; Davis and Davis 1989, 1995; Asencio 1999), agency and identity (Sharp 2002; Stephens 1995; Amit-Talai and Wulff 1995; Guboglo 1999; Maira 1999; Dole and Csordas 2003), violence (Allison 2001; Scheper-Hughes and Sargent 1998; Korbin 1981), religion (Stambach 2000; Csordas 2009; Cornelio 2016), ethnicity (Burton 1997; Young 1997), the role of social peer groups (Condon 1988, 1995; Gable 2000), work and labor (Mills 1999), poverty (Miles 2000), teenage childbearing and parenting (Konner and Shostak 1986), and adolescent transition from dependence to autonomy (Lebra 1995; Hollos and Leis 1989; Leis and Hollos 1995; Martínez-Hernáez et al 2016), and includes several edited volumes (Fuchs 1976; Schlegel and Barry 1991; James, Jenks, and Prout 1998; Skelton and Valentine 1998).

3. For discussion of a comparable dialectic of environment-self creation in urban South Asia, where women use the slum environment as a tool for personal and social redefinition, see Snell-Rood (2013).

4. In this book, we work with the term "precarity" as an alternative to "vulnerability" because it is more precise from the standpoint of the person's immediate experience: the phenomenology of mental illness, it seems, is less that of vulnerability than of precarity. More than arguing that the mentally ill are not victims, this is an assertion that the afflicted live precariously on the edge of experience. More to the point, from the standpoint of subjective experience, persons are less likely to express themselves or act in terms of vulnerability than to live in anticipation of trouble or the possibility that things may fall apart. This includes recognition of their own volatility as well as the volatility of their immediate surrounding (Jenkins 2015a: 13), and of their capacity for struggle. Anne Lovell (2013) advances compelling formulations of the ontological and social precarity of persons experiencing psychosis under extraordinary circumstances or spectacular eruptions as a "crisis of the uncanny" (Lovell and Diagne 2019: 671–678).

5. This is standard for university-sponsored research, in which confidentiality is required for all research team members in accord with approved UCSD protocols, practices, and research ethics for work with human subjects. All research interviews were transcribed using a coded numbering system without the actual name of the youth, parent, or others interviewed.

CHAPTER 2

1. "Emo" (or emotional hardcore), "goth" (or gothic), and "scene" are youth stylistic subcultures associated with certain music, dress, and attitudes. Emo in particular cultivates an ethos of brooding cynicism, goth leans toward dark nihilism, and scene is more upbeat and colorful.

CHAPTER 3

1. A larger problem for epigenetic researchers is that the majority of studies are carried out with rodent populations, for which application to humans is questionable at best. Theoretically there is good reason for interest in epigenetics; however, the research agendas in this field today are often driven by available funding. For decades now, the problem has not been the transformative possibilities of neuroscience but the paradigmatic imbalance that renders neuroscience dominant and reductive rather than equivalent and complementary to social and behavioral scientific research (Jenkins 2015a: 4–7). For an elegant formulation of subjectivity and meaning entailed here, see Martínez-Hernáez 2000, 2020).

2. During its post-structuralist and postmodernist phases, anthropology in particular became so self-consciously susceptible to this unmooring that ethnographers had to defensively refer to cultural reality as always shifting or contested, or both, with the additional defense of pluralizing "reality" as "realities" without feeling required to specify how many such realities might be in question.

CHAPTER 4

1. This analysis of emotional tone draws on the phenomenological method of "imaginative variation" (Husserl 2013 [1931]), which consists of fleshing out the permutations of a given situation or phenomenon. It is the intellectual

equivalent of glancing at a stone as one turns it over in one's hand to grasp its being as a thing from as many perspectives as possible.

CLOSING REMARKS

1. Anthropologist Sarah Willen has weighed in on the notion of dignity, making observations and raising questions such as these: "Anthropologists, for the most part, have been quiet. Some might find this anthropological silence strange. Doesn't our field presume an incipient link among all ἄνθρωποι (anthropoi), whether wealthy or indigent, modal or transgressive, living or dead? If so, might something like dignity not name that link?" (Dedios and Anderson 2014). In this book we have touched upon such questions, but further reflection and anthropological analysis are clearly indicated.

Works Cited

Achenbach, Thomas M. 1991. "The Deviation of Taxonomic Constructs: A Necessary Stage in the Development of Developmental Psychopathology." In Dante Cicchette and S. L. Toth (Eds.), Rochester Symposium on Developmental Psychopathology, vol. 3: Models and Integrations. Rochester, NY: University of Rochester Press.

Adams, Gerald R. 2005. "Adolescent Development." In Thomas P. Gullotta and Gerald R. Adams (Eds.), Handbook of Adolescent Behavioral Problems: Evidence-Based Approaches to Prevention and Treatment. Boston: Springer. pp. 3–16.

Alanen, Leena. 2005. "Women's Studies/Childhood Studies: Parallels, Links, and Perspectives." In Jan Mason and Toby Fattore (Eds.), Children Taken Seriously in Theory, Policy, and Practice. London: Jessica Kingsley. pp. 31–46.

Allison, Anne. 2001. "Cyborg Violence: Bursting Borders and Bodies with Queer Machines." Cultural Anthropology 16(2): 237–65.

Amit-Talai, Vered, and Helena Wulff (Eds.). 1995. Youth Cultures: A Cross-Cultural Perspective. New York: Routledge.

Anderson, Irina. 2017. "Sexual Violence and Rape." In Bryan S. Turner (Ed.), The Wiley Blackwell Encyclopedia of Social Theory. London: Wiley Blackwell.

Anderson-Fye, Eileen, and Jill Korbin (Eds.). 2011. "Special Issue, Psychological Anthropology and Adolescent Well-being: Steps toward Bridging Research, Practice, and Policy." Ethos 39(4).

Ariès, Philippe. 1996. Centuries of Childhood: A Social History of Family Life. London: Pimlico.

Aristizabal, Maria J., Ina Anreiter, Thorhildur Halldorsdottir, Candice L. Odgers, Thomas W. McDade, Anna Goldenberg, Sara Mostafavi, Michael S. Kobor, Elisabeth B. Binder, Marla B. Sokolowski, and Kieran J. O'Donnell. 2019. "Biological Embedding of Experience: A Primer on Epigenetics."

Proceedings of the National Academy of Sciences USA. www.pnas.org/cgi /doi/10.1073/pnas.1820838116.

Asencio, Marysol. 1999. "Machos and Sluts: Gender, Sexuality and Violence among a Cohort of Puerto Rican Adolescents." Medical Anthropology Quarterly: International Journal for the Analysis of Health 13(1): 107–26.

Avenevoli, Shelli, Erin Knight, Ronald C. Kessler, and Kathleen R. Merikangas. 2008. "Epidemiology of Depression in Children and Adolescents." In John R. Z. Abela and Benjamin L. Hankin (Eds.), Handbook of Depression in Children and Adolescents. New York: Guilford Press. pp. 6–32.

Badiou, Alain. 2003. Saint Paul: The Foundation of Universalism. Palo Alto, CA: Stanford University Press.

Barthes, Roland. 1986 [1967]. "The Discourse of History." In The Rustle of Language, translated by Richard Howard. New York: Hill and Wang. pp. 127–40.

Becker, A. E., and Kleinman, A. 2013. "Mental Health and the Global Agenda." New England Journal of Medicine 369(1): 66–73.

Behere, Prakash B., Anweshak Das, Aniruddh P. Behere, and Richa Yadav. 2018. "Psychotropic Drugs in Children and Adolescents." In Kamal N. Kalita and Angshuman Kalita (Eds.), Psychiatry Update: Psychopharmacology. Assam, India: Bhabani Books.

Benedict, Ruth. 1934. "Anthropology and the Abnormal." Journal of General Psychology 10: 59–82.

———. 1938. "Continuities and Discontinuities in Cultural Conditioning." Psychiatry: Interpersonal and Biological Processes 1(2): 161–67.

Benoit, Laelia. 2016. L'Adolescent "Fragile:" Peut-on prédire en Psychiatrie? Paris: Editions Recherches.

Berlant, Lauren. 2011. Cruel Optimism. Durham, NC: Duke University Press.

Berthelot, Jean-Michel. 1995. "The Body as a Discursive Operator: Or the Aporias of a Sociology of the Body." Body and Society 1(1): 13–23.

Biehl, João. 2013. Vita: Life in a Zone of Social Abandonment, Updated with a New Afterword and Photo Essay [photographs by Torben Eskerod]. Oakland: University of California Press.

Biehl, João, Byron Good, and Arthur Kleinman (Eds.). 2007. Subjectivity: Ethnographic Investigations. Berkeley: University of California Press.

Bird, Hector R. 1996. "Epidemiology of Childhood Disorders in a Cross-Cultural Context." Journal of Child Psychology and Psychiatry and Allied Disciplines 37: 35–49.

Bleuler, Eugen. 1950 [1911]. Dementia Praecox or the Group of Schizophrenias. Translated by J. Zinkin. New York: International Universities Press.

Bloch, Ernst. 1986 [1959]. The Principle of Hope, vol. 1. Cambridge, MA: MIT Press.

Bluebond-Langner, Myra, and Jill Korbin. 2007. "Challenges and Opportunities in the Anthropology of Childhoods: An Introduction to 'Children, Childhoods, and Childhood Studies.'" American Anthropologist 109(2): 241–46.

Bogdan, Robert, and Steven J. Taylor. 1998. Introduction to Qualitative Research Methods: A Guidebook and Resource. New York: John Wiley & Sons.

Boon, James A. 1972. "Further Operations of 'Culture' in Anthropology: A Synthesis of and for Debate." Social Science Quarterly 53(2): 221–52.

Boozary, Andrew, and Kaveh G. Shojania. 2017. "Pathology of Poverty: The Need for Quality Improvement Efforts to Address Social Determinants of Health." BMJ Quality and Safety 27(6).

Bourdieu, Pierre. 1990 [1980]. The Logic of Practice. Translated by Richard Nice. Palo Alto, CA: Stanford University Press.

Briggs, Jean L. 1970. Never in Anger: Portrait of an Eskimo Family. Cambridge, MA: Harvard University Press.

Brodwin, Paul. 2013. Everyday Ethics: Voices from the Frontline of Community Psychiatry. Berkeley: University of California Press.

Brown, George W., and Tirril O. Harris. 1978. Social Origins of Depression: A Study of Psychiatric Disorder in Women. New York: Free Press.

Brown, Julia E. H., and S. Dennis. 2017. "Actively Negotiating the Mind-Body Divide: How Clozapine-Treated Schizophrenia Patients Make Health for Themselves." Culture, Medicine and Psychiatry 41(3): 368–81.

Burbank, Victoria. 1988. Aboriginal Adolescence: Maidenhood in and Australian Community. Piscataway, NJ: Rutgers University Press.

———. 1995. "Gender Hierarchy and Adolescent Sexuality: The Control of Female Reproduction in an Australian Aboriginal Community." Ethos 23(1): 33–46.

Burton, Linda M. 1997. "Ethnography and the Meaning of Adolescence in High-Risk Neighborhoods." Ethos 25(2): 208–17.

Canguilhem, Georges. 1989. The Normal and the Pathological. New York: Zone Books.

Carpenter-Song, Elizabeth. 2009. "Caught in the Psychiatric Net: Meanings and Experiences of ADHD, Pediatric Bipolar Disorder and Mental Health Treatment among a Diverse Group of Families in the United States." Culture, Medicine, and Psychiatry 33(1): 61–85.

———. 2015. "Putting Meaning into Medicine: Why Context Matters in Psychiatry." Epidemiology and Psychiatric Sciences 24: 1–4.

———. 2019. "'The Kids Were My Drive': Shattered Families, Moral Striving, and the Loss of Parental Selves in the Wake of Homelessness." Ethos 47(1): 54–72.

Cavalluzzo, Virginia A. 1991. "The Educational Process as Ego Enhancement in Inpatient Settings." In Robert L. Hendren and Irving N. Berlin (Eds.), Psychiatric Inpatient Care of Children and Adolescents: A Multicultural Approach. New York: John Wiley & Sons. pp. 161–75.

CDC [Centers for Disease Control and Prevention]. 2018. "Drug Overdose Mortality by State." www.cdc.gov/nchs/pressroom/sosmap/drug_poisoning_mortality/drug_poisoning.htm.

Chiedi, Joanne. 2019. "Provider Shortages and Limited Availability of Behavioral Health Services in New Mexico's Medicaid Managed Care." US Department of Health and Human Services Office of Inspector General Report OEI-02-17-00490.

Choudhury, Suparna, Kelly A. McKinney, and Laurence J. Kirmayer. 2015. "'Learning How to Deal with Feelings Differently': Psychotropic Medications as Vehicles of Socialization in Adolescence." Social Science & Medicine 143: 311–19.

Chubinsky, Peter, and Horacio Hojman. 2013. "Psychodynamic Perspectives on Psychotropic Medications for Children and Adolescents." Child and Adolescent Psychiatric Clinics of North America 22(2): 351–66.

Condon, Richard G. 1988. Inuit Youth: Growth and Change in the Canadian Arctic. Piscataway, NJ: Rutgers University Press.

———. 1995. "The Rise of the Leisure Class: Adolescence and Recreational Acculturation in the Canadian Arctic." Ethos 23(1): 47–68.

Cornelio, Jayeel S. 2016. Being Catholic in the Contemporary Philippines: Young People Reinterpreting Religion. London: Routledge.

Corrigan, Patrick W., and Amy C. Watson. 2002. "The Paradox of Self-Stigma and Mental Illness." Clinical Psychology: Science and Practice 9(1): 35–53.

Crapanzano, Vincent. 2003. "Reflections on Hope as a Category of Social and Psychological Analysis." Cultural Anthropology 18(1): 3–32.

Csordas, Thomas J. 2002. Body/Meaning/Healing. New York: Palgrave.

———. 2008. "Intersubjectivity and Intercorporeality." Subjectivity 22: 110–21.

———. 2009. "Growing Up Charismatic: Morality and Spirituality among Children in a Religious Community." Ethos 37(4): 414–40.

———. 2013. "Inferring Immediacy in Adolescent Accounts of Depression." Journal of Consciousness Studies 20(7–8): 239–53.

———. 2015. "Cultural Phenomenology of Psychiatric Illness." In L. Kirmayer, R. Lemelson, and C. Cummings (Eds.), Revisioning Psychiatry: Cultural Phenomenology, Critical Neuroscience, and Global Mental Health. New York: Cambridge University Press. pp. 117–40.

Csordas, Thomas J., Christopher Dole, Allen Tran, Matthew Strickland, and Michael G. Storck. 2010. "Ways of Asking, Ways of Telling: A Methodological Comparison of Ethnographic and Research Diagnostic Interviews." Culture, Medicine and Psychiatry 34: 29–55.

Csordas, Thomas J., and Janis H. Jenkins. 2018. "Living with a Thousand Cuts: Self-Cutting, Agency, and Mental Illness among Adolescents." Ethos 46(2): 206–29.

Csordas, Thomas J., and Arthur Kleinman. 1996. "The Therapeutic Process." In Carolyn Sargent and Thomas Johnson (Eds.), Medical Anthropology: Contemporary Theory and Method, revised ed. New York: Praeger. pp. 3–21.

Csordas, Thomas J., Michael Storck, and Milton Strauss. 2008. "Diagnosis and Distress in Navajo Healing." Journal of Nervous and Mental Disease 196(8): 585–96.

Danely, Jason. 2017. "Carer Narratives of Fatigue and Endurance in Japan and England." Subjectivity 10(4): 411–26.

Davis, Susan S., and Douglas A. Davis. 1989. Adolescence in a Moroccan Town: Making Social Sense. Piscataway, NJ: Rutgers University Press.

———. 1995. "'The Mosque and the Satellite': Media and Adolescence in a Moroccan Town." Journal of Youth and Adolescence 24(5): 577–93.

Dedios, Maria C., and Ekaterina Anderson. 2014. "Top of the Heap: Sarah Willen." Somatosphere. http://somatosphere.net/2014/top-of-the-heap-sarah-willen.html/.

Denzin, Norman, and Yvonna Lincoln. 1998. Strategies of Qualitative Inquiry. Thousand Oaks, CA: SAGE.

Desjarlais, Robert. 1997. Shelter Blues: Sanity and Selfhood among the Homeless. Philadelphia: University of Pennsylvania Press.

Desjarlais, Robert, and C. Jason Throop. 2011. "Phenomenological Approaches in Anthropology." Annual Review of Anthropology 40: 87–102.

Dole, Christopher, and Thomas J. Csordas. 2003. "Trials of Navajo Youth." Ethos 31: 357–84.

Dumit, Joseph. 2012. Drugs for Life: How Pharmaceutical Companies Define Our Health. Durham, NC: Duke University Press.

Duncan, Whitney L. 2015. "Gendered Trauma and Its Effects: Domestic Violence and 'PTSD' in Oaxaca." In Devon Hinton and Byron Good (Eds.), Culture and PTSD. Philadelphia: University of Pennsylvania Press.

———. 2018. Transforming Therapy: Mental Health Practice and Cultural Change in Mexico. Nashville, TN: Vanderbilt University Press.

Duranti, Alessandro. 2010. "Husserl, Intersubjectivity, and Anthropology." Anthropological Theory 10(1–2): 16–35.

Eagleton, Terry. 2015. Hope without Optimism. Charlottesville: University of Virginia Press.

Ecks, Stefan. 2013. Eating Drugs: Psychopharmaceutical Pluralism in India. New York: NYU Press.

Erikson, Erik H. 1963. Childhood and Society. New York: Norton.

Fabrega, Horacio J., and Barbara D. Miller. 1995a. "Toward a More Comprehensive Medical Anthropology: The Case of Adolescent Psychopathology." Medical Anthropology Quarterly: International Journal for the Cultural and Social Analysis of Health 9(4): 431–61.

———. 1995b. "Cultural and Historical Foundations." In Vincent B. Van Hasselt and Michel Hersen (Eds.), Handbook of Adolescent Psychology: A Guide to Diagnosis and Treatment. New York: Lexington Books. pp. 3–68.

Farmer, Paul. 2004a. "An Anthropology of Structural Violence." Current Anthropology 45(3): 305–25.

———. 2004b. Pathologies of Power: Health, Human Rights, and the New War on the Poor. Berkeley: University of California Press.

Fattore, Tobia, Jan Mason, and Elizabeth Watson. 2016. Children's Understandings of Well-being: Towards a Child Standpoint. New York: Springer.

Fields, M.J. 1960. Search for Security: An Ethno-Psychiatric Study of Rural Ghana. New York: Norton.

Floersch, Jerry, Lisa Townsend, Jeffrey Longhofer, Michelle Munson, Victoria Winbush, Derrick Kranke, Rachel Faber, Jeremy Thomas, Janis H. Jenkins, and Robert L. Findling. 2009. "Adolescent Experience of Psychotropic Treatment." Transcultural Psychiatry 46(1): 157–79.

Foltz, Robert, and Jonathan C. Huefner. 2014. "The Subjective Experience of Being Medicated in Troubled Youth: A Sample from Residential Treatment." Journal of Child and Family Studies 23(4): 752–63.

Ford, Tamsin, Robert Goodman, and Howard Meltzer. 2003. "The British Child and Adolescent Mental Health Survey 1999: The Prevalence of DSM-

IV Disorders." Journal of the American Academy of Psychiatry 42(10): 1203–11.

Foster, George M. 1976. "Disease Etiologies in Non-Western Medical Systems." American Anthropologist New Series 78(4): 773–82.

Fuchs, Estelle (Ed.). 1976. Youth in a Changing World: Cross-Cultural Perspectives on Adolescence. Chicago: Aldine.

Furlong, Michael J., and Douglas C. Smith. 1998. "Raging Rick to Tranquil Tom: An Empirically Based Multidimensional Anger Typology for Adolescent Males." Psychology in the Schools 35(3): 229–45.

Gable, Eric. 2000. "The Culture Development Club: Youth, Neo-tradition, and the Construction of Society in Guinea-Bissau." Anthropological Quarterly 73(4): 195–203.

Garcia, Angela. 2010. The Pastoral Clinic: Addiction and Dispossession along the Rio Grande. Berkeley: University of California Press.

Gilligan, Carol. 1977. "In a Different Voice: Women's Conceptions of Self and of Morality." Harvard Educational Review 47(4): 481–517.

———. 1982. In a Different Voice: Psychological Theory and Women's Development. Cambridge, MA: Harvard University Press.

Godfrey, J. 1987. A Philosophy of Human Hope. Dordrecht, Netherlands: Martinus Nijhoff.

Goffman, Erving. 1961. Asylums. New York: Anchor Books.

Goldston, David, Stephanie Daniel, Beth Reboussin, David Reboussin, Patricia Frazier, and Ashley Harris. 2001. "Cognitive Risk Factors and Suicide Attempts among Formerly Hospitalized Adolescents: A Prospective Naturalistic Study." Journal of the American Academy of Child and Adolescent Psychiatry 40(1): 91–99.

Good, Byron. 1992. "Culture and Psychopathology: Directions for Psychiatric Anthropology." In Theodore Schwartz, Geoffrey White, and Catherine Lutz (Eds.), New Directions in Psychological Anthropology. Cambridge: Cambridge University Press. pp. 181–205.

———. 1994. "Medicine, Rationality, and Experience." In Medicine, Rationality and Experience: An Anthropological Perspective. Cambridge: Cambridge University Press.

———. 2010. "The Complexities of Psychopharmaceutical Hegemonies in Indonesia." In Janis H. Jenkins (Ed.), Pharmaceutical Self: The Global Shaping of Experience in an Age of Psychopharmacology. Santa Fe, NM: School for Advanced Research Press. pp. 117–44.

———. 2012. "Theorizing the 'Subject' of Medical and Psychiatric Anthropology." Journal of the Royal Anthropological Institute 18: 515–35.

Good, Mary-Jo D. 1995. American Medicine: The Quest for Competence. Berkeley: University of California Press.

———. 2007. "The Biotechnical Embrace and the Medical Imaginary." In João Biehl, Byron Good, and Arthur Kleinman (Eds.), Subjectivity: Ethnographic Investigations. Berkeley: University of California Press. pp. 362–80.

———. 2010. "Trauma in Postconflict Aceh and Psychopharmaceuticals as a Medium of Exchange." In Janis H. Jenkins (Ed.), Pharmaceutical Self. Santa Fe, NM: School for Advanced Research Press.

Good, Mary-Jo D., Byron J. Good, Cynthia Schaffer, and Stuart E. Lind. 1990. "American Oncology and the Discourse on Hope." Culture, Medicine and Psychiatry 14: 59–79.

Good, Mary-Jo D., Seth D. Hannah, and Sarah S. Willen. 2011. "Shattering Culture: An Introduction." In Mary-Jo D. Good et al. (Eds.), Shattering Culture: American Medicine Responds to Cultural Diversity. New York: Russell Sage Foundation.

Good, Mary-Jo D., Cara James, Byron J. Good, and Anne E. Becker. 2005. "The Culture of Medicine and Racial, Ethnic, and Class Disparities in Healthcare." In Mary Romero and Eric Margolis (Eds.), The Blackwell Companion to Social Inequalities. Hoboken, NJ: Wiley-Blackwell. pp. 396–423.

Guboglo, M.N. 1999. "The Formation of a Civil Identity: The Experience of Russian Youth." Anthropology & Archaeology of Eurasia 38(3): 38–56.

Gullotta, Thomas P., and Gerald R. Adams (Eds.). 2005. Handbook of Adolescent Behavioral Problems: Evidence-Based Approaches to Prevention and Treatment. Boston: Springer.

Haas, Bridget M. 2017. "Citizens-in-Waiting, Deportees-in-Waiting: Power, Temporality and Suffering in the U.S. Asylum System." Ethos 45(1): 75–97.

———. 2019a. "Adjudicators, Suspicion, and the Ambivalent Production of Authoritative Knowledge." In Bridget M. Haas and Amy Shuman (Eds.), Technologies of Suspicion and the Ethics of Obligation in Political Asylum. Athens: Ohio University/Swallow Press.

———. 2019b. "Therapeutic Interventions amid Immigration Limbo." Paper presented to the Psychological and Medical Anthropology Seminar, University of California San Diego.

Habermas, Tilman, and Susan Block. 2000. "Getting a Life: The Emergence of the Life Story in Adolescence." Psychological Bulletin 126(5): 748–69.

Hage, Ghassan. 2003. Against Paranoid Nationalism: Searching for Hope in a Shrinking Society. Annandale, Australia: Pluto Press.

Haidt, Jonathan. 2003. "The Moral Emotions." In Richard J. Davidson, Klaus R. Scherer, and H. Hill Goldsmith (Eds.), Handbook of Affective Sciences. Oxford: Oxford University Press.

Hall, Granville S. 1904. Adolescence: Its Psychology and Its Relations to Physiology, Anthropology, Sociology, Sex, Crime, Religion and Education. New York: D. Appleton.

Hallowell, A. Irving. 1955. Culture and Experience. Philadelphia: University of Pennsylvania Press.

Hannah, Seth D. 2011. "Clinical Care in Environments of Hyperdiversity." In Mary-Jo D. Good et al. (Eds.), Shattering Culture: American Medicine Responds to Cultural Diversity. New York: Russell Sage Foundation. pp. 35–69.

Harding, Sandra. 1991. "Strong Objectivity and Socially Situated Knowledge." In Whose Science? Whose Knowledge? Ithaca, New York: Cornell University Press.

———. 2015. Objectivity and Diversity: Another Logic of Scientific Research. Chicago: University of Chicago Press.

Harvey, David. 2000. Spaces of Hope. Berkeley: University of California Press.

Heidegger, Martin. 1962 [1927]. Being and Time. New York: Harper and Row.

———. 1978 [1947]. "Letter on Humanism." In Basic Writings: Nine Key Essays, Plus the Introduction to Being and Time. Translated by David Farrell Krell. London: Routledge.

Hein, D., F. Matzner, M. First, R. Spitzer, J. Williams, and M. Gibbon. 1998. Structured Clinical Interview for DSM-IV Childhood Diagnoses, KID-SCID. New York: Columbia University Medical School.

Hejtmanek, Katherine. 2014. "Practicing and Resisting Constraint: Ethnography of 'Counter Response' in American Adolescent Psychiatric Custody." Culture, Medicine, and Psychiatry 38: 578–96.

———. 2016. "Care, Closeness, and Becoming 'Better': Transformation and Therapeutic Process in American Adolescent Psychiatric Custody." Ethos 44(3): 313–32.

Hendren, Robert L., and Irving N. Berlin (Eds.). 1991. Psychiatric Inpatient Care of Children and Adolescents: A Multicultural Approach. New York: John Wiley & Sons.

Hollan, Douglas. 2008. "Being There: On the Imaginative Aspects of Understanding Others and Being Understood." Ethos 36(4): 475–89.

Hollan, Douglas, and C. Jason Throop. 2008. "Whatever Happened to Empathy? Introduction." Ethos 36(4): 385–401.

Hollifield, Michael, Teddy D. Warner, Janis Jenkins, Nityamo Sinclair-Lian, Barry Krakow, Valorie Eckert, Pary Karadaghi, and Joseph Westermeyer. 2006. "Assessing War Trauma in Refugees: Properties of the Comprehensive Trauma Inventory-104." Journal of Traumatic Stress 19(4): 527–40.

Hollifield, Michael, Teddy D. Warner, Nityamo Lian, Barry Krakow, Janis H. Jenkins, James Kesler, Jayne Stevenson, and Joseph Westermeyer. 2001. "Measuring Trauma and Health Status in Refugees: A Critical Review." Journal of the American Medical Association 288: 611–21.

Hollos, Marida, and Philip E. Leis. 1989. Becoming Nigerian in Ijo Society. New Brunswick, NJ: Rutgers University Press.

Hunner-Kreisel, Christine, and Melanie Kuhn. 2010. "Children's Perspectives: Methodological Critique and Empirical Studies." In Sabine Andresen, Isabell Diehm, Uwe Sander, and Holger Ziegler (Eds.), Children and the Good Life: New Challenges for Research on Children. Dordrecht, Netherlands: Springer. pp. 115–18.

Husserl, Edmund. 2013 [1931]. Ideas: General Introduction to Pure Phenomenology. New York: Routledge.

Hydén, Lars-Christer. 1997. "Illness and Narrative." Sociology of Health & Illness 19(1): 48–69.

Jackson, Michael (Ed.). 1996. Things as They Are: New Directions in Phenomenological Anthropology. Bloomington: Indiana University Press.

James, Allison. 2007. "Giving Voice to Children's Voices: Practices and Problems, Pitfalls and Potentials." American Anthropologist 109(2): 261–72.

James, Allison, Chris Jenks, and Alan Prout. 1998. Theorizing Childhood. Cambridge, MA: Polity Press.

Jenkins, Janis H. 1996. "Culture, Emotion, and Post-Traumatic Stress Disorder." In Anthony J. Marsella, Matthew J. Friedman, Ellen T. Gerrity, and Raymond M. Scurfield (Eds.), Ethnocultural Aspects of Posttraumatic Stress Disorder. Washington, DC: American Psychological Association Press. pp. 165–82.

———. 1997. "Subjective Experience of Persistent Schizophrenia and Depression among US Latinos and Euro-Americans." British Journal of Psychiatry 171(1): 20–25.

———. 2010a. "Introduction." In Janis H. Jenkins (Ed.), Pharmaceutical Self: The Global Shaping of Experience in an Age of Psychopharmacology. Santa Fe, NM: School for Advanced Research Press. pp. 3–16.

———. 2010b. "Pharmaceutical Self and Imaginary in the Social Field of Psychiatric Treatment." In Janis H. Jenkins (Ed.), Pharmaceutical Self: The Global Shaping of Experience in an Age of Psychopharmacology. Santa Fe, NM: School for Advanced Research Press. pp. 17–40.

———. 2015a. Extraordinary Conditions: Culture and Experience in Mental Illness. Berkeley: University of California Press.

———. 2015b. "Straining Psychic and Social Sinew: Trauma among Adolescent Psychiatric Patients in New Mexico." Medical Anthropology Quarterly 29(1): 42–60.

———. In press. "Intimate and Social Spheres of Mental Illness." In João Biehl and Vincanne Adams (Eds.), Arc of Interference: Medical Anthropology for Worlds on the Edge. Durham, NC: Duke University Press.

Jenkins, Janis H., and Robert J. Barrett. 2004. "Introduction." In Janis H. Jenkins and Robert J. Barrett (Eds.), Schizophrenia, Culture, and Subjectivity: The Edge of Experience. New York: Cambridge University Press. pp. 29–61.

Jenkins, Janis H., and Elizabeth Carpenter-Song. 2005. "The New Paradigm of Recovery from Schizophrenia: Cultural Conundrums of Improvement without Cure." Culture, Medicine, and Psychiatry 29(4): 379–413.

———. 2008. "Stigma Despite Recovery: Strategies for Living in the Aftermath of Psychosis." Medical Anthropology Quarterly 22(4): 381–409.

———. 2009. "Awareness of Stigma among Persons with Schizophrenia: Marking the Contexts of Lived Experience." Journal of Nervous and Mental Disease 197(7): 520–29.

Jenkins, Janis H., and Mary-Jo D. Good. 2014. "Women and Global Mental Health: Vulnerability and Empowerment." In Samuel O. Opakpu (Ed.), Essentials of Global Mental Health. New York: Cambridge University Press.

Jenkins, Janis H., and Bridget M. Haas. 2015. "Trauma in the Lifeworlds of Adolescents." In Devon Hinton and Byron Good (Eds.), Culture and PTSD. Philadelphia: University of Pennsylvania Press. pp. 215–45.

Jenkins, Janis H., and Marvin Karno. 1992. "The Meaning of 'Expressed Emotion': Theoretical Issues Raised by Cross-Cultural Research." American Journal of Psychiatry 149: 9–21

Jenkins, Janis H., and Ellen E. Kozelka. 2017. "Global Mental Health and Psychopharmacology in Precarious Ecologies: Anthropological Considerations for Engagement and Efficacy." In Ross G. White, Sumeet Jain, David M.R. Orr, and Ursula M. Read (Eds.), The Palgrave Handbook of Sociocultural Perspectives on Global Mental Health. New York: Palgrave Press.

Jenkins, Janis H., Giselle Sanchez, and Olga L. Olivas-Hernández. 2019. "Loneliness, Adolescence, and Global Mental Health: *Soledad* and Structural Violence in Mexico." Transcultural Psychiatry. https://doi.org/10.1177/1363461519880126.

Jenkins, Janis H., and Annika Stone. 2017. "Global Mental Health and Adolescent Anxiety: Kin, Care, and Struggle in New Mexico." Culture, Medicine and Psychiatry 41(4): 609–29.

Jenkins, Janis H., Milton E. Strauss, Elizabeth Carpenter-Song, Dawn Miller, Jerry Floersch, and Martha Sajatovic. 2005. "Subjective Experience of Recovery from Schizophrenia with Atypical Antipsychotic Medications." International Journal of Social Psychiatry 51(3): 211–27.

Jordan, Jessica, Niti Patel, and Kia J. Bentley. 2017. "Emerging Adult Identity Following Adolescent Experiences with Psychotropic Medications: A Retrospective Study." Journal of Human Behavior in the Social Environment 27(7): 694–705.

Kaiser, Bonnie N., C. Ticao, C. Anoje, J. Minto, J. Boglosa, and B.A. Kohrt. 2019a. "Adapting Culturally Appropriate Mental Health Screening Tools for Use among Conflict-Affected and Other Vulnerable Adolescents in Nigeria." Global Mental Health 6: e10.

Kaiser, Bonnie N., Saiba Varma, Elizabeth Carpenter-Song, Rebecca Sareff, Sauharda Rai, and Brandon A. Kohrt. 2019b. "Eliciting Recovery Narratives in Global Mental Health: Benefits and Potential Harms in Service User Participation." Psychiatric Rehabilitation Journal. https://doi.org/10.1037/prj0000384.

Kano, Miria, Cathleen Willging, and Barbara Rylko-Bauer. 2009. "Community Participation in New Mexico's Behavioral Health Carew Reform." Medical Anthropology Quarterly 23(3): 277–97.

Karno, Marvin, Janis H. Jenkins, Aurora De La Selva, Felipe Santana, Cynthia Telles, Steven Lopez, and Jim Mintz. 1987. "Expressed Emotion and Schizophrenic Outcome among Mexican-American Families." Journal of Nervous and Mental Disease 175(3): 143–51.

Kashani, Javad, Lourdes Suarez, Wesley Allen, and John C. Reid. 1997. "Hopelessness in Inpatient Youths: A Closer Look at Behavior, Emotional Expression, and Social Support." Journal of the American Academy of Child and Adolescent Psychiatry 36(11): 1625–31.

Katz, Jack, and Thomas J. Csordas. 2003. "Phenomenological Ethnography in Sociology and Anthropology." Ethnography 4(3): 275–88.

Kazdin, Alan E., Nancy French, Alan Unis, Karen Esveldt-Dawson, and Rosanna Sherick. 1983. "Hopelessness, Depression, and Suicidal Intent among Psychiatrically Disturbed Inpatient Children." Journal of Counseling and Clinical Psychology 51(4): 504–10.

Kerlinsky, Daniel. 1991. "Integrating Interdisciplinary Team-Centered Treatment." In Robert L. Hendren and Irving N. Berlin (Eds.), Psychiatric Inpatient Care of Children and Adolescents: A Multicultural Approach. New York: John Wiley & Sons. pp. 93–111.

Kessler, Ronald C. 2003. "Epidemiology of Women and Depression." Journal of Affective Disorders 74(1): 5–13.

Kessler, Ronald C., Patricia Berglund, Olga Delmer, Robert Jin, Kathleen R. Merikangas, and Ellen E. Walters. 2005. "Lifetime Prevalence and Age-of-Onset Distribution of DSM-IV Disorders in the National Co-Morbidity Survey Replication." Archives of General Psychiatry 62: 593–602.

Kessler, Ronald C., Katie A. McLaughlin, Jennifer Greif Green, and Michael J. Gruber. 2010. "Childhood Adversities and Adult Psychopathology in the WHO World Mental Health Surveys." British Journal of Psychiatry 197(5): 378–85.

Kieling, Christian, Helen Baker-Henningham, Myron Belfer, Gabriella Conti, Ilgi Ertem, Olayinka Omigbodun, Luis A. Rohde, Shoba Srinath, Nurper Ulkuer, and Atif Rahman. 2011. "Child and Adolescent Health Worldwide: Evidence for Action." Lancet 378: 1515–25.

Kirmayer, Laurence J. 2008. "Empathy and Alterity in Cultural Psychiatry." Ethos 36(4): 457–74.

Kirmayer, Laurence J., Robert Lemelson, and Constance A. Cummings. 2015. Re-visioning Psychiatry: Cultural Phenomenology, Critical Neurosciences, and Global Mental Health. Cambridge: Cambridge University Press.

Kleinman, Arthur. 1980. Patients and Healers in the Context of Culture: An Exploration of the Borderland between Anthropology, Medicine, and Psychiatry. Berkeley: University of California Press.

———. 1988a. Rethinking Psychiatry: From Cultural Category to Personal Experience. New York: Free Press.

———. 1988b. The Illness Narratives: Suffering, Healing, and the Human Condition. New York: Basic Books.

———. 1999. "Experience and Its Moral Modes: Culture, Human Conditions and Disorder." In Grethe B. Peterson (Ed.), The Tanner Lectures on Human Values, vol. 20. Salt Lake City: University of Utah Press. pp. 357–420.

———. 2006. What Really Matters: Living a Moral Life amidst Uncertainty and Danger. New York: Oxford University Press.

———. 2019. The Soul of Care: The Moral Education of a Husband and Doctor. New York: Penguin Random House.

Kleinman, Arthur, Veena Das, and Margaret Lock (Eds). 1997. Social Suffering. Berkeley: University of California Press.

Kleinman, Arthur, and Joan Kleinman. 1991. "Suffering and Its Professional Transformation: Toward an Ethnography of Interpersonal Experience." Culture, Medicine and Psychiatry 15(3): 275–300.

Kohrt, Brandon, Mark J. D. Jordans, Wietse A. Tol, Em Perera, Rohit Karaki, Suraj Koirala, and Nawaraj Upadhaya. 2010. "Social Ecology of Child Soldiers: Child, Family, and Community Determinants of Mental Health, Psychosocial Well-being, and Reintegration in Nepal." Transcultural Psychiatry 47: 727–53.

Kohrt, Brandon, Mark J. D. Jordans, Wietse A. Tol, Rebecca A. Speckman, Sujen M. Maharjan, Carol M. Worthman, and Ivan H. Komproe. 2008.

"Comparison of Mental Health between Former Child Soldiers and Children Never Conscripted by Armed Groups in Nepal." Journal of the American Medical Association 300(6): 691–702.

Kohrt, Brandon, and Emily Mendenhall (Eds.). 2015. Global Mental Health (Anthropology and Global Public Health). Walnut Creek, CA: Left Coast Press.

Kokanović, Renata, and Jacinthe Flore (Guest Eds.). 2017. "Subjectivity and Illness Narratives" [Special issue]. Subjectivity 10(4).

Konner, Melvin, and Marjorie Shostak. 1986. "Adolescent Pregnancy and Childbearing: An Anthropological Perspective." In Jane B. Lancaster and Beatrix A. Hamburg (Eds.), School-Age Pregnancy and Parenthood: Biosocial Dimensions. New York: Aldine de Gruyter. pp. 325–46.

Korbin, Jill (Ed.). 1981. Child Abuse and Neglect: Cross-Cultural Perspectives. Berkeley: University of California Press.

Korbin, Jill, and Eileen P. Anderson-Fye. 2011. "Adolescence Matters: Practice- and Policy-Relevant Research and Engagement in Psychological Anthropology." Ethos 39(4): 415–25.

Koss, Mary, Lori Heise, and Nancy Russo. 1994. "The Global Health Burden of Rape." Psychology of Women Quarterly 18: 509–37.

Kranke, Derrick A., Jerry Floersch, Bridget O. Kranke, and Michelle R. Munson. 2011. "A Qualitative Investigation of Self-Stigma among Adolescents Taking Psychiatric Medication." Psychiatric Services 62(8): 893–99.

Kranke, Derrick A., Sally E. Jackson, Debbie A. Taylor, Joan Landguth, and Jerry Floersch. 2015. "'I'm Loving Life': Adolescents' Empowering Experiences of Living with a Mental Illness." Qualitative Social Work 14(1): 102–18.

Lakoff, George, and Zoltan Kovecses. 1987. "The Cognitive Model of Anger Inherent in American English." In Dorothy Holland and Naomi Quinn (Eds.), Cultural Models and Language in Thought. Cambridge: Cambridge University Press.

Lear, Jonathan. 2006. Radical Hope: Ethics in the Face of Cultural Devastation. Cambridge, MA: Harvard University Press.

Lebra, Takie. 1995. "Skipped and Postponed Adolescence of Aristocratic Women in Japan: Resurrecting the Culture/Nature Issue." Ethos 23(1): 79–102.

Leis, Philip E., and Marida Hollos. 1995. "Intergenerational Discontinuities in Nigeria." Ethos 23(1): 103–18.

Lende, Daniel H. 2012. "Poverty Poisons the Brain." Annals of Anthropological Practice 36(1): 183–201.

Leocata, Angela. 2018. Reconsidering Care: Subjectivities, Technologies, and Caregiving among Lay-Counselors in Goa, India. Honor's thesis, Department of Anthropology, Harvard University.

Leocata, Angela, Vikram Patel, and Arthur Kleinman. In review. "When the Trial Ends: Moral Experiences of Caregiving in a Randomized Controlled Trial in Goa, India." Presented by Angela Leocata at UC San Diego Seminar Series for the Program in Psychological and Medical Anthropology, November 1, 2019.

Lester, Rebecca. 2011. "How Do I Code for Black Fingernail Polish? Finding the Missing Adolescent in Managed Mental Health Care." Ethos 39(4): 481–96.

LeVine, Robert. 2007. "Ethnographic Studies of Childhood: A Historical Overview." American Anthropologist 109(2): 247–60.

———. 2011. "Traditions in Transition: Adolescents Remaking Culture." Ethos 39(4): 426–31.

Lindemann, Hilde. 2006. An Invitation to Feminist Ethics. Boston: McGraw-Hill.

Linger, Daniel. 2010. "What Is It Like to Be Someone Else?" Ethos 38(2): 205–29.

Lofland, John, and Lyn H. Lofland. 1995. Analyzing Social Settings: A Guide to Qualitative Observation and Analysis. Belmont, CA: Wadsworth.

Longhofer, Jeffrey, and Jerry Floersch. 2010. "Desire and Disappointment: Adolescent Psychotropic Treatment and Adherence." Anthropology & Medicine 17(2): 159–72.

Lovell, Anne M. 2013 Tending to the unseen in extraordinary circumstances. On Arendt's natality and severe mental illness after hurricane Katrina. Iride 26(70):563–580 DOI: 10.1414/75074

———. 2019. Falling, Dying Sheep, and the Divine: Notes on Thick Therapeutics in Peri-Urban Senegal. Culture, Medicine, and Psychiatry https://doi.org/10.1007/s11013-019-09657-2. In Genealogies and Anthropologies of Global Mental Health, Anne M. Lovell, Ursula M. Read, and Claudia Lang, Eds. Culture, Medicine, and Psychiatry 43:519–547 https://doi.org/10.1007/s11013-019-09660-7

Lowe, Edward. 2003. "Identity, Activity, and the Well-being of Adolescents and Youth: Lessons from Young People in a Micronesian Society." Culture, Medicine, and Psychiatry 27: 187–219.

Lu, Chunling, Zhihui Li, and Vikram Patel. 2018. "Global Child and Adolescent Mental Health: The Orphan of Development Assistance for Health." PLoS Medicine 15(3): e1002524.

Luborsky, Mark, and Robert Rubinstein. 1995. "Sampling in Qualitative Research: Rationale, Issues, and Methods." Research on Aging SAGE 17(1): 89–113.

Lund, Crick. 2012. "Poverty and Mental Health: A Review of Practice and Policies." Neuropsychiatry 2(3): 1–7.

Lutz, Catherine A. 1988. Unnatural Emotions: Everyday Sentiments on a Micronesian Atoll and Their Challenge to Western Theory. Chicago: University of Chicago Press.

Macartney, Suzanne E. 2011. Child Poverty in the United States 2009 and 2010 Selected Race Groups and Hispanic Origin. Washington, DC: US Department of Commerce, Economics and Statistics Administration, US Census Bureau.

Maira, Sunaina. 1999. "Identity Dub: The Paradoxes of an Indian American Youth Subculture (New York Mix)." Cultural Anthropology 14(1): 29–60.

Marcel, Gabriel. 1951. Homo Viator: Introduction to a Metaphysic of Hope. Translated by Emma Craufurd. New York: Harper and Row.

Marcia, James. 1980. "Identity in Adolescence." In Joseph Adelson (Ed.), Handbook of Adolescent Psychology. New York: John Wiley & Sons.

Marett, Robert R. 1933. Sacraments of Simple Folk. Oxford: Clarendon Press.

Marmot, Michael, Sharon Friel, Ruth Bell, Tanja A. J. Houweling, and Sebastian Taylor. 2008. "Closing the Gap in a Generation: Health Equity through Action on the Social Determinants of Health." Lancet 372: 1661–69.

Marmot, Michael, and Richard Wilkinson (Eds.). 2006. Social Determinants of Health, 2nd ed. Oxford: Oxford University Press.

Martin, Emily. 2009. Bipolar Expeditions: Mania and Depression in American Culture. Princeton, NJ: Princeton University Press.

———. 2010. "Self-Making and the Brain." Subjectivity 3(4): 366–81

———. 2018. "Playing with Fire: Imagining Anthropology and Science." Distinguished Lecture, American Anthropological Association, San Jose, CA.

Martínez-Hernáez, Angel. 2000. What's Behind the Symptom? On Psychiatric Observation and Anthropological Understanding. Oxfordshire, England: Routledge.

———. 2020. Neuronarratives of Affliction: Antidepressants, Neuropolitics and the "Entrepreneur of Oneself." Culture Medicine and Psychiatry 44(2): 230-248 DOI: 10.1007/s11013-019-09651-8

Martínez-Hernáez, Angel, Natàlia Carceller-Maicas, Susan M. DiGiacomo, Santiago Ariste. 2016. Social support and gender differences in coping with depression among emerging adults: A mixed-methods study. Child and Adolescent Psychiatry and Mental Health 10(2):1-11. DOI: 10.1186/s13034-015-00880x.

Mattingly, Cheryl. 2010. "The Paradox of Hope: Journeys through a Clinical Borderland." Berkeley: University of California Press.

Mattingly, Cheryl, and Linda Garro. 2000. Narrative and the Cultural Construction of Illness and Healing. Berkeley: University of California Press.

Mayall, Berry. 2002. Towards a Sociology of Childhood: Thinking from Children's Lives. Buckingham, UK: Open University Press.

McLaughlin, Katie A., Jennifer G. Green, Margarita Alegría, E. Jane Costello, Michael J. Gruber, Nancy A. Sampson, Ronald C. Kessler. 2012. "Food Insecurity and Mental Disorders in a National Sample of U.S. Adolescents." Journal of the American Academy of Child and Adolescent Psychiatry 51(12): 1293–1303.

McMillan, Dean, Simon Gilbody, Emma Beresford, and Liz Neilly. 2007. "Can We Predict Suicide and Non-fatal Self-harm with the Beck Hopelessness Scale?" Psychological Medicine 37(6): 769–78.

Mead, Margaret. 1928. Coming of Age in Samoa: A Psychological Study of Primitive Youth for Western Civilization. New York: William Morrow.

Menon, Usha, and Richard A. Shweder. 1994. "Kali's Tongue: Cultural Psychology and the Power of Shame in Orissa, India." In Shinobu Kitayama and Hazel R. Markus (Eds.), Emotion and Culture: Empirical Studies of Mutual Influence. Washington, DC: American Psychological Association.

Merleau-Ponty, Maurice. 1962 [1945]. Phenomenology of Perception. Translated by Colin Smith. New York: Routledge.

———. 1968 [1964]. The Visible and the Invisible. Translated by Alhonsi Lingis. Edited by Claude Lefort. Evanston, IL: Northwestern University Press.

Meyers, Todd. 2013. The Clinic and Elsewhere: Addiction, Adolescents, and the Afterlife of Therapy. Seattle: University of Washington Press.

Miles, Ann. 2000. "Poor Adolescent Girls and Social Transformations in Cuenca, Ecuador." Ethos 28(1): 54–74.

Mills, Mary Beth. 1999. "Enacting Solidarity: Unions and Migrant Youth in Thailand." Critique of Anthropology 19(2): 175–92.

Minkowski, Eugene. 1970 [1933]. Lived Time: Phenomenological and Psycho-pathological Studies. Evanston, IL: Northwestern University Press.

Miyazaki, Hirokazu. 2004. The Method of Hope: Anthropology, Philosophy, and Fijian Knowledge. Palo Alto, CA: Stanford University Press.

———. 2006. "Economy of Dreams: Hope in Global Capitalism and Its Critiques." Cultural Anthropology 21(2): 147–72.

Mundy, Peter, Julia Robertson, Milton Greenblatt, and Marjorie Robertson. 1989. "Residential Instability in Adolescent Inpatients." Journal of the American Academy of Child & Adolescent Psychiatry 28(2): 176–81.

Murphy, Andrea L., David M. Gardner, Steve Kisely, Charmaine Cooke, Stanley P. Kutcher, and Jean Hughes. 2013. "Youth, Caregiver, and Prescriber Experiences of Antipsychotic-Related Weight Gain." ISRN Obesity: 390130.

———. 2015. "A Qualitative Study of Antipsychotic Medication Experiences of Youth." Journal of the Canadian Academy of Child and Adolescent Psychiatry 24(1): 61.

Myers, Neely L. 2015. Recovery's Edge: An Ethnography of Mental Health Care and Moral Agency. Nashville, TN: Vanderbilt University Press.

Narendorf, Sarah C., Michelle R. Munson, and Jerry Floersch. 2015. "Perspectives on Psychotropic Medication Treatment among Young Adults Formerly Served in Public Systems of Care: A Thematic and Narrative Analysis." Journal of the Society for Social Work and Research 6(1): 121–43.

Nasser, Elizabeth H., Natalie Walders, and Janis H. Jenkins. 2002. "The Experience of Schizophrenia: What's Gender Got to Do with It? A Critical Review of the Current Status of Research on Schizophrenia." Schizophrenia Bulletin 28(2): 351–62.

New Mexico Department of Health. 2018. "New Mexico Substance Use Epidemiology." https://nmhealth.org/data/view/substance/2201/.

Nissen, Nina, and Mette Bech Risor. 2018. Diagnostic Fluidity: Working with Uncertainty and Mutability. Tarragona, Spain: Publicacions Universitat Rovira i Virgili.

Nolen-Hoeksema, Susan. 1990. Sex Differences in Depression. Stanford, CA: Stanford University Press.

———. 1995. "Epidemiology and Theories of Gender Differences in Unipolar Depression." In Mary V. Seeman (Ed.), Gender and Psychopathology. Arlington, VA: American Psychiatric Association. pp. 63–87.

Obeyesekere, Gananath. 1990. The Work of Culture: Symbolic Transformation in Psychoanalysis and Anthropology. Chicago: University of Chicago Press.

Ochs, Elinor, and Lisa Capps. 1996. "Narrating the Self." Annual Review of Anthropology 25: 19–43.

———. 2001. Living Narrative: Creating Lives in Everyday Storytelling. Cambridge, MA: Harvard University Press.

Olfson, Mark, Marissa King, and Michael Schoenbaum. 2015. "Treatment of Young People with Antipsychotic Medications in the United States." JAMA Psychiatry 72(9): 867–74.

Opakpu, Samuel O. (Ed.). 2014. Essentials of Global Mental Health. New York: Cambridge University Press.

Panter-Brick, Catherine. 2002. "Street Children, Human Rights, and Public Health: A Critique and Future Directions." Annual Review of Anthropology 31: 147–71.

Parish, Steven M. 2008. Subjectivity and Suffering in American Culture: Possible Selves. New York: Palgrave Macmillan.

———. 2014. "Between Persons: How Concepts of the Person Make Moral Experience Possible." Ethos: Journal of the Society for Psychological Anthropology 42(1): 31–50.

Patel, Vikram. 2005. "Poverty, Gender and Mental Health Promotion in a Global Society." Promotion & Education 12(Supplement 2): 26–29.

Patel, Vikram, Alan Flisher, Sarah Hetrick, and Patrick McGorry. 2007a. "Mental Health of Young People: A Global Public-Health Challenge." Lancet 369: 1302–13.

Patel, Vikram, Alan Flisher, Anula Nikapota, and Savita Malhotra. 2007b. "Promoting Child and Adolescent Mental Health in Low- and Middle-Income Countries." Child Psychology and Psychiatry 49(3): 313–34.

Perreault, Marc, and Gilles Bibeau. 2003. La Gang: une chimère à apprivoiser: marginalité et transnationalité chez les jeunes Québécois d'origine afro-antillaise. Montreal, Canada: Boreal.

Pescosolido, Bernice A., Brea L. Perry, J.K. Martin, Jane D. McLeod, Peter S. Jensen. 2007. "Stigmatizing Attitudes and Beliefs about Treatment and Psychiatric Medications for Children with Mental Illness." Psychiatric Services 58(5): 613–18.

Pratt, Laura A., Debra J. Brody, and Qiuping Gu. 2017. "Antidepressant Use among Persons Aged 12 and Over: United States, 2011–2014." NCHS Data Brief 283. Hyattsville, MD: National Center for Health Statistics.

Ram, Kalpana, and Chris Houston (Eds.). 2015. Phenomenology in Anthropology: A Sense of Perspective. Bloomington: Indiana University Press. pp. 50–67.

Ratcliffe, Matthew. 2012. "Phenomenology as a Form of Empathy." Inquiry 55(5): 473–95.

Read, Ursula. 2012. "'I Want the One That Will Heal Me Completely So It Won't Come Back Again': The Limits of Antipsychotic Medication in Rural Ghana." Transcultural Psychiatry 49(3–4): 438–60.

Resnick, M.D., R.W. Blum, and L. Harris. 1989. Technical Report on the Adolescent Health Survey, Adolescent Health Database Project, University of Minnesota Adolescent Health Program. Minneapolis: University of Minnesota Press.

Ricoeur, Paul. 1984. Time and Narrative, vol. 1. Chicago: University of Chicago Press.

Rorty, Richard. 1999. Philosophy and Social Hope. London: Penguin.

Rosaldo, Michelle. 1984. "Toward an Anthropology of Self and Feeling." In Richard A. Shweder and Robert A. LeVine (Eds.), Culture Theory: Essays on Mind, Self, and Emotion. New York: Cambridge University Press. pp. 137–57.

Rosaldo, Renato. 1993 [1989]. "Introduction: Grief and a Headhunter's Rage." In Culture and Truth: The Remaking of Social Analysis. Boston: Beacon Press.

Sapir, Edward. 1932. "Cultural Anthropology and Psychiatry." Journal of Abnormal and Social Psychology 27: 229–42.

Scheper-Hughes, Nancy, and Carolyn Sargent (Eds.). 1998. Small Wars: The Cultural Politics of Childhood. Berkeley: University of California Press.

Schepis, Ty S., Timothy E. Wilens, Sean E. McCabe. 2019. "Prescription Drug Misuse Sources of Controlled Medications in Adolescents." Journal of the American Academy of Child & Adolescent Psychiatry 58(7): 670–80.

Schlegel, Alice. 1995. "A Cross-Cultural Approach to Adolescence." Ethos 23(1): 15–32.

Schlegel, Alice, and Herbert Barry. 1991. Adolescence: An Anthropological Inquiry. New York: Free Press.

Seidman, Jerome M. (Ed.) 1953. The Dryden Press Publications in Interpersonal Relations. The Adolescent: A Book of Reading. Ft. Worth, TX: Dryden Press.

Shaffer, David, Madelyn S. Gould, James R. Brasic, Paul Ambrosini, Prudence Fisher, Hector Bird, and Satwant Aluwahlia. 1983. "A Children's Global Assessment Scale (CGAS)." Archives of General Psychiatry 40: 1228–31.

Sharp, Lesley. 2002. The Sacrificed Generation: Youth, History, and the Colonized Mind in Madagascar. Berkeley: University of California Press.

Shimazono, Yosuke. 2005. Narrative Analysis in Medical Anthropology. M. Phil. dissertation, Institute of Social and Cultural Anthropology, University of Oxford.

Shohet, Merav. 2018. "Beyond the Clinic? Eluding a Medical Diagnosis of Anorexia through Narrative." Transcultural Psychiatry 55(4): 495–515.

Skelton, Tracey, and Gill Valentine (Eds.). 1998. Cool Places: Geographies of Youth Cultures. London: Routledge.

Snell-Rood, Claire. 2013. "To Know the Field: Shaping the Slum Environment and Cultivating the Self." Ethos 41(3): 271–91.

Snyder, C.R. 2002. "Hope Theory: Rainbows in the Mind." Psychological Inquiry 13(4): 249–75.

Snyder, C.R., Betsy Hoza, William Pelham, Michael Rapoff, Leanne Ware, Michael Danovsky, Lori Highberger, Howard Rubinstein, and Kandy Stahl. 1997. "The Development and Validation of the Children's Hope Scale." Journal of Pediatric Psychology 22(3): 399–421.

Spitzer, Robert L., Janet B.W. Williams, Miriam Gibbon, and Michael B. First. 1992. "The Structured Clinical Interview for DSM-III-R (SCID): I. History, Rationale, and Description." Archives of General Psychiatry 49(8): 624–29.

Stambach, Amy. 2000. Lessons from Mount Kilimanjaro: Schooling, Community, and Gender in East Africa. New York: Routledge.

Stearns, F.A. 1991. "Inpatient Group Treatment of Children and Adolescents." In Robert L. Hendren and Irving M. Berlin (Eds.), Psychiatric Inpatient Care of Children and Adolescents. New York: John Wiley & Sons. pp. 112–26.

Stephens, Sharon (Ed.). 1995. Children and the Politics of Culture, Princeton, NJ: Princeton University Press.

Storck, Michael, Thomas J. Csordas, and Milton E. Strauss. 2000. "Depressive Illness and Navajo Healing." In Thomas J. Csordas (Guest Editor), "Ritual Healing in Contemporary Navajo Society" [Special issue]. Medical Anthropology Quarterly 14: 360–81.

Stroul, Beth, and Robert M. Friedman. 1986. A System of Care for Severely Emotionally Disturbed Children and Youth. Washington, DC: Georgetown

University Center for Child Development, National Technical Assistance Center for Children's Mental Health.

Suárez-Orozco, Carola, and Marcelo Suárez-Orozco. 1995. Transformations: Immigration, Family Life, and Achievement Motivation among Latino Adolescents. Palo Alto, CA: Stanford University Press.

Sullivan, Harry Stack. 1953. The Interpersonal Theory of Psychiatry. New York: Norton.

Swaffer, Tracey, and Clive R. Hollin. 1997. "Adolescents' Experiences of Anger in a Residential Setting." Journal of Adolescence 20: 567–75.

Te Riele, Kitty. 2010. "Philosophy of Hope: Concepts and Applications for Working with Marginalized Youth." Journal of Youth Studies 13(1): 35–46.

Thomas, Cindy P., Peter Conrad, Rosemary Casler, and Elizabeth Goodman. 2006. "Trends in the Use of Psychotropic Medications among Adolescents, 1994–2001." Psychiatric Services 57(1): 63–69.

Throop, C. Jason. 2008. "On the Problem of Empathy: The Case of Yap, Federated States of Micronesia." Ethos 36(4): 402–26.

Todorov, Tzvetan. 1969. "Structural Analysis of Narrative" (translated by Arnold Weinstein). Novel: A Forum on Fiction 3(1): 70–76.

Valle, Michael, E. Scott Huebner, and Shannon Suldo. 2006. "An Analysis of Hope as a Psychological Strength." Journal of School Psychology 44: 393–406.

Van Hasselt, Vincent B., and Michel Hersen. 1995. Handbook of Adolescent Psychology: A Guide to Diagnosis and Treatment. New York: Lexington Books.

Venning, Anthony J., Jaklin Eliott, Lisa Kettler, and Anne Wilson. 2009. "Normative Data for the Hope Scale Using Australian Adolescents." Australian Journal of Psychology 61(2): 100–106.

Ventura, Joseph, Robert P. Liberman, Michael F. Green, Andrew Shaner, and Jim Mintz. 1998. "Training and Quality Assurance with the Structured Clinical Interview for DSM-IV (SCID-I/P)." Psychiatry Research 79(2): 163–73.

Verhulst, Frank C. 1995. "A Review of Community Studies." In Frank C. Verhulst and Hans M. Koot (Eds.), The Epidemiology of Child and Adolescent Psychopathology. Oxford: Oxford University Press. pp. 146–77.

Waterworth, Jayne M. 2004. A Philosophical Analysis of Hope. New York: Palgrave Macmillan.

Watson, Marnie, Caroline Bonham, Cathleen Willging, and Richard Hough. 2011. "'An Old Way to Solve an Old Problem': Provider Perspectives on Recovery-Oriented Services and Consumer Capabilities in New Mexico." Human Organization 70(2): 107–17.

Wells, Karen. 2015. Childhood in a Global Perspective. Hoboken, NJ: John Wiley & Sons.

White, Geoffrey. 1990. "Emotion Talk and Social Inference: Disentangling in Santa Isabel, Solomon Islands." In Karen A. Watson-Gegeo and Geoffrey M. White (Eds.), Disentangling: Conflict Discourse in Pacific Societies. Palo Alto, CA: Stanford University Press.

White, Ross G., Sumeet Jain, David M.R. Orr, and Ursula M. Read (Eds.). 2017. The Palgrave Handbook of Sociocultural Perspectives on Global Mental Health. New York: Palgrave Press.

Willen, Sarah S. 2012. "How Is Health-Related 'Deservingness' Reckoned? Perspective from Unauthorized Immigrants in Tel Aviv." Social Science and Medicine 74: 812–21.

Willging, Cathleen, and Rafael Semansky. 2010. "It's Never Too Late to Do It Right: Lessons from Behavioral Health Reform in New Mexico." Psychiatric Services 61(7): 646–48.

Willging, Cathleen E., and Elise M. Trott. 2018. "Outsourcing Responsibility: State Stewardship of Behavioral Health Care Services." In Jessica Mulligan and Heiede Castaneda (Eds.), Unequal Coverage: The Experience of Health Care Reform in the United States. New York: NYU Press. pp. 231–53.

Willging, Cathleen, Howard Waitzkin, and Louise Lamphere. 2009. "Transforming Administrative and Clinical Practice in a Public Behavioral Health System: An Ethnographic Assessment of the Context of Change." Journal of Health Care for the Poor and Underserved 20: 866–83.

Woods, Angela. 2011. "The Limits of Narrative: Provocations for the Medical Humanities." Medical Humanities 37: 73–78.

———. 2012. "Beyond the Wounded Storyteller: Rethinking Narrativity, Illness and Embodied Self-Experience." In Havi Carel and Rachel Cooper (Eds.), Health, Illness and Disease: Philosophical Essays. Newcastle, UK: Acumen. pp. 113–28.

World Health Organization. 2005. Child and Adolescent Mental Health Policies and Plans. Geneva: World Health Organization.

———. 2012. Adolescent Mental Health: Mapping Actions of Nongovernmental Organizations and Other Development Organizations. Geneva: World Health Organization.

———. 2013. "Child and Adolescent Health." www.who.int/mental_health /maternal-child/child_adolescent/en/.

Young, Allan. 1997. The Harmony of Illusions: Inventing Post-Traumatic Stress Disorder. Princeton, NJ: Princeton University Press.

Zigon, Jarrett. 2009. "Hope Dies Last: Two Aspects of Hope in Contemporary Moscow." Anthropological Theory 9(3): 253–71.

Zournazi, Mary (Ed.). 2002. Hope: New Philosophies for Change. Annandale, Australia: Pluto Press.

Zournazi, Mary, and Isabelle Stengers. 2002. "A 'Cosmo-Politics'—Risk, Hope, Change." In Mary Zournazi (Ed.), Hope: New Philosophies for Change. Annandale, Australia: Pluto Press. pp. 244–72.

Index

GENERAL INDEX

Note: Pages in italics refer to illustrative matter.

Founded in 1893,
UNIVERSITY OF CALIFORNIA PRESS
publishes bold, progressive books and journals
on topics in the arts, humanities, social sciences,
and natural sciences—with a focus on social
justice issues—that inspire thought and action
among readers worldwide.

The UC PRESS FOUNDATION
raises funds to uphold the press's vital role
as an independent, nonprofit publisher, and
receives philanthropic support from a wide
range of individuals and institutions—and from
committed readers like you. To learn more, visit
ucpress.edu/supportus.

Ingram Content Group UK Ltd.
Milton Keynes UK
UKHW010232170623
423577UK00007B/630